Congenital malformations worldwide

Congenital malformations worldwide

A Report from The International Clearinghouse for Birth Defects Monitoring Systems

A Non-Governmental Organization of the World Health Organization

1991
ELSEVIER-AMSTERDAM-NEW YORK-OXFORD

ISBN 0 444 89137 4

This book is printed on acid-free paper.

Published by:

Elsevier Science Publishers B.V.
P.O. Box 181
1000 AD Amsterdam

Sole distributors for the USA and Canada:

Elsevier Science Publishers Co. Inc.
655 Avenue of the Americas
New York, NY 10010

Contents

The International Clearinghouse for Birth Defects Monitoring Systems: What's in the name?

A *clearinghouse*, a term borrowed from the world of banking, is a central office for receiving and distributing data.

The terms *birth defects* and *congenital malformations* are often used interchangeably in the following text, although technically differences exist. "Birth defects" is the more general and all-inclusive term, referring to many kinds of abnormal development that originated in the prenatal period, whether present at birth or expressed later (like mental retardation). Some birth defects, such as certain inborn errors of metabolism, can be diagnosed only with specialized techniques, while others are obvious to the naked eye. The term "congenital malformations", on the other hand, usually refers to gross structural anomalies, internal or external, and either severe or mild.

Monitoring involves systematic observations of certain events, evaluation of their frequency against a pre-set standard of occurrences (baseline data), and a short time interval between the occurrence of the events and their observation and evaluation. Implied in monitoring is the ability and commitment to investigate deviations from the expected or usual level of occurrence in order to find the causes of the deviations and prevent further occurrences. The term "surveillance" is often used synonymously with monitoring. On the other hand, a distinction can be made between a monitoring system and a registry. A *registry* is a database or collection of information on individual events, often compiled from multiple sources in order to achieve more complete ascertainment and fuller detail. Broad time limits (or none at all) are often allowed between occurrence of an event and its inclusion in the registry, and the contents of a registry are likely to be updated with additional information as it becomes available. Registry data often have several uses, one of which can be monitoring, provided that there is a way to identify cases diagnosed within a defined short time interval so they can be compared to baseline data similarly compiled. While registries often exist without the monitoring function, a monitoring system set up independently, apart from a registry, is less likely to be efficient.

Foreword

This book was written to summarize the experience of a unique experiment in international cooperation in the field of public health. The International Clearinghouse for Birth Defects Monitoring Systems has operated successfully for nearly two decades through the voluntary cooperation of a number of private and public institutions and individuals throughout the world.

The *Clearinghouse* was initiated and mainly supported during its first ten years by the March of Dimes Birth Defects Foundation, a voluntary nongovernmental association dedicated to the prevention of birth defects and related forms of suboptimal pregnancy outcome. First organized in 1938 as the National Foundation for Infantile Paralysis, it sponsored the research that led to the development of vaccines and the elimination of poliomyelitis as a public health problem wherever vaccination was widely employed. The Foundation entered the field of birth defects in 1958 and today administers a variety of research, health service, and educational programs in that field.

The great epidemic of congenital rubella in the early 1950s followed in 1958-59 by the outbreak of phocomelia caused by thalidomide focused interest on the search for mechanisms for the rapid detection of significant changes in the geographic and temporal distribution of birth defects. In response to complaints heard from professionals, research scientists, and clinicians about delays in the transmission of such information, the March of Dimes sponsored a meeting in 1974 of interested parties who were active in birth defects prevention in their respective countries and initiated a survey to assess the possibility of establishing a uniform mechanism for the timely exchange of statistical data on the incidence of birth defects. Out of these efforts the International Clearinghouse for Birth Defects Monitoring Systems was born.

This book not only documents the origins, organization, and functions of the *Clearinghouse*, but presents research findings and systematically organized data, much of it previously unpublished, on 22 types of congenital malformations reported from all around the world making them available to researchers and health planners alike. The book was prepared by Bengt Källén and Sylvia Hay, who were involved in the *Clearinghouse* from the beginning, but it can also be thought of as the joint effort of all the people who represent the various monitoring systems that belong to the *Clearinghouse*.

The *Clearinghouse* has succeeded in enlisting its members in a variety of collaborative investigations of "alarms" generated by its reporting system. (These are described elsewhere in this volume.) The fact that most of these studies have yielded negative results render them no less important. In this era of concern with environmental hazards to human health, especially reproductive health, we tend to conjure up an apocalypse. I believe that those responsible for the protection of human health have to learn to balance the fear of missing hidden hazards against the harm of inflating non-hazards.

The International Clearinghouse for Birth Defects Monitoring Systems can contribute to this end.

Gabriel Stickle, Senior Vice President (Retired)
March of Dimes Birth Defects Foundation

Chapter I
The Clearinghouse: Origins, objectives, and achievements

Origins

The International Clearinghouse for Birth Defects Monitoring Systems was conceived in 1974, at a meeting in Helsinki, where representatives of monitoring systems in ten countries decided to exchange routine information on the current reported incidence of congenital malformations. From today's perspective such a decision may not seem remarkable; it is necessary to review some history in order to recognize its full significance.

By 1974 about 15 years had elapsed since the well-known thalidomide disaster stunned medical and health professionals, as well as the general public, throughout the world. This disaster demonstrated that not only could a prescribed therapeutic drug cause severe and devastating birth defects, but that national borders could be as irrelevant in an epidemic of birth defects as they were in epidemics of infectious diseases. When thalidomide was released, birth defects were not being monitored on a current and ongoing basis, and even if they had been the standard coding system then in use (7th Revision of the International Statistical Classification of Diseases, Injuries and Causes of Death, ICD) was too crude to isolate the specific conditions involved. Furthermore, there was no method for rapid notification between countries. It has been pointed out that the delays in the exchange of information about the suspected teratogenicity of thalidomide resulted in its continued sale in several countries six months or more after it was withdrawn from the market in Germany, Sweden, and England.

Although by 1970 at least ten countries had initiated programs to identify, quantify, and, it was hoped, prevent malformations, there was still no mechanism for communicating findings from one program to the others except through the traditional channels of scientific publications or, in the worst case scenario, through the public media. In that year James Miller, head of the British Columbia Birth Defects Registry, recommended to the World Health Organization (WHO) that it look into international monitoring and registration of congenital malformations.

In 1972 WHO held a formal consultation to get advice on its possible activities in this field. The eleven consultants were directors of birth defects monitoring systems and registries, among whom were several who later took part in the

Clearinghouse: Philip Banister (four provinces of Canada), Andrew Czeizel (Hungary), William Flynt (Atlanta, U.S.A.), Sylvia Hay (31 states, U.S.A.), Jiří Kučera (Czechoslovakia), and Josephine Weatherall (England and Wales). The group recommended that WHO take immediate steps to initiate a collaborative monitoring system and that information on individual cases be forwarded to Geneva for compilation and dissemination. In other words, the surveillance and analysis would be done centrally by an international organization.

About a year later, data from Atlanta, Canada, Hungary, and Jerusalem were sent to the Statistics Section of WHO in Geneva, but were unusable, having arrived in a variety of formats: incompatible magnetic tapes, punched cards with round holes, and punched cards with rectangular holes. By 1974 - two years after the consultation - more data from Atlanta, Canada, and England-Wales were obtained on purportedly compatible tapes, but by then WHO had no staff available to work on them. In retrospect, it seems obvious that neither the consultants nor the World Health Organization had fully appreciated the complexity and cost of the project they had undertaken.

Meanwhile, at a workshop at the 4th International Conference on Birth Defects in Vienna, organized in 1973 under the auspices of the March of Dimes Birth Defects Foundation, an extensive and elaborate, though purely hypothetical, computerized system was proposed whose task would be to meld a wide range of information from a multitude of sources into specialized international data banks, where the data would pass through an advisory panel en route to the output. The output would include everything from unevaluated raw data to scientific publications. The possibility of connecting different existing national monitoring systems through computer technology was also discussed at the workshop and felt by some to be feasible, though requiring that "compromises" be made in the existing monitoring systems.

For most of the proponents of such complicated proposals, a birth defects monitoring system was only an abstract concept. However, some people present at the workshop had years of actual, hands-on experience with monitoring systems, and while welcoming the idea of international cooperation, they found the proposed methods rather alarming and potentially unworkable. It disturbed them that the initiative in international monitoring was being taken by the proponents of enormous banks of pooled data that would be dealt with centrally, far from the sources of the data. They considered it impractical to believe that all the compromises necessary to standardize the existing systems - most of which were integral parts of governmental programs - could ever be made. And they feared that the energies spent on trying to develop such complex systems would only further delay the advent of international monitoring; perhaps the experience with WHO's relatively modest attempts was still fresh in their minds.

Stimulated by the discussions at the workshop as well as by the concerns expressed to him about those discussions, Gabriel Stickle, Vice President of the

March of Dimes, offered to organize a meeting of representatives of as many birth defects monitoring systems and registries as possible, as well as the World Health Organization, to explore practical approaches to international collaboration. The meeting, which later became known as the "First Working Conference on Birth Defects Monitoring", was held in Helsinki on June 7, 1974. Among the 20 participants were representatives of ten of the programs that are presently members of the *Clearinghouse*: Philip Banister, Canada; Tor Bjerkedal, Norway, Eduardo Castilla, South America; Andrew Czeizel, Hungary; Madeleine Dessemond, France; William Flynt, United States; A. Härö, Finland; Bengt Källén, Sweden; Marcus Klingberg, Israel; Josephine Weatherall, England-Wales.

At this meeting the pros and cons of monitoring were debated and philosophical differences were expressed, again with some people favoring pooled data and standardized models and others contending that each country should decide the structure of its own system. Some wanted an objective outsider to evaluate the systems; others felt each system should evaluate itself. While it was the consensus that an exchange of information was a good idea, the form and methods could not be agreed upon. Finally, Gabriel Stickle suggested that if an exchange of information was wanted, "Let's just do it". He offered the March of Dimes to serve for at least one year as a clearinghouse, with the hope that an international body could take over in the future. The suggestion was welcomed, and WHO was asked to work on the data they already had and to develop standards and guidelines (e.g., standardized definitions, coding, diagnosis, etc.). The WHO representative cautioned that it would require negotiations with the individual governments and at least three or four years to get a new program underway.

It was agreed that each program should send its regular monitoring reports on a quarterly basis to the March of Dimes, where they would be reproduced and distributed to the participants. It should be pointed out that at that time not all of the birth defects programs represented at this meeting put out regular quarterly (or more frequent) reports on their data.

Five months later, in November 1974, the March of Dimes distributed copies of the reports received from Canada, England-Wales, Norway, Sweden, and the United States. Although no attempt was made to standardize the formats or content, these reports represented the first exchange of data through the *International Clearinghouse for Birth Defects Monitoring Systems.* At about this time the March of Dimes asked Sylvia Hay, a public health statistician who from 1962 to 1973 had run a large study of congenital malformations, including both descriptive epidemiology and monitoring, to survey the existing monitoring systems in order to determine their similarities and differences and to identify the factors that might facilitate or impede international collaboration. She was also asked to make recommendations for a standardized reporting system based on the outcome of the survey.

In the summer of 1975, she visited 15 monitoring systems, registries, and some research projects in Europe, North America, and Israel, meeting with the program directors and their associates. She also met with representatives of WHO's Statistics Section. The survey consisted of informal and relatively open-ended interviews, albeit with a set of specific questions.

During the survey, the same two schools of thought as expressed in Vienna and Helsinki were apparent. One group wanted a central body - preferably WHO - to collect, pool, and analyze raw data, while the other group wanted a "clearinghouse" to disseminate summarized data in an easily readable standard format. The majority shared the latter view.

At the 2nd Working Conference in Geneva, September 1975, Hay presented a specific, detailed plan for exchanging information on a quarterly basis. In devising the plan, she was greatly influenced by practical considerations; that is, she did not feel it advisable to wait until an ideal system could be developed, but that "something" was better than "nothing" and "sooner" was preferable to "later". She also felt that whatever international program might emerge, its ultimate success or failure would depend on whether the needs and desires of the participating monitoring systems were respected.

At this meeting, which was well-represented by the World Health Organization - its Maternal and Child Health and Genetics Divisions, as well as the Statistics Section, were invited - a central registry of individual cases was still being discussed as a viable option. However, most of the program people wanted the March of Dimes to continue to operate a clearinghouse for at least another year, or until WHO was ready to take over in a smooth transition. While the WHO representatives expressed interest in taking over the exchange of data and developing a coding system, standardized diagnoses, etc., they said they could do it only if they could get money from an "outside source".

A committee composed of William Flynt, Gabriel Stickle, and representatives of WHO was appointed to consider Hay's report and "the problems arising from the recommendations and to make a study of the ways in which standardization of reporting can be implemented". A couple of months later, WHO wrote to the March of Dimes that it would be "premature" for WHO to "introduce central processing of individual records" and that their role should be to promote exchange of data and standardization of methodology.

The upshot was to proceed with the quarterly reporting as recommended. In August 1976, the first compiled report, which included data from the first three months of that year, was produced and distributed. The format of this first Quarterly Report was generally similar to that still in use: i.e., quarterly data on the reported incidence of selected malformations in each monitoring system; reports of unusual events, suspected outbreaks of birth defects, suspected teratogens, or any other relevant information thought to be of interest; and copies of lists of relevant pre-publication articles. Because of their provisional nature, these reports have never been available to anyone except the participating programs.

The 3rd Working Conference of the *Clearinghouse* was held in Gardone, Italy, in September 1976. All of the recommendations were presented, discussed and prioritized. Two of them - the quarterly data exchange and the idea of annual working conferences - were already being implemented, both of them supported financially by the March of Dimes. Committees were formed to give immediate attention to some of the other recommendations, including the reporting and following up of alarms, the reporting and analysis of multiple malformations, and improvement of classification of malformations with the idea of influencing the ICD.

No immediate action would be taken on the remaining recommendations, which included developing a cross-indexed compilation of synonyms of various malformations, preparation of a handbook describing in detail each monitoring system and a manual for helping new monitoring systems get started, and development of guidelines for the optimal size and other characteristics of a monitoring program.

By 1976 the *Clearinghouse* was quite firmly established and interest in it was extending beyond the original participants. Nevertheless, the desire for association with the World Health Organization persisted in many members of the *Clearinghouse* and eventually led to the structure it has today.

In 1977 it was decided to seek a formal relationship with WHO as a recognized nongovernmental organization (NGO). By 1981, having repeatedly been unsuccessful in this effort, the *Clearinghouse* determined to become more autonomous and less informally structured in order to satisfy WHO's requirements for establishing an official relation with a nongovernmental organization. To this end, the officers (Godfrey Oakley, Bengt Källén, and Gabriel Stickle) and the Coordinator (Sylvia Hay) met in 1982 to draft a set of bylaws which were adopted at the annual meeting later that year. The special relationship with the March of Dimes Birth Defects Foundation was in effect severed, although the Foundation continued to provide gradually diminishing financial support for four more years.

Finally, in 1986, after nearly 10 years of efforts, the *Clearinghouse* obtained its desired NGO status with the World Health Organization.

Three years later, in 1989, the *Clearinghouse* formed an association with the newly-created International Centre for Birth Defects (ICBD), an organization that is fully funded by the Norwegian government and located in Bergen. By agreement, the Centre presently coordinates the activities of the *Clearinghouse*, produces its routine reports, and serves as its general office.

At the present time, 26 monitoring programs participate in the *Clearinghouse* (see table on next page).

Participating programs and program directors

Year of entry	Program	Program Director
The Formative Period: 1974-1976	Hungary	Andrew Czeizel until 1989 Csaba Elek 1989 to present
	Israel	Marcus Klingberg until 1983 Paul Merlob 1983 to present
	United States and Atlanta	William Flynt until 1979 Godfrey Oakley 1979-1985 David Erickson 1985 to present
	Czechoslovakia	Jiří Kučera to present
	Canada	Philip Banister until 1979 Francine Lortie-Monette 1979-1981 Donald Wigle 1981 to present
	Norway	Tor Bjerkedal until 1985 Lorentz Irgens 1985 to present
	Central-East France	Madeleine Dessemond until 1980 Pierre Guibaud 1982-1983 Elisabeth Robert 1983 to present
	England-Wales	Josephine Weatherall until 1982 Michael MacDowall 1982-86 Beverley Botting 1986 to present
	Finland	Anneli Ruusinen until 1981, 1983 to present Maarit Heikkinen 1981-1983
	Sweden	Bengt Källén until 1982 Anders Ericson 1982 to present
1977	South America	Eduardo Castilla to present
1978	Tokyo	Masami Ashizawa to present
	Northern Ireland	Norman Nevin to present
1979	New Zealand	Frank Foster until 1984 John Findlay 1984-1990 Barry Borman 1990 to present
	Spain	María Luisa Martínez-Frías to present
1980	Denmark	Lisbeth B. Knudsen to present
	Italy	Pierpaolo Mastroiacovo to present
	Mexico	Osvaldo Mutchinick to present
1982	Australia	Paul Lancaster to present
	Paris	Janine Goujard to present
	Strasbourg	Claude Stoll to present
1983	Belgium (withdrew in 1984)	Roger Beckers
1985	Emilia-Romagna	Guido Cocchi to present
	Sichuan	Xiao Kunze to present
1988	Japan	Shoichi Sakamoto to present
	Thailand	Saree Chitinand to present

Objectives and achievements

The mission of the *Clearinghouse* is to prevent birth defects, particularly any widespread outbreaks or epidemics. The *Clearinghouse* has proposed to accomplish this by means of three objectives: **exchange of information, collaborative research,** and **consultation and assistance**.

The *Clearinghouse* was designed to provide a means whereby monitoring systems, wherever they exist in the world, could in a timely manner **exchange information** about possible or suspected outbreaks of congenital malformations or other relevant information so that preventive action could be taken, if indicated. This remains the primary and most enduring goal of the *Clearinghouse*.

The system of information exchange has been shown to work, or at least it has not been shown to have failed. Some alarms have been reported and the *Clearinghouse* has reacted. Three examples readily come to mind: an "outbreak" of femur hypoplasia and the relationship between spina bifida and maternal use of valproic acid – both reported to the *Clearinghouse* from the Central-East France program – and the teratogenicity of Accutane (isotretinoin) reported from Atlanta. Fortunately, these were all limited problems for one reason or another. However, if a new teratogen had been introduced that was widely used by pregnant women, like thalidomide, and its adverse fetal effects had been detected by at least one of the member monitoring programs, evidence suggests that the present system of information exchange would have halted or prevented a widespread outbreak of malformations.

Regularly since 1976, Quarterly Reports containing abundant information have been produced and distributed. However, the input to the Quarterly Reports has been largely routine data, uninterpreted and without comment, contrary to the original purpose of these reports. The participation in this process has been more passive than was hoped for, in spite of more than a decade of prodding and cajoling by coordinators, chairpersons, and others.

A significant achievement in the area of information exchange is the development of a seemingly workable method for monitoring multiple malformations. For more than 20 years the importance of multiple malformations as indicators of possible teratogenicity was talked about, but it was only under the auspices of the *Clearinghouse* that a practical methodology was finally devised. There is evidence that a thalidomide-like outbreak would be detected through the collaborative monitoring of multiple malformations in the method developed and implemented by Bengt Källén and continued by Pierpaolo Mastroiacovo. That is, it would be detected if the event occurred in one or more monitoring systems that have data sufficiently precise to participate in this activity.

The methods, uses, and problems associated with the exchange of information among the various monitoring systems are discussed in Chapters III through VII.

Since at least 1980, **collaborative epidemiological research** has become an increasingly important aspect of the *Clearinghouse*. Joint studies have attempted to understand endemic occurrence as well as outbreaks of malformations. In order to conduct joint research, the *Clearinghouse* has had to tackle some of the problems of comparability and standardization that have impeded the development of international data banks. Chapter VII describes some of the collaborative research conducted by participants in the *Clearinghouse*. It is highly unlikely that these projects could have been done as timely or efficiently, if at all, had agencies of five or six different governments, rather than the nongovernmental *Clearinghouse*, tried to share and integrate their data.

Like the quarterly information exchange, joint studies have sometimes suffered from a lack of active participation by all programs. Some of this has been unavoidable because of inherent characteristics of the programs themselves. However, in some instances non-participation may have been for other reasons - perhaps lack of interest or unwillingness to spend the necessary extra time on the projects or perhaps this kind of activity is not seen by everyone as essential to the basic aims of the *Clearinghouse*.

The *Clearinghouse*'s third approach to the prevention of birth defects is through expert **consultation and assistance**; that is, helping existing monitoring systems investigate outbreaks and helping new monitoring systems get established. The *Clearinghouse* has not been aggressive in developing this objective, though the very existence of the organization has without question stimulated the formation of new monitoring systems. The *Clearinghouse* has made efforts to help many of these new programs avoid pitfalls.

Another achievement - which to some extent meets all three objectives, being partly information exchange, partly collaborative research, and partly assistance - is the Annual Report, eight of which have thus far been published. Much more than summaries of collected statistics, these reports contain practical, original discussions of methodology that probably deserve a larger audience than they have received.

Perhaps the major achievement of the *Clearinghouse* is its very survival for all of 17 years. This is, in all seriousness, no small accomplishment and is a tribute to the program directors - past and present - and to their governments and sources of funding and to Gabriel Stickle and the March of Dimes who provided so much early encouragement and support. In Chapter VIII we will look at the future of the organization.

Chapter II

The organization of the Clearinghouse

During its early years the *Clearinghouse* had a very informal structure. In 1981, it was decided to formalize the organization, in part to meet the World Health Organization's requirements for official recognition as a Non-Governmental Organization. Bylaws were drawn up and accepted at the Annual Meeting in London the following year.

Membership

Members of the *Clearinghouse* are malformation monitoring programs, not persons, though each program is represented in all activities by a designated person, usually the program director. The programs must be actively engaged in the systematic collection and analysis of data for the comprehensive monitoring of birth defects. In addition to monitoring, the programs must also be capable of undertaking epidemiologic investigations of birth defects.

Excluded from membership are any research programs designed merely to describe the occurrence of birth defects in a restricted population during a restricted period of time. Also excluded are "passive" programs that only collect and report health statistics data without continual and systematic surveillance. Obviously, it is sometimes difficult to draw a line for acceptable activity.

If a malformation monitoring program fulfills the criteria laid down in the bylaws and outlined above, it can apply for membership by letter. The program director is then asked to complete a questionnaire in order to describe the program. The questionnaire is scrutinized by the officers of the *Clearinghouse* and by the directors of the current member programs. Additional clarifying information is frequently requested. Acceptance of the new program as a member is made after a majority of votes cast by the present program directors have declared that the eligibility requirements have been met.

There are two classes of membership: full and associate. Full members must be able to submit quarterly data according to an agreed-upon format, and the population monitored must include at least 20,000 births per year. Furthermore, the program must have used its current methods of monitoring to collect baseline data on birth defects occurring in a minimum of 100,000 births during at least two years.

The only special requirement for associate membership is that the population monitored must include at least 5,000 births per year. In this way, small but active monitoring systems may participate in the *Clearinghouse*. Often a new monitoring system with the potential for full membership will be admitted to the *Clearinghouse* with associate member status while it is in the process of accumulating the necessary baseline material.

Occasionally complications arise because an applicant for membership monitors a population that overlaps a population already being monitored by a full member. Under such circumstances the consent of the full member in question is required.

Responsibilities of members

The basic function of the *Clearinghouse* is to share information among monitoring programs around the world. Such information may take many forms, including routine reports on certain defined conditions, observations of unusual events, such as clusters of malformations or associations between specific exposures and specific malformations, and pre-publication results of scientific studies.

Full members are required to participate in this sharing of information by submitting quarterly reports in a prescribed form, by submitting reports on special studies, and by submitting relevant pre-publication articles. While associate members are not required to submit quarterly reports, they are encouraged to submit reports on special studies and pre-publication articles. Representatives of both full and associate member programs are expected to serve on committees as needed and to respond to specific requests from the *Clearinghouse*. Data from all members, both full and associate, are included in annual reports.

Annual meeting and executive committee

A meeting of all members is held annually, usually in September or October, and usually at the site of one or another of the member programs. Each program is represented at the meetings by the program director and/or a representative selected by the program director.

At the annual meeting the past year's achievements are reviewed and analyzed, goals are set for the year ahead, committees are appointed and officers elected. Decisions affecting the operation of the *Clearinghouse* are made by voting; each full member has one vote and each associate member half a vote. During recent years a supplementary "scientific session" has been held where representatives of member programs have a chance to report on their own studies and discuss their results.

Prior to the adoption of the bylaws in 1982, officers were elected each year at the annual meeting and their responsibilities did not extend beyond planning and conducting the next annual meeting. Under the bylaws, the officers - chairperson, vice chairperson and secretary-treasurer - form the Executive Committee, which represents the *Clearinghouse* in relations with other organizations, is responsible for preparing the annual budgets and making financial commitments, initiates investigations of alarms, and carries out other assignments given them at the annual meeting.

Other committees

Since its inception, much of the work of the *Clearinghouse* has been assigned to small committees or work groups, usually appointed at the annual meetings. A number of *ad hoc* committees of limited duration have been formed during the past fifteen years to work on specific methodological problems or to conduct special projects. One of the earliest and most long-lived groups was the "Emergency" or "Epidemiology" Committee, which was formed to develop protocols and methodology for investigating possible clusters or increases in occurrence of specific malformations reported from one or more of the member monitoring systems. The functions of this committee were eventually taken over by the Executive Committee, and in its place the Statistical Committee was formed whose task is to work on statistical methodological problems in birth defects monitoring. Another committee of relatively long duration has been involved in the monitoring of multiple malformations. A third long-standing committee, the Classification Committee, has been working on classification problems and has been consulted by WHO for the chapter on malformations in the 10th edition of the ICD.

In addition to such formally constituted committees, more informal collaboration on projects of mutual interest occurs among various member programs. Results of their collaboration are usually reported at the annual meetings.

Central office functions

From the beginning, the central office functions of the *Clearinghouse* were performed by a part-time coordinator (first Sylvia Hay and later Lisbeth B. Knudsen) who collected data for quarterly and annual reports and for special studies, served as *de facto* secretary, and provided the official address of the *Clearinghouse*. Since 1989, these functions have been performed for the *Clearinghouse* by the International Centre for Birth Defects in Norway, which is operating under a three-year grant from the Norwegian Government. The Centre is run by a board of directors consisting of the Executive Committee of the *Clearinghouse* and representatives of the University of Bergen and the Norwegian government.

Chapter III

The monitoring programs participating in the Clearinghouse

Structure of a monitoring program

Each monitoring system is created within a unique political, social, geographic, economic, and historical context. It also will reflect the particular philosophy, training, and interests of its founders. Many programs utilize databases and methodologies that were already in place long before the *Clearinghouse* was created. It is, therefore, not surprising that each monitoring program has a unique structure. The *Clearinghouse* has always recognized and accepted the differences among programs and has never insisted on conformity to a model as a prerequisite for participation in its activities. In fact, the *Clearinghouse* subscribes to the notion that there can be no single ideal model with universal applicability.

This variability in structure among the programs obviously results in variability in the registration systems and, inevitably, in the quality of data. This problem will be more fully discussed in a later chapter. The present chapter will point out some important sources of variability in the data and briefly describe each of the participating monitoring systems according to some rather simple characteristics.

Size of the monitoring system

The size of a monitoring system refers to the number of births it includes rather than the size of the general population. In large programs the effects of random fluctuations on the recorded rates of a malformation are minimized. Rare malformations, such as cyclopia which occurs about once in 100,000 births, can only be effectively monitored in a large system; it would be rather hopeless to try to follow changes in prevalence of such a rare condition in a monitoring system based on only 10,000 annual births. A very large system, however, also has its drawbacks: information in such a system has to be encoded and handled by computers, and there is often less opportunity to get the detailed descriptions needed to correctly identify rare and complex conditions.

If a monitoring system covers an entire nation, its size is irrelevant, because all births occurring in the country are monitored and undetected changes in the risk of very rare malformations will be of little practical significance. If only a portion of the population of a large country is monitored, the sample may be too small to detect changes in the rate of rather infrequent conditions which - in the total population - may have significant effects.

A small monitoring system may be more suitable for studying relatively common but indistinct minor birth defects that are difficult to define and therefore also to register in a uniform way. The Israeli monitoring system, for example, includes only a few hospitals but has intensively studied the occurrence and significance of minor anomalies.

Population-based and hospital-based programs

A population-based monitoring system tries to identify all births of malformed infants within a population living in a given geographic area, often a country, but sometimes a smaller region. Thus, it is possible to relate the births to a more or less closed population whose characteristics and environment can be defined. Where home births are rare, population-based programs will include almost exclusively all delivery units within the defined area. In practice, however, it is not always possible to maintain a perfect population-based program, because some births in the defined area will always be to women who are temporary visitors, and some births to women belonging to the population will occur outside the area. Although the risk of misclassified births is greatest in small geographic areas, it also exists when the defined area is an entire country.

Another advantage of population-based registries is that it is often possible to follow repeated births among the same women and to follow up the infants born in the area. Again, the smaller the geographic area is, the larger is the risk that people will move from the area and be lost for follow-up. When national registries are effective, this problem gets further reduced but never disappears.

In many areas of the world only a hospital-based system is at all feasible. In such cases the monitoring program samples from the births in the population by recording all births that take place in a selected group of hospitals. Ideally, the hospitals should be selected in such a way that the sample of births is totally representative of the births in the general population. In practice this is seldom possible. Hospitals are often selected because of their willingness to participate in the program and sometimes also because of characteristics such as size, location, type of ownership, etc. There will always be the question of a particular sample's representativeness.

An extremely large population of births may be too cumbersome to monitor in its entirety. The task may be made more manageable by sampling, either from a number of defined geographic areas or from a network of hospitals. A combination of several small population-based registries and an umbrella registry sampling from hospitals may be one possible solution to the problem of how to monitor a large population.

Governmental programs and research projects

Monitoring programs can be dichotomized in yet another way. The typical program in one group is run by a governmental body and is usually part of a centralized health registration system. In the other group the typical program began as a research activity, with the registry supported by research grants. There are advantages and disadvantages with both types. Direct governmental operation probably results in better longterm stability and may also facilitate communication between the registry and other governmental offices, which may be important in case an epidemic of birth defects (and perhaps even its cause) is detected. On the other hand, this type of organization risks the disadvantages of a bureaucracy and may have fewer opportunities for active research utilizing the data. A research-based registry has the opposite characteristics: dependence on research grants makes the longterm stability more uncertain and possible findings may be more difficult to communicate to decision-making authorities, but the opportunity and competence for using data for research are usually greater than in a governmental registry. A hybrid is also possible - a research program located within a governmental agency.

A related issue is the characteristics and qualifications of the program director. If the registry is part of a national health statistics system, he or she is likely to be a governmental representative, often with a strong background in health statistics or epidemiology, but without specific expertise in teratology. In a research program the program director is more likely to have academic training in genetics, teratology or related disciplines, resulting in a more case-oriented, rather than statistical, approach to monitoring. These different approaches will be discussed in a later chapter.

Single or multiple sources of ascertainment

In many programs information on malformations present in the newborn can only be collected within the first few hours or days after birth. While this may be adequate for identifying and recording gross external malformations, it can result in significant underreporting of internal malformations, even serious ones such as cardiac defects, which may not give symptoms until later. Experience has also taught that even for easily recognized conditions ascertainment is never complete. Ascertainment can be increased by using multiple sources of information, but the additional time involved may reduce the effectiveness of the monitoring, where timeliness is a virtue. In some programs, in Atlanta and Sweden, for example, provisional monitoring is done using information from immediate sources such as delivery and neonatal pediatric units, with more complete ascertainment achieved later by utilizing multiple sources.

Exposure information

Some programs, e.g., Sweden, Australia, and Atlanta, do not routinely record possible exposures during pregnancy. Such programs are usually found in areas where it is relatively easy to go back later to medical records and to contact the parents of the damaged infant if exposure information is thought to be of interest. In others, such as the Central-East France program and the large hospital-based program in Italy, information on possible exposures during pregnancy is collected at the same time the malformed infant is reported, but no similar data are collected on normal infants. A third group, including programs in Mexico, Spain, and South America, have ongoing case-control data collection, in which possible exposure information is obtained for each malformed infant and for a control (normal) infant born at the same hospital. Each technique has its advantages and disadvantages, but in areas of the world where it may not be possible to follow up an observation by interview at some time after birth, an ongoing case-control data collection seems the most effective way to obtain exposure data.

Background information

For basic monitoring of a specific malformation one needs only to be able to calculate rates of prevalence at birth, based upon the number of cases of the malformation and the total number of births from which these cases came. For the evaluation of changes in prevalence at birth of conditions that are strongly dependent on maternal age (like Down syndrome) one also should know, or be able to estimate, the maternal age distribution of the referent population and, of course, of the cases. When the data are used for epidemiological studies beyond the simple monitoring for changes in prevalence, more details from the background population are necessary. This can be a problem in countries where population statistics are not easily available or reliable. The control material in the case-control studies mentioned above may help provide this background information. Sometimes, however, the needed data must be specially collected.

Description of individual member programs

Each of the member programs will be briefly characterized according to the various aspects outlined above. Further details can be obtained from the correspondent given for each program.

The programs are listed in alphabetic order according to their standard abbreviations, which are used in the tables and graphs.

Atlanta

Metropolitan Atlanta Congenital Defects Program.

History: The program started in 1967. The program was a founding member of the *Clearinghouse* and is a full member.

Size and coverage: The program covers all births in Metropolitan Atlanta, USA. The approximate annual number of births is 35,000. Stillbirths of 20 weeks or more gestation and/or at least 500g birthweight are included.

Legislation and funding: The program is run and funded by the governmental Centers for Disease Control (CDC). Data are retrieved by personnel from CDC.

Sources of ascertainment: Multiple sources are used to ascertain malformed infants born in the defined area with a follow-up to one year's age using records from delivery units, pediatric departments and other specialities dealing with malformed infants.

Exposure information: Through 1980, exposure information was obtained by interviews of mothers of reported malformed infants.

Background information: Number of births and some basic epidemiological information are obtained from vital statistics.

Address for further information: David Erickson, Centers for Disease Control - Birth Defects Branch, 1600 Clifton Road, Atlanta, Georgia 30333, USA.

Australia

Australian Congenital Malformation Monitoring System.

History: National monitoring of malformations began in 1981, but not all States and Territories were collecting data at that stage. Subsequently, perinatal data systems have been introduced in all States and Territories. The program became an associate member of the *Clearinghouse* in 1982 and a full member in 1984.

Size and coverage: All births in Australia are nowadays covered, at the present approximately 250,000 annual births. Coverage increased from about 50% in 1981 to 100% in 1986. Stillbirths of 20 weeks or more gestation are registered. Incomplete data for the Northern Territory were excluded from this report.

Legislation and funding: State and Territory health departments report to the central registry. Central registration is funded by a grant from the Australian Institute of Health, which is a statutory body within the national Department of Community Services and Health.

Sources of ascertainment: Reports are obtained from birth notifications, referral hospitals, death certificates, pathology departments and cytogenetic laboratories.

Exposure information: Except in South Australia, exposure information is not routinely recorded but has to be obtained *ad hoc*.

Background information: General perinatal statistics are obtained from notification of birth to health departments and from birth and perinatal death registrations compiled by the Australian Bureau of Statistics.

Address for further information: Paul A.L. Lancaster, National Perinatal Statistics Unit, Building A27, The University of Sydney, Sydney N.S.W. 2006, Australia.

Canada

Canadian Congenital Anomalies Surveillance System.

History: The program was started in 1966, and revised in 1973, 1978, and 1987. The program was a founding member of the *Clearinghouse* and was a full member until 1987, when it became an associate member.

Size and coverage: In 1973 the register covered all births in five Canadian provinces (New Brunswick, Ontario, Manitoba, Alberta, British Columbia). Prince Edward Island was added in 1977, and New Brunswick left the system in 1980. The system presently monitors about 215,000 births annually, which represents about 60% of all births in Canada. Stillbirths of at least 20 weeks gestation and/or 500g birthweight are included.

Legislation and funding: Reporting is based on an agreement between provinces that choose to participate in the registration and the central registry, which is run by and funded by Health and Welfare Canada.

Sources of ascertainment: Reporting is based on birth and death notifications and information obtained from Hospital Insurance Admission-Separation summary records. Follow-up continues to one year of age.

Exposure information: No exposure information is routinely collected in the central registry.

Background information: Background information, based on birth notifications of all livebirths, is obtained from Statistics Canada.

Address for further information: Kenneth C. Johnson, Room A7 HPB Bldg, Bureau of Chronic Disease Epidemiology, Laboratory Centre for Disease Control, Tunney's Pasture, Ottawa, Ontario K1A OL2, Canada.

Central-East France

Central-East France Register of Congenital Malformations.

History: The registry began in 1973 within the Rhône-Alps area - the Auvergne region was added in 1983, and the Jura area in 1985. The program was a founding member of the *Clearinghouse* and is a full member.

Size and coverage: The registry covers all births in the area, approximately 90,000 annually, which represents about 12% of all births in France. Stillbirths of 28 weeks or more gestation are included.

Legislation and funding: Reporting is voluntary. The system is run by a privately funded research organization.

Sources of ascertainment: Reports are received from delivery units, pediatric and child surgery clinics, pathology departments, and cytogenetic laboratories. Infants up to the age of one are registered.

Exposure information: Information on maternal and paternal occupation, drug use, diseases, etc. are collected by interviews of the mothers of the malformed infants. No controls are interviewed.

Background information: Some background information is available from the general population statistics.

Address for further information: Elisabeth Robert, Institut Européen des Génomutations, 86 Rue Edmond Locard, F-69005 Lyon, France.

Czechoslovakia

Czechoslovakian Registry and Monitor of Congenital Malformations.

History: A registration of malformation began in 1961, but actual monitoring started in 1975. The program was a founding member of the *Clearinghouse* and is a full member.

Size and coverage: All births occurring in Bohemia and Moravia are covered, at present comprising about 130,000 annual births, or about 65% of all births in Czechoslovakia. Stillbirths weighing at least 1,000g are included.

Legislation and funding: Reporting is compulsory. The registry is financed and run by the government at the Institute of Health Statistics, Ministry of Health.

Sources of ascertainment: Reports are obtained from delivery units, pediatricians in neonatology wards, pathologists, infant death certificates, and perinatal mortality certificates. Reporting to the central registry occurs via District Health Units and Regional Health Offices.

Exposure information: Some exposure information is available on malformed infants, none on controls.

Background information: Some general demographic background data can be obtained from general birth statistics.

Address for further information: Jiří Kučera, Department of Population Teratology and Epidemiology, nábř. Podolské 157, 147 10 Prague 4 - Podolí, CSR.

Denmark

The Danish Registry of Congenital Malformations and the Medical Birth Registry.

History: Since 1968, all births have been registered in the Medical Birth Registry with malformation diagnoses given by midwives. The Registry of Congenital Malformations started in 1983. The program became a full member of the *Clearinghouse* in 1980.

Size and coverage: All births in Denmark are covered, at the present approximately 60,000 annual births. Stillbirths of 28 weeks or more gestation are registered.

Legislation and funding: Reporting is compulsory. Registries are run and financed by the governmental National Board of Health.

Sources of ascertainment: Reports to the Registry of Congenital Malformations are received from various sources, e.g., delivery units, pediatric clinics, pathology departments, and cytogenetic laboratories. Malformations detected before the age of one are reported.

Exposure information: Some exposure information is available in the Registry for Congenital Malformations: maternal and paternal occupation, drugs, X-rays, infections.

Background information: Epidemiological background data are available on all births in the Medical Birth Registry.

Address for further information: Lisbeth B. Knudsen, National Board of Health, Box 2020, DK-1012 Copenhagen K, Denmark.

Emilia-Romagna

Emilia-Romagna Registry of Congenital Malformations (IMER).

History: The registry was started in 1978 in a few hospitals and has increased in size to now include 45 delivery units. The program became an associate member of the *Clearinghouse* in 1985.

Size and coverage: The program is based on approximately 90% of all births in the Emilia-Romagna region, or approximately 23,000 annual births (4% of all births in Italy). Stillbirths of 28 weeks or more gestation are included.

Legislation and funding: The program is recognized and financed by the health authorities, the National Research Council, and the Regional Health Council. Hospital participation is voluntary.

Sources of ascertainment: Reporting is made by neonatologists and pediatricians during the first week of the infant's life. Selected malformations are followed up.

Exposure information: Detailed exposure information is obtained by interviews of the mothers of malformed infants. For each malformed infant, a control is chosen (the baby born before or after the malformed case in the same hospital) and its mother is interviewed in a similar way.

Background information: Some general demographic information is known for all births in the area. For each participating hospital, the number of livebirths and stillbirths are known.

Address for further information: Guido Cocchi, Instituto Clinico di Pediatria Preventiva e Neonatologia, Università di Bologna, Via Massarenti N.11, 40138 Bologna, Italy.

England-Wales

Congenital Malformation Monitoring Program of England and Wales.

History: The monitoring program was started in 1964. It was a founding member of the *Clearinghouse* and is a full member.

Size and coverage: All births in England and Wales are covered, at present approximately 700,000 annually. Stillbirths of 28 weeks or more gestation are registered.

Legislation and funding: Reporting is voluntary. The system is financed by the governmental Office of Population Censuses and Surveys.

Sources of ascertainment: Reports are mainly based on notifications of births prepared by attendants at birth, either physicians or midwives, supplemented by other reports from neonatal intensive care units, special care baby units, etc.

Exposure information: Parents' occupation is known. No information on other exposures is available but can be retrieved *ad hoc* from general practitioners.

Background information: Information on all births is available from birth certificates.

Address for further information: Beverley J. Botting, Office of Population Censuses & Surveys, St. Catherines House, 10 Kingsway, London WC2B 6JP, England.

Finland

The Finnish Register of Congenital Malformations.

History: The registry was established in 1963 and regular monitoring began in 1977. The program was a founding member of the *Clearinghouse* and is a full member. At present, stillbirths of at least 22 weeks gestation are registered; prior to 1987, stillbirths of 28 weeks or more were registered.

Size and coverage: All births in Finland are covered, approximately 64,000 annually.

Legislation and funding: Reporting is compulsory. The registry is run and financed by the National Board of Health.

Sources of ascertainment: Reports are obtained from delivery units and pediatric hospitals.

Exposure information: Until 1986, extensive exposure information was obtained from maternity health centers and by personal interview but only for some selected malformations and their controls, i.e., the baby born immediately before the proband at the same hospital.

Background information: Some general background information is obtained from birth notifications. Since 1987, a special Medical Birth Registry exists that provides more detailed information on each birth.

Address for further information: Anneli Ruusinen, The National Board of Health, Siltasaarenkatu 18A, PB 221, SF-00531 Helsinki 53, Finland.

Hungary

Hungarian Congenital Malformation Registry.

History: Centralized registration of congenital malformations was begun in 1970, and monitoring began in 1973. The program was a founding member of the *Clearinghouse* and is a full member.

Size and coverage: The registry covers all births in Hungary, approximately 125,000 annually. Stillbirths of 28 weeks or more gestation are included.

Legislation and funding: Reporting is compulsory. The registry is run and financed by the governmental National Institute of Hygiene.

Sources of ascertainment: Reports are obtained from delivery units, neonatal and pediatric wards, and institutes of cardiology, ophthalmology, pediatric surgery, and pathology.

Exposure information: Exposure information is available only since 1980, when a case-control system was initiated in which mothers of malformed infants and controls are interviewed.

Background information: General background information on all births is available from central statistics.

Address for further information: Csaba Elek, Center for Congenital Anomaly Control, National Institute of Hygiene, Budapest, IX Gyáli út 2-6, 1966 Hungary.

Israel

Israel Birth Defects Monitoring System.

History: The program started in one hospital in 1966 and was a founding member of the *Clearinghouse.* It was a full member until 1986, when it became an associate member.

Size and coverage: Reports are now obtained from four hospitals, with approximately 18,000 annual births or nearly 20% of all births in Israel. Stillbirths of 28 weeks or more gestation are included.

Legislation and funding: The program is a research program supported by research grants without any governmental support.

Sources of ascertainment: Reports are obtained from delivery units and pediatric departments in the participating hospitals.

Exposure information: All women admitted for delivery are interviewed on occupation, parental chronic diseases, oral contraceptives, etc.

Background information: Epidemiological information on all births occurring in the participating hospitals is available.

Address for further information: Paul Merlob, Neonatal Department, Beilinson Medical Center, 49100 Petah Tikva, Israel.

Italy

Italian Multicentric Register of Congenital Malformations (IPIMC).

History: The registry started in 1977. The program became a full member of the *Clearinghouse* in 1980.

Size and coverage: The program is based on reporting from hospitals distributed all over Italy. Initially, 28 hospitals reported and the annual number of births was 38,000. At the present time, 147 hospitals participate, covering approximately 140,000 annual births or approximately 25% of all Italian births. Stillbirths of 180 days or more gestation are included.

Legislation and funding: The program is a research program supported by grants from the National Research Council, Ministry of Health, and Regional Health Authorities. Participation in the program is voluntary.

Sources of ascertainment: Reports are obtained from delivery units and pediatric clinics at the participating hospitals.

Exposure information: For each malformed infant reported, information is given on certain exposures, including maternal drug usage and parental occupation. No information on controls is available.

Background information: Little background information is available beyond the number of births and maternal age distribution.

Address for further information: Pierpaolo Mastroiacovo, Clinica Pediatrica, Università Cattolica, Largo Gemelli 8, 00168 Rome, Italy.

Japan

Japan Association for Maternal Welfare.

History: The program started in 1972 and became a full member of the *Clearinghouse* in 1988.

Size and coverage: The program is based on reports from 270 hospitals throughout Japan (excluding the 16 Tokyo hospitals which report to the Tokyo program). At present approximately 115,000 births are covered, representing about 10% of all Japanese births. Stillbirths of 28 weeks or more gestation are included.

Legislation and funding: The program is a research program acknowledged by the Ministry of Welfare and supported by the Japanese Association for Maternal Welfare.

Sources of ascertainment: Reports are obtained from delivery units and pediatric clinics of the participating hospitals.

Exposure information: No exposure information is available.

Background information: Basic epidemiological information on all births is available from each participating hospital.

Address for further information: Shoichi Sakamoto, Hokken Kaikan, 1-2, Sadohara-cho, Ichigaya, Shinjuku-ku, Tokyo, 162, Japan.

Mexico

Mexican Registry and Epidemiological Surveillance of External Congenital Malformations (RYVEMCO).

History: The program was started in 1978. The program became a full member of the *Clearinghouse* in 1980.

Size and coverage: Reports are obtained from 21 hospitals in 11 cities in Mexico. Participation is voluntary. The annual number of births is approximately 50,000, about 2% of all births in Mexico. Stillbirths of 20 weeks or more gestation and/or at least 500g birthweight are included.

Legislation and funding: The program is a research program and is funded by research grants.

Sources of ascertainment: Reports are obtained from the delivery units and pediatric departments of the participating hospitals.

Exposure information: The mother of each reported infant and the mother of a control infant - the next non-malformed infant born at that hospital with the same sex as the proband - are interviewed on various exposures, including drug usage and parental occupation.

Background information: The total number of births in the hospitals is known.

Address for further information: Osvaldo Mutchinick, Departamento de Genética, Instituto Nacional de Nutrición, Salvador Zubirán, Vasco de Quiroga 15, Tlalpan, 14000 Mexico, D.F., Mexico.

New Zealand

New Zealand Congenital Anomalies Monitoring Program.

History: The program began in 1975 and became a full member of the *Clearinghouse* in 1979.

Size and coverage: The program covers all births in New Zealand, approximately 55,000 annual births. Stillbirths of 28 weeks or more gestation are included.

Legislation and funding: The program is run and funded by the governmental Department of Health. Reporting is compulsory.

Sources of ascertainment: Reports are based on birth notification forms for deliveries inside or outside hospitals and on discharge diagnoses.

Exposure information: No exposure information is routinely available.

Background information: General epidemiological characteristics for all births are available.

Address for further information: Barry Borman, Health Statistical Services, Private Bag 2, Upper Willis Street, Wellington, New Zealand.

Northern Ireland

Northern Ireland Malformation Registry.

History: Malformation registration began in Belfast in 1957 and was extended to all Northern Ireland in 1970. The program became a full member of the *Clearinghouse* in 1978.

Size and coverage: All births in Northern Ireland are covered, approximately 28,000 annual births. Stillbirths of 28 weeks or more gestation are included.

Legislation and funding: The program is a research program funded by the Department of Health.

Sources of ascertainment: Reports from delivery units, pediatric clinics, and departments of pathology and medical genetics.

Exposure information: No exposure information is routinely collected.

Background information: Extensive epidemiological data are available on all births.

Address for further information: Norman C. Nevin, Dept. of Medical Genetics, Queens's University, Institute of Clinical Science, Grosvenor Road, Belfast BT12 6BJ, Northern Ireland.

Norway

Medical Birth Registry of Norway.

History: The program was started in 1967. The program was a founding member of the *Clearinghouse* and is a full member.

Size and coverage: The program covers all births in Norway, approximately 55,000 annual births. Stillbirths of 16 weeks or more gestation are included.

Legislation and funding: The program is run and funded by the governmental National Institute of Public Health. Reporting is compulsory.

Sources of ascertainment: The registry is based on the notification of births from the delivery units.

Exposure information: Some basic information, such as maternal diseases, is collected on all infants, malformed or not.

Background information: All information available for the reported malformed infants is also available for the total population of births.

Address for further information: Lorentz Irgens, Medical Birth Registry of Norway, Haukeland Sykehus, N-5021 Bergen, Norway.

Paris

Paris Register of Congenital Malformations.

History: The program began in Paris in 1975 and was extended to the Department of Yvelines during the period 1978-1987. The program became an associate member of the *Clearinghouse* in 1982.

Size and coverage: All births in Paris are eligible for inclusion, but actual coverage is estimated at 95%. The approximate annual number of births is

40,000, 6% of all births in France. Stillbirths of 28 weeks or more gestation are included.

Legislation and funding: Reporting is voluntary. The registry is associated with the National Institute of Health and partly funded by Institut National de la Santé et de la Recherche Médicale (INSERM).

Sources of ascertainment: Reports are obtained from delivery units and pediatric departments (to the age of one year) and are linked to birth certificates. Information is also received from cytogenetic and pathology laboratories.

Exposure information: Exposure information, such as contraceptive practice and maternal diseases and occupation, is obtained for reported malformed infants.

Background information: Information from birth certificates is available.

Address for further information: Janine Goujard, INSERM - Unité 149 123, Bd. de Port Royal, 75014 Paris, France.

Sichuan

Birth Defects Monitoring Program of Sichuan Province, China.

History: The program began in 1984. It became an associate member of the *Clearinghouse* in 1985 and a full member in 1987.

Size and coverage: In 1984, reports were obtained from 100 hospitals but participation has increased. In 1985, 205 hospitals participated. At present, the program covers approximately 65,000 births annually, or about 5% of all births in the province - less than 0.4% of all births in China.

Legislation and funding: Participation is voluntary. Funding is mainly from local health authorities.

Sources of ascertainment: Reports are obtained from delivery units, pediatric clinics, and pathology departments of the participating hospitals.

Exposure information: Exposure information is obtained by interviews of mothers of the reported malformed infants. No information is available on exposures in controls.

Background information: Total number of births from each participating hospital is known.

Address for further information: Xiao Kunze, National Center for Birth Defects Monitoring, West China University of Medical Sciences, Chengdu, China.

South America

Latin American Collaborative Study of Congenital Malformations (ECLAMC).

History: The program started in 1967 and has grown in size and coverage. The program became a full member of the *Clearinghouse* in 1977.

Size and coverage: The number of participating hospitals has grown from 20 in 1980 to 70 at the present time, distributed over all South American countries. The annual number of births covered is at present approximately 215,000, less than 1% of all births. Stillbirths of at least 500g birthweight have been included since 1978.

Legislation and funding: The program is a research program with voluntary participation of hospitals and is funded by research grants.

Sources of ascertainment: Reporting is made by delivery units and pediatric departments of participating hospitals.

Exposure information: The mother of each reported infant and the mother of a control infant - the next non-malformed infant born at that hospital with the same sex as the proband - are interviewed on various exposures, including drug usage and parental occupation.

Background information: Background information is obtained partly from summarizing tables of births in each participating hospital, partly from the control material.

Address for further information: Eduardo Castilla, ECLAMC/GENETICA/FIOCRUZ, C.P. 926, 21.040 Rio de Janeiro, Brazil.

Spain

Spanish Collaborative Study of Congenital Malformations (ECEMC).

History: The program started in 1976. It became a full member of the *Clearinghouse* in 1979.

Size and coverage: Reports are obtained from hospitals distributed all over Spain. In 1980, 27 hospitals participated; at present there are 51. The annual number of births is approximately 60,000, representing almost 15% of all Spanish births. Stillbirths of at least 500g birthweight have been included since 1980.

Legislation and funding: The program is a research program with voluntary participation of hospitals and is financed by research grants.

Sources of ascertainment: Reports are obtained from delivery units and pediatric departments of the participating hospitals.

Exposure information: The mother of each reported infant and the mother of a control infant - the next non-malformed infant born at that hospital with the same sex as the proband - are interviewed on various exposures, including drug usage and parental occupation.

Background information: Total number of births by sex and number of twin pairs in each participating hospital are known. Other background information is obtained from the control material collected.

Address for further information: María Luisa Martínez-Frías, ECEMC, Facultad de Medicina, Universidad Complutense, 28040 Madrid, Spain.

Strasbourg

Strasbourg Prospective Study of Congenital Malformations.

History: The registry was started in 1979. The program became an associate member of the *Clearinghouse* in 1982.

Size and coverage: All births in an area including and around Strasbourg and the Bas-Rhin are covered - approximately 13,000 annually, or less than 2% of all births in France.

Legislation and funding: The program is a research program, recognized by the local health authorities and funded by Social Security, Ministry of Health, and INSERM.

Sources of ascertainment: Reports are obtained from pediatricians examining the newborn infants. A control infant is selected for each malformed one: the next infant of the same sex as the proband born at that hospital.

Exposure information: Detailed information on various exposures is obtained by interview of the mothers of the malformed infants and their controls. The children are followed to the age of one year.

Background information: General demographic information is obtained from the National Institute of Statistics. Further information is obtained from Social Security Records and Health Sheets.

Address for further information: Claude Stoll, Institut de Puericulture - Hospices Civils, F-67000 Strasbourg, France.

Sweden

The Swedish Registry of Congenital Malformations and the Medical Birth Registry.

History: The Registry of Congenital Malformations started in 1964, the Medical Birth Registry in 1973. The program was a founding member of the *Clearing-house* and is a full member.

Size and coverage: All births in Sweden are included, approximately 120,000 annual births.

Legislation and funding: Reporting is compulsory. Registries are run by and funded by the National Board of Health and Social Welfare (governmental).

Sources of ascertainment: Reports are received from delivery units, pediatric clinics, pathology departments, child cardiology clinics, and cytogenetic laboratories.

Exposure information: Some exposure information for all births is available in the Medical Birth Registry: maternal occupation, socioeconomic factors, maternal smoking, contraceptive usage, maternal diseases. Additional information, on drugs for instance, can be obtained *ad hoc* from medical records where the information is recorded prospectively.

Background information: Epidemiological background data are available on all births in the Medical Birth Registry.

Address for further information: Anders Ericson, Department of Epidemiology, National Board of Health, S-106 30 Stockholm, Sweden.

Thailand

Thailand Malformation Registry.

History: The program began in 1987 and became an associate member of the *Clearinghouse* in 1988. The program has ceased monitoring.

Size and coverage: Reports were obtained from five hospitals, three of which were located in Bangkok. The approximate annual number of births was 30,000, representing about 3% of the births in Thailand. Stillbirths of 28 weeks or more gestation were included.

Legislation and funding: The program was a research program, funded by research grants.

Sources of ascertainment: Reports were obtained from delivery units, pediatric departments, and pathology departments of the participating hospitals.

Address for further information: Saree P. Chitinand, Neonatal Unit, Pediatric Department, Chulalongkorn Hospital, Bangkok 10500, Thailand.

Tokyo

Tokyo Area Birth Defects Monitoring Programs.

History: The registry started in 1976, became a full member of the *Clearinghouse* in 1978, and changed to an associate member in 1988.

Size and coverage: The program is based on reports from 16 hospitals in the Tokyo area which cover about 20% of the births in that area. The approximate annual number of births is 17,000, about 1% of all births in Japan. Stillbirths of 28 weeks or more gestation in five hospitals and 16 weeks or more gestation in 11 hospitals are included.

Legislation and funding: The program is a research program funded by research grants but acknowledged by the Ministry of Health and Welfare.

Sources of ascertainment: Reports are obtained from delivery units and pediatric clinics in the participating hospitals.

Exposure information: Information, including occupation and drugs, is recorded for each malformed infant and its three controls.

Background information: Total number of births in participating hospitals is known. Further information is available from the control material.

Address for further information: Masami Ashizawa, The Institute of Public Health, 6-1, Shirokanedai 4, Minato-ku, Tokyo, 108 Japan.

United States

Birth Defects Monitoring Program, United States.

History: The program started in 1974. The program was a founding member of the *Clearinghouse* and is a full member.

Size and coverage: Information is collected from approximately 1,200 hospitals distributed all over the United States. The annual number of births is currently approximately 575,000, about 15% of all births in the nation. Stillbirths of 20 weeks or more gestation are included.

Legislation and funding: The program is run and funded by the governmental Centers for Disease Control.

Sources of ascertainment: Computerized discharge diagnoses from the participating hospitals are obtained.

Exposure information: No exposure information is available.

Background information: Some limited epidemiological information on all births in the participating hospitals is available.

Address for further information: David Erickson, Centers for Disease Control - Birth Defects Branch, 1600 Clifton Road, Atlanta, Georgia 30333, USA.

Chapter IV

Congenital malformations registered in the Clearinghouse programs, 1974-1988

Introduction

When the *Clearinghouse* was being designed, it was decided to require routine reporting of a few selected congenital malformations in order to ensure that data are tabulated and analyzed at least every three months, both in the individual monitoring systems and in the *Clearinghouse* itself. Eleven congenital malformations were selected for inclusion in the first Quarterly Report issued in 1976. Most of these malformations were still being reported each quarter 15 years later. (One malformation - congenital hip dislocation - was dropped during the period and another one - omphalocele - added.) These particular conditions were selected for routine reporting because they are reasonably common and easily diagnosed, and in the mid-1970s there existed either special interest in them or the belief that exogenous factors seemed to play a role in their etiologies.

Unfortunately, this selection of certain malformations has sometimes led to the fallacious assumption that they represent the only malformations that should be monitored. All types of congenital defects that potentially can be monitored should be monitored, and the fundamental purpose of the Quarterly Reports is not the reporting of the selected malformations but the reporting of unusual events irrespective of what type of malformation is involved.

Nevertheless, the accumulation of data on these selected malformations has provided an opportunity to tabulate and compare their rates as recorded in different parts of the world. The quarterly data are provisional and incomplete, but from 1980 through 1987 Annual Reports were published that contain updated and more complete data. For the following analyses these annual figures have been supplemented by the addition of year 1988 and, when available, 1974-1979. A few corrections to the published data have also been made.

Some malformations that had not been reported quarterly were included in the Annual Reports. The material that follows contains these plus a few additional malformations that on one occasion or another have caused concern because either an apparent increase in their rate of occurrence or a clustering has been observed.

In this Chapter, 22 selected malformations reported in 25 of the 26 monitoring programs have been tabulated and annual rates have been calculated. For each malformation the rates can be compared in two ways: between programs and over time.

In interpreting these data many precautions must be taken. Some sources of variation are listed below.

Definition

Each condition has been briefly defined in order to provide the monitoring programs with some rough guidelines for reporting. However, the extent to which the definition is applied at data collection depends both on local conditions and philosophy. Many malformations exhibit a range in severity, and the inclusion or exclusion of mild forms may be a source of variation. This is obviously of greatest consequence for widely variable conditions like hypospadias, where the very mild forms that represent a large proportion of all cases may or may not be counted. Even less ambiguous malformations, such as cleft lip and cleft palate, represent a spectrum from severe forms that are easily diagnosed and reported to slight defects that may go unnoticed or at least unreported.

Another source of variation is the definition and inclusion or exclusion of stillbirths. As malformed infants have a tendency to be born prematurely and to be stillborn, the inclusion or exclusion of stillbirths will affect the reported rates. Although stillbirths are included in the data of a majority of programs in the *Clearinghouse*, they are defined variably by a minimum of 16, 20, or 28 weeks of gestation or, less frequently, by birthweight limits of at least 500 or 1,000 grams.

Prenatal diagnosis

During recent decades the development of various prenatal diagnostic techniques has made it possible to identify and selectively abort fetuses having some types of birth defects, especially neural tube defects, abdominal wall defects, and chromosome anomalies, notably Down syndrome. The use of prenatal diagnosis followed by selective abortion varies widely among the *Clearinghouse* programs and thus can be a source of variation in the reported rates of infants born with these defects. It might be possible to collect data on aborted fetuses and add them to the number of malformed infants born, but this would overestimate the malformation rates because a considerable proportion of such induced abortions would have been spontaneous abortions or miscarriages at gestational ages too young to be reported.

The interpretation of "syndromes"

In the tables in this Chapter each malformation is counted once; if an infant has both cleft lip and omphalocele, for example, it enters both tables. If an infant is multimalformed, the description of its individual malformations may be less complete than when they appear isolated, and furthermore, the infant may be reported or classified with a syndrome designation. If, for instance, an infant with trisomy 18 and omphalocele is recorded in one program as having both the trisomy and the omphalocele, while in another program a similar infant is counted only as a trisomy 18, different rates of omphalocele will result. From a monitoring point of view it might seem reasonable not to count the omphalocele that occurs in a trisomy 18 infant because the trisomies form an entity of their own, but for the tabulation of the number of infants with omphalocele that are born in the population, it is reasonable to include it. The reporting practice varies from program to program.

Ascertainment

Differences in ascertainment are probably the major source of interprogram variations in malformation rates. Overall ascertainment probably never reaches 100%, and its degree depends on a program's methods of data collection, the time period after birth during which data are collected, autopsy rates (for internal malformations), etc. Programs using multiple sources will reach a higher level of ascertainment than programs relying on only one source, typically the delivery unit. While these differences are most marked for less severe malformations, they are probably always present.

Changes within a program can easily occur over time. Changes in the coverage of the program, inclusion criteria, etc. may occur. Prenatal diagnosis may be introduced and its use may gradually increase. Therefore, great care must be taken in the interpretation of temporal changes within a program as well as in comparisons of the rates between programs.

Data on some types of malformations

On the following pages, data for 1974-1988 (as available) are presented for 22 malformations. Minor differences may exist between data presented here and previously published data, as most programs have provided new information for this report. Two programs - New Zealand and Northern Ireland - did not submit new data, so their information has been taken from the 1980-1988 Annual Reports of the *Clearinghouse* (the 1988 report is being prepared). No data are available from Thailand.

Total births

Monitoring program	1974	1975	1976	1977	1978	1979	1980	1981
Atlanta	24,775	23,026	22,679	23,505	24,396	25,541	27,342	26,835
Australia								113,514
Canada	226,070	230,636	228,110	232,264	247,615	252,152	239,504	242,929
Central-East France			66,642	68,602	68,514	70,676	74,760	76,943
Czechoslovakia	194,215	191,776	187,378	181,763	178,901	172,112	153,801	144,438
Denmark								
Emilia-Romagna					7,042	6,365	12,471	14,322
England-Wales	647,060	609,740	589,979	574,664	601,526	643,153	661,007	638,697
Finland	62,277	65,343	66,484	65,278	63,576	63,015	63,064	63,469
Hungary	187,957	195,847	186,916	179,152	169,524	161,677	149,829	144,062
Israel	7,035	7,450	8,472	8,156	18,372	18,813	18,601	18,217
Italy					44,177	71,981	82,318	107,121
Japan						158,874	156,759	139,495
Mexico							41,748	34,500
New Zealand							46,180	49,763
Northern Ireland							28,835	27,543
Norway	60,335	57,026	54,118	51,454	52,268	52,127	51,528	51,061
Paris								39,000
Sichuan								
South America	84,961	65,214	77,992	67,432	73,041	69,415	55,412	55,752
Spain			12,234	27,426	35,533	68,785	56,910	56,102
Strasbourg								
Sweden	110,606	104,235	98,890	96,549	93,738	96,700	97,500	94,445
Tokyo							18,850	18,067
United States	1,085,047	1,068,246	1,049,798	1,077,090	974,151	1,030,270	769,742	864,659

Monitoring program	1982	1983	1984	1985	1986	1987	1988	Total
Atlanta	27,866	27,937	29,240	30,995	32,790	35,004	36,648	418,579
Australia	238,684	241,015	236,794	241,126	241,583	241,818	244,194	1,798,728
Canada	252,724	242,626	251,853	261,962	262,485	247,686	215,128	3,633,744
Central-East France	75,135	85,843	86,300	90,160	91,327	89,618	91,231	1,035,751
Czechoslovakia	141,738	137,431	136,941	135,881	133,356	130,921	132,667	2,353,319
Denmark		51,087	52,030	53,989	55,554	56,509	59,136	328,305
Emilia-Romagna	18,362	21,767	23,155	24,016	22,868	22,741	22,794	195,903
England-Wales	629,870	632,765	640,461	660,062	644,567	684,934	696,959	9,555,494
Finland	66,106	66,892	65,076	62,796	60,632	59,827	59,944	953,779
Hungary	134,579	128,160	126,158	131,008	129,032	126,726	125,060	2,275,687
Israel	17,963	18,325	18,181	17,820	17,550	16,640	17,479	229,074
Italy	125,754	139,625	136,732	131,144	141,847	136,921	138,209	1,255,829
Japan	121,375	125,579	125,424	130,004	157,584	144,272	138,318	1,397,684
Mexico	34,610	38,167	33,597	24,088	24,647	40,751	40,903	313,011
New Zealand	48,229	50,521	50,147	51,254	52,409	54,592	54,903	457,998
Northern Ireland	27,215	27,459	27,857	27,813				166,722
Norway	51,676	50,289	50,609	51,472	52,791	54,383	57,885	799,022
Paris	38,922	39,754	39,986	41,009	40,753	40,357	41,376	321,157
Sichuan				62,998	79,449	84,663	65,100	292,210
South America	144,374	154,324	169,289	182,454	211,192	195,348	188,363	1,794,563
Spain	61,333	71,816	69,513	66,720	58,244	51,051	52,685	688,352
Strasbourg	13,532	12,428	12,693	12,973	12,855	12,922	13,346	90,749
Sweden	93,122	92,120	94,280	98,851	102,373	105,111	112,502	1,491,022
Tokyo	19,203	18,903	19,547	19,157	18,296	17,573	16,320	165,916
United States	823,271	813,844	742,282	722,790	683,053	600,372	509,189	12,813,804

The annual number of births in each program are shown in a table on the previous pages.

Each malformation is introduced with a short description of its appearance and clinical significance.

For each malformation, two tables are presented - one showing the actual number of infants with the malformation in question, the other giving the rate per 10,000 births. The rates are plotted in a set of figures with the programs grouped according to geographic relationship. These graphs are based on three-year moving averages (except for the first and last years when only two years are averaged).

The average rates are compared in a second set of figures. As different programs have data for different periods and marked time-trends exist for some malformations, most comparisons have been restricted to the period 1985-1988. For particularly rare malformations (epispadias, bladder exstrophy, conjoined twins) the whole time period has been used. As Northern Ireland did not report data after 1985, the period 1981-1985 was used for that program. The programs have been grouped into sets according to geographic relationship.

Anencephaly

Anencephaly (acrania) is a lethal malformation that originates early in development and is related to the non-closure of the anterior neuropore. As a result, the cranial vault is deficient and the main part of the brain does not develop properly but lies as a disorganized, usually vessel-rich, mass on the exterior of the head. The face and neck are often markedly abnormal. Many anencephalic infants also have malformations in other parts of the body.

An anencephalic infant is stillborn or expires soon after birth - survival to one week's life is unusual but happens.

The condition can with rather high accuracy be detected at prenatal diagnosis, either by ultrasound or by studies on alphafetoprotein (AFP) in maternal blood or in amniotic fluid.

A genetic background to the malformation exists but various exogenous causes leading to anencephaly have been discussed. A certain risk exists for recurrence in a later child.

Anencephaly

Definition: A congenital malformation characterized by total or partial absence of the cranial vault, the covering skin, and the brain.

A. Number of infants born with anencephaly

Monitoring program	1974	1975	1976	1977	1978	1979	1980	1981	1982	1983	1984	1985	1986	1987	1988	Total
Atlanta	15	8	12	11	13	18	17	9	7	10	12	9	12	9	12	174
Australia								103	140	139	99	122	102	91	88	884
Canada	183	166	179	158	142	116	113	99	101	106	88	98	89	92	75	1805
Central-East France			5	6	7	4	4	9	8	10	9	7	1	5	5	80
Czechoslovakia	62	45	66	61	62	35	69	56	47	35	47	21	19	16	14	655
Denmark										5	7	5	5	8	17	47
Emilia-Romagna					1	1	2	2	3	4	3	2	2	2	1	23
England-Wales	849	775	644	568	525	455	342	253	162	117	89	61	52	31	41	4964
Finland	11	18	22	20	16	13	19	14	17	4	6	7	6	7	4	184
Hungary	195	148	139	102	86	95	74	130	84	82	48	41	31	28	22	1305
Israel	1	4	8	8	5	10	6	12	9	9	7	6	5	4	3	97
Italy					26	28	27	40	30	40	23	25	27	18	12	296
Japan					87	160	178	112	100	127	106	110	116	98	90	1284
Mexico							73	67	66	71	56	44	53	79	68	577
New Zealand							32	29	34	19	14	18	19	17	9	191
Northern Ireland							48	48	35	25	13	22				191
Norway	20	27	18	26	19	25	18	23	15	18	10	22	19	16	15	291
Paris								8	7	7	8	4	3	7	3	47
Sichuan												34	59	50	41	184
South America	31	11	22	19	21	20	10	24	89	109	121	114	107	142	108	948
Spain			4	7	9	27	35	25	29	24	27	38	14	14	13	266
Strasbourg									1	4	8	3	3	6	5	30
Sweden	42	29	38	37	18	23	17	11	14	17	10	7	13	20	8	304
Tokyo							8	10	16	21	9	8	14	19	15	120
United States	478	463	437	401	360	371	253	302	270	245	194	194	177	120	106	4371

B. Rate per 10,000 infants.

Monitoring program	1974	1975	1976	1977	1978	1979	1980	1981	1982	1983	1984	1985	1986	1987	1988	Average
Atlanta	6.1	3.5	5.3	4.7	5.3	7.0	6.2	3.4	2.5	3.6	4.1	2.9	3.7	2.6	3.3	4.2
Australia								9.1	5.9	5.8	4.2	5.1	4.2	3.8	3.6	4.9
Canada	8.1	7.2	7.8	6.8	5.7	4.6	4.7	4.1	4.0	4.4	3.5	3.7	3.4	3.7	3.5	5.0
Central-East France			0.8	0.9	1.0	0.6	0.5	1.2	1.1	1.2	1.0	0.8	0.1	0.6	0.5	0.8
Czechoslovakia	3.2	2.3	3.5	3.4	3.5	2.0	4.5	3.9	3.3	2.5	3.4	1.5	1.4	1.2	1.1	2.8
Denmark										1.0	1.3	0.9	0.9	1.4	2.9	1.4
Emilia-Romagna					1.4	1.6	1.6	1.4	1.6	1.8	1.3	0.8	0.9	0.9	0.4	1.2
England-Wales	13.1	12.7	10.9	9.9	8.7	7.1	5.2	4.0	2.6	1.8	1.4	0.9	0.8	0.5	0.6	5.2
Finland	1.8	2.8	3.3	3.1	2.5	2.1	3.0	2.2	2.6	0.6	0.9	1.1	1.0	1.2	0.7	1.9
Hungary	10.4	7.6	7.4	5.7	5.1	5.9	4.9	9.0	6.2	6.4	3.8	3.1	2.4	2.2	1.8	5.7
Israel	1.4	5.4	9.4	9.8	2.7	5.3	3.2	6.6	5.0	4.9	3.9	3.4	2.8	2.4	1.7	4.2
Italy					5.9	3.9	3.3	3.7	2.4	2.9	1.7	1.9	1.9	1.3	0.9	2.4
Japan						10.1	11.4	8.0	8.2	10.1	8.5	8.5	7.4	6.8	6.5	9.2
Mexico							17.5	19.4	19.1	18.6	16.7	18.3	21.5	19.4	16.6	18.4
New Zealand							6.9	5.8	7.0	3.8	2.8	3.5	3.6	3.1	1.6	4.2
Northern Ireland							16.6	17.4	12.9	9.1	4.7	7.9				11.5
Norway	3.3	4.7	3.3	5.1	3.6	4.8	3.5	4.5	2.9	3.6	2.0	4.3	3.6	2.9	2.6	3.6
Paris								2.1	1.8	1.8	2.0	1.0	0.7	1.7	0.7	1.5
Sichuan												5.4	7.4	5.9	6.3	6.3
South America	3.6	1.7	2.8	2.8	2.9	2.9	1.8	4.3	6.2	7.1	7.1	6.2	5.1	7.3	5.7	5.3
Spain			3.3	2.6	2.5	3.9	6.2	4.5	4.7	3.3	3.9	5.7	2.4	2.7	2.5	3.9
Strasbourg									0.7	3.2	6.3	2.3	2.3	4.6	3.7	3.3
Sweden	3.8	2.8	3.8	3.8	1.9	2.4	1.7	1.2	1.5	1.8	1.1	0.7	1.3	1.9	0.7	2.0
Tokyo							4.2	5.5	8.3	11.1	4.6	4.2	7.7	10.8	9.2	7.2
United States	4.4	4.3	4.2	3.7	3.7	3.6	3.3	3.5	3.3	3.0	2.6	2.7	2.6	2.0	2.1	3.4

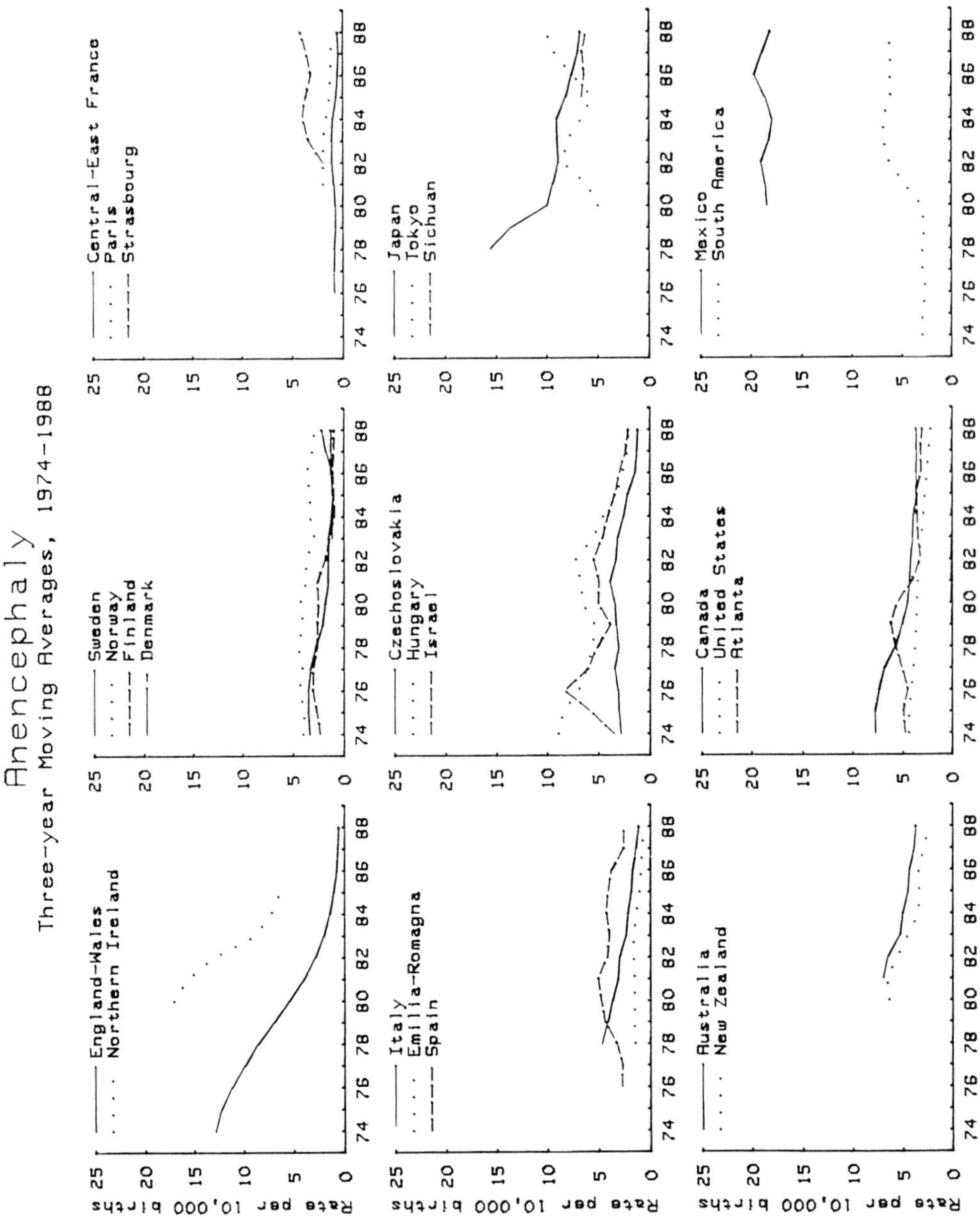

Anencephaly
Three-year Moving Averages, 1974-1988
England-Wales
Northern Ireland
Sweden
Norway
Finland
Denmark
Central-East France
Paris
Strasbourg
Italy
Emilia-Romagna
Spain
Czechoslovakia
Hungary
Israel
Japan
Tokyo
Sichuan
Australia
New Zealand
Canada
United States
Atlanta
Mexico
South America
Rate per 10,000 births
25 20 15 10 5 0
74 76 78 80 82 84 86 88

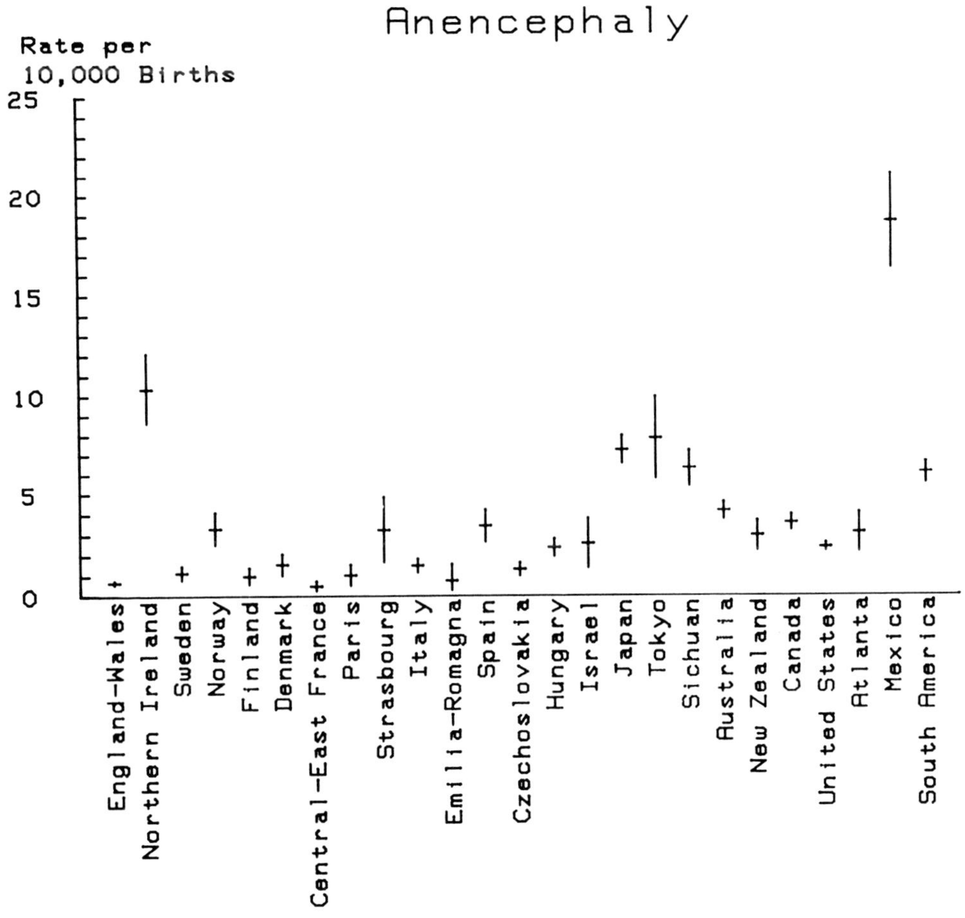

Diagram showing average rates of anencephaly in different programs for the years 1985-1988. Vertical lines indicate 95% confidence intervals of the recorded rates.

Comments

There is marked variability in the rates of anencephaly among the programs. In many but not all programs the rates have declined during the observation period.

A remarkably high rate is seen in Mexico, but not in South America. In the latter program, an increase in rate is seen which occurs after the time when stillbirths began to be included in the reporting. South America, the Asian programs, and Northern Ireland have slightly elevated rates compared with the majority of the programs. The higher rate in Norway compared with other Nordic countries can be an effect of a much lower stillbirth limit in the former program than in the others (16 vs. 28 weeks).

Both the declining time trends and the differences in rates between the programs may largely be the result of prenatal diagnosis followed by elective abortion.

Spina bifida

Spina bifida (aperta) is an inclusive name for various conditions with non-closure of the spine and a neurological deficit as a result of a defect in the spinal cord development. A completely open spinal cord (myeloschisis) may exist; more often there is a myelomeningocele with a herniated sac of meninges and sometimes also neural tissue. The defect is often in the lumbosacral area, but sometimes higher up in the spine. The origin of the defect is a disturbance in the normal closure of the neural walls and related developmental processes. As a direct result of the spina bifida, hydrocephaly and positional foot defects often exist. Other malformations may also exist.

Infants with spina bifida can be operated on and usually survive, but neurological handicap of varying severity may remain. Hydrocephaly may lead to mental handicap.

Spina bifida can usually, but not always, be detected with prenatal diagnosis: ultrasound and/or alphafetoprotein investigation.

A genetic background to the malformation exists and there may be a recurrence in a subsequent child. Various exogenous factors are thought to contribute, including maternal use of specific drugs (e.g., valproic acid) and folic acid deficiency. Spina bifida may occur with chromosome anomalies, such as trisomy 18. High and low defects may have different etiology.

Spina bifida

Definition: A congenital malformation characterized by herniation or exposure of the spinal cord and/or meninges through an incompletely closed spine. Not counted when present with anencephaly.

A. Number of infants born with spina bifida

Monitoring program	1974	1975	1976	1977	1978	1979	1980	1981	1982	1983	1984	1985	1986	1987	1988	Total
Atlanta	22	16	13	19	16	15	18	16	14	21	20	20	23	17	19	269
Australia								80	184	193	153	157	155	175	168	1265
Canada	271	249	222	212	242	243	206	172	199	245	208	237	222	237	179	3344
Central-East France			28	29	24	22	29	24	28	27	30	37	28	23	29	358
Czechoslovakia	86	82	76	84	67	67	70	55	56	59	49	52	55	33	46	937
Denmark										20	17	18	26	26	17	124
Emilia-Romagna					2	2	10	3	6	12	9	9	11	7	5	76
England-Wales	1185	1101	880	881	841	851	757	665	511	424	380	361	267	209	157	9470
Finland	16	14	8	16	10	13	11	15	12	19	12	10	8	5	5	174
Hungary	294	223	217	168	128	119	110	152	107	112	91	84	117	82	75	2079
Israel	3	1	4	4	2	5	8	11	9	9	14	10	13	12	4	109
Italy					19	16	43	52	49	38	54	58	52	45	52	478
Japan						39	34	27	37	37	22	57	46	38	42	396
Mexico							63	56	44	52	55	27	46	78	78	499
New Zealand							58	54	50	58	53	37	39	50	26	425
Northern Ireland							58	56	56	43	48	31				292
Norway	33	31	28	29	22	15	34	29	33	24	26	24	26	30	26	410
Paris								24	18	19	9	11	18	8	6	113
Sichuan												28	37	25	17	107
South America	53	30	42	47	43	40	32	54	76	97	119	116	132	153	132	1166
Spain			4	13	16	24	24	20	29	31	37	37	27	20	27	309
Strasbourg									8	6	8	5	12	2	3	44
Sweden	70	68	51	42	49	51	38	49	42	41	38	54	58	65	44	760
Tokyo							4	1	4	6	5	7	3	7	5	42
United States	646	592	538	525	501	516	403	437	396	383	368	327	310	267	180	6389

B. Rate per 10,000 infants.

Monitoring program	1974	1975	1976	1977	1978	1979	1980	1981	1982	1983	1984	1985	1986	1987	1988	Average
Atlanta	8.9	6.9	5.7	8.1	6.6	5.9	6.6	6.0	5.0	7.5	6.8	6.5	7.0	4.9	5.2	6.4
Australia								7.0	7.7	8.0	6.5	6.5	6.4	7.2	6.9	7.0
Canada	12.0	10.8	9.7	9.1	9.8	9.6	8.6	7.1	7.9	10.1	8.3	9.0	8.5	9.6	8.3	9.2
Central-East France			4.2	4.2	3.5	3.1	3.9	3.1	3.7	3.1	3.5	4.1	3.1	2.6	3.2	3.5
Czechoslovakia	4.4	4.3	4.1	4.6	3.7	3.9	4.6	3.8	4.0	4.3	3.6	3.8	4.1	2.5	3.5	4.0
Denmark										3.9	3.3	3.3	4.7	4.6	2.9	3.8
Emilia-Romagna					2.8	3.1	8.0	2.1	3.3	5.5	3.9	3.7	4.8	3.1	2.2	3.9
England-Wales	18.3	18.1	14.9	15.3	14.0	13.2	11.5	10.4	8.1	6.7	5.9	5.5	4.0	3.1	2.3	9.9
Finland	2.6	2.1	1.2	2.5	1.6	2.1	1.7	2.4	1.8	2.8	1.8	1.6	1.3	0.8	0.8	1.8
Hungary	15.6	11.4	11.6	9.4	7.6	7.4	7.3	10.6	8.0	8.7	7.2	6.4	9.1	6.5	6.0	9.1
Israel	4.3	1.3	4.7	4.9	1.1	2.7	4.3	6.0	5.0	4.9	7.7	5.6	7.4	7.2	2.3	4.8
Italy					4.3	2.2	5.2	4.9	3.9	2.7	3.9	4.4	3.7	3.3	3.8	3.8
Japan						2.5	2.2	1.9	3.0	2.9	1.8	4.4	2.9	2.6	3.0	2.8
Mexico							15.1	16.2	12.7	13.6	16.4	11.2	18.7	19.1	19.1	15.9
New Zealand							12.6	10.9	10.4	11.5	10.6	7.2	7.4	9.2	4.7	9.3
Northern Ireland							20.1	20.3	20.6	15.7	17.2	11.1				17.5
Norway	5.5	5.4	5.2	5.6	4.2	2.9	6.6	5.7	6.4	4.8	5.1	4.7	4.9	5.5	4.5	5.1
Paris								6.2	4.6	4.8	2.3	2.7	4.4	2.0	1.5	3.5
Sichuan												4.4	4.7	3.0	2.6	3.7
South America	6.2	4.6	5.4	7.0	5.9	5.8	5.8	9.7	5.3	6.3	7.0	6.4	6.3	7.8	7.0	6.5
Spain			3.3	4.7	4.5	3.5	4.2	3.6	4.7	4.3	5.3	5.5	4.6	3.9	5.1	4.5
Strasbourg									5.9	4.8	6.3	3.9	9.3	1.5	2.2	4.8
Sweden	6.3	6.5	5.2	4.4	5.2	5.3	3.9	5.2	4.5	4.5	4.0	5.5	5.7	6.2	3.9	5.1
Tokyo							2.1	0.6	2.1	3.2	2.6	3.7	1.6	4.0	3.1	2.5
United States	6.0	5.5	5.1	4.9	5.1	5.0	5.2	5.1	4.8	4.7	5.0	4.5	4.5	4.4	3.5	5.0

Spina bifida
Three-year Moving Averages, 1974-1988

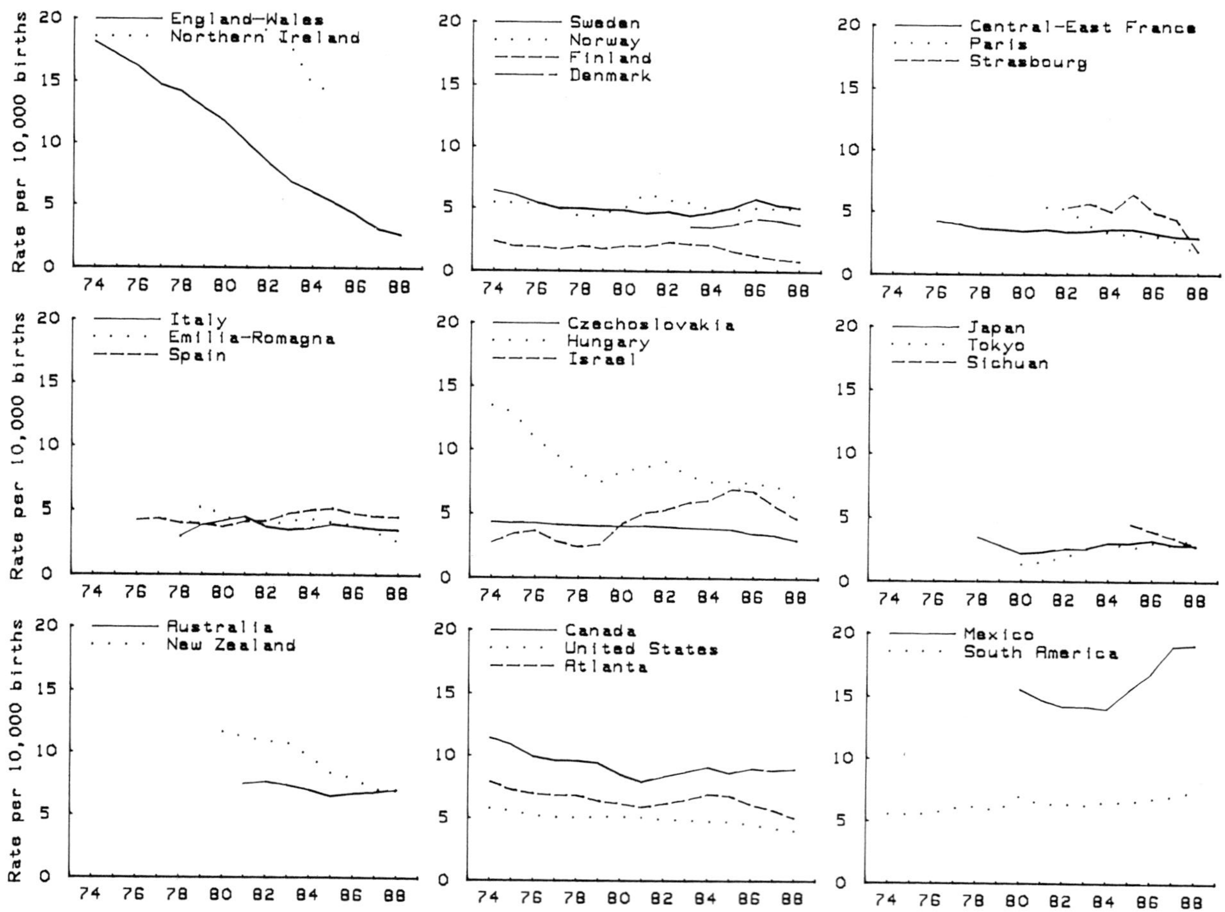

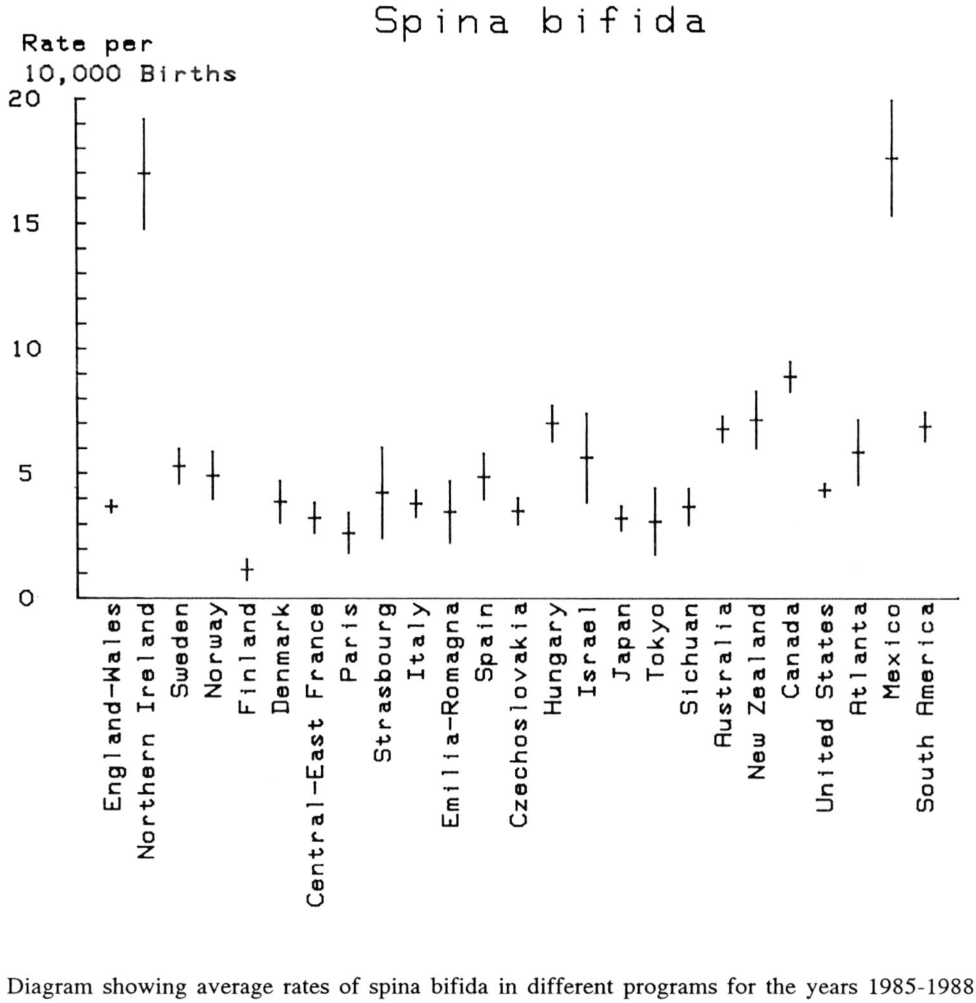

Diagram showing average rates of spina bifida in different programs for the years 1985-1988. Vertical lines indicate 95% confidence intervals of the recorded rates.

Comments

The majority of the programs report rates between 3 and 6 per 10,000 births, but higher rates are seen in Hungary, Australia, New Zealand, Canada, South America, and especially in Northern Ireland and Mexico. A lower rate is reported from Finland.

Clearly declining rates are seen in England-Wales, Northern Ireland, Hungary, and New Zealand, while an increasing trend is seen in Mexico and possibly in Israel. For most programs with a low rate, no marked changes are seen during the observation period.

Prenatal diagnosis and elective abortion play a role in the reduction of the spina bifida rate, but the impact is less than for anencephaly.

Encephalocele

Encephalocele is included among the neural tube defects. It consists of a defect in the skull through which a skin-covered hernia of meninges, sometimes containing brain substance, emerges. Its size may vary and in the most extreme forms a large part of the brain is included in the hernia. The most common location is the occipital region, but frontonasal ones are not rare.

Encephalocele is often combined with other malformations, including hydrocephaly and microcephaly. Small and moderate encephaloceles can be operated on successfully. Survival is good if no other serious malformation jeopardizes the child's life, but if the brain is involved in the malformation, neurological or mental deficit may occur.

Some encephaloceles occur in hereditary syndromes (e.g., the autosomal recessive Meckel syndrome) with a high recurrence risk. Others have a relatively low recurrence risk, but a genetic component is often present. Exogenous factors may play a role.

Prenatal ultrasound investigation can detect encephaloceles and elective abortion can be made.

Encephalocele

Definition: A congenital malformation characterized by herniation of the brain and/or meninges through a defect in the skull. Not counted when present with spina bifida.

A. Number of infants born with encephalocele

Monitoring program	1974	1975	1976	1977	1978	1979	1980	1981	1982	1983	1984	1985	1986	1987	1988	Total
Atlanta	3	4	4	4	10	3	10	7	7	5	6	8	8	6	7	92
Australia								23	44	39	40	30	40	25	30	271
Canada	37	36	43	36	37	39	36	26	49	44	36	46	38	36	40	579
Central-East France			1	6	4	3	6	6	3	11	2	4	4	5	5	60
Czechoslovakia	7	6	6	17	9	5	15	9	9	14	12	4	4	3	5	125
Denmark										5	0	4	2	3	5	19
Emilia-Romagna					1	1	0	0	1	0	0	2	5	1	0	11
England-Wales	139	146	135	150	138	84	77	76	67	51	47	40	43	24	30	1247
Finland										3	2	1	3	2	2	13
Hungary					18	20	28	30	31	15	19	21	19	27	17	245
Israel	0	1	0	0	1	1	0	0	1	1	1	1	0	0	1	8
Italy					4	12	3	17	11	13	14	14	15	14	5	122
Japan					7	17	24	8	13	16	8	18	24	23	15	173
Mexico							18	8	13	9	12	6	16	14	4	100
New Zealand										4	2	4	4	4	4	22
Northern Ireland										4	5	4				13
Norway	2	3	2	4	1	1	2	6	6	4	3	10	3	6	0	53
Paris								0	5	5	7	4	1	3	4	29
Sichuan												9	29	21	19	78
South America	16	8	7	8	12	3	12	19	30	35	35	24	24	24	42	299
Spain			0	2	3	5	6	11	7	8	5	8	2	2	2	61
Strasbourg									4	2	3	1	0	1	3	14
Sweden	8	12	7	9	8	12	3	7	9	8	4	10	6	8	7	118
Tokyo										1	2	4	0	2	0	9
United States	137	152	129	135	125	108	90	84	86	97	85	72	91	58	48	1497

B. Rate per 10,000 infants.																
Monitoring program	1974	1975	1976	1977	1978	1979	1980	1981	1982	1983	1984	1985	1986	1987	1988	Average
Atlanta	1.2	1.7	1.8	1.7	4.1	1.2	3.7	2.6	2.5	1.8	2.1	2.6	2.4	1.7	1.9	2.2
Australia								2.0	1.8	1.6	1.7	1.2	1.7	1.0	1.2	1.5
Canada	1.6	1.6	1.9	1.5	1.5	1.5	1.5	1.1	1.9	1.8	1.4	1.8	1.4	1.5	1.9	1.6
Central-EastFrance			0.2	0.9	0.6	0.4	0.8	0.8	0.4	1.3	0.2	0.4	0.4	0.6	0.5	0.6
Czechoslovakia	0.4	0.3	0.3	0.9	0.5	0.3	1.0	0.6	0.6	1.0	0.9	0.3	0.3	0.2	0.4	0.5
Denmark										1.0	0	0.7	0.4	0.5	0.8	0.6
Emilia-Romagna					1.4	1.6	0	0	0.5	0	0	0.8	2.2	0.4	0	0.6
England-Wales	2.1	2.4	2.3	2.6	2.3	1.3	1.2	1.2	1.1	0.8	0.7	0.6	0.6	0.4	0.4	1.3
Finland										0.4	0.3	0.2	0.5	0.3	0.3	0.3
Hungary					1.1	1.2	1.9	2.1	2.3	1.2	1.5	1.6	1.5	2.1	1.4	1.6
Israel	0	1.3	0	0	0.5	0.5	0	0	0.6	0.5	0.6	0.6	0	0	0.6	0.3
Italy					0.9	1.7	0.4	1.6	0.9	0.9	1.0	1.1	1.1	1.0	0.4	1.0
Japan						1.1	1.5	0.6	1.1	1.3	0.6	1.4	1.5	1.6	1.1	1.2
Mexico							4.3	2.3	3.8	2.4	3.6	2.5	6.5	3.4	1.0	3.2
New Zealand										0.8	0.4	0.8	0.8	0.7	0.7	0.7
Northern Ireland										1.5	1.8	1.4				1.6
Norway	0.3	0.5	0.4	0.8	0.2	0.2	0.4	1.2	1.2	0.8	0.6	1.9	0.6	1.1	0	0.7
Paris								0	1.3	1.3	1.8	1.0	0.2	0.7	1.0	0.9
Sichuan												1.4	3.7	2.5	2.9	2.7
South America	1.9	1.2	0.9	1.2	1.6	0.4	2.2	3.4	2.1	2.3	2.1	1.3	1.1	1.2	2.2	1.7
Spain			0	0.7	0.8	0.7	1.1	2.0	1.1	1.1	0.7	1.2	0.3	0.4	0.4	0.9
Strasbourg									3.0	1.6	2.4	0.8	0	0.8	2.2	1.5
Sweden	0.7	1.2	0.7	0.9	0.9	1.2	0.3	0.7	1.0	0.9	0.4	1.0	0.6	0.8	0.6	0.8
Tokyo										0.5	1.0	2.1	0	1.1	0	0.8
Unites States	1.3	1.4	1.2	1.3	1.3	1.0	1.2	1.0	1.0	1.2	1.1	1.0	1.3	1.0	0.9	1.2

Encephalocele
Three-year Moving Averages, 1974–1988

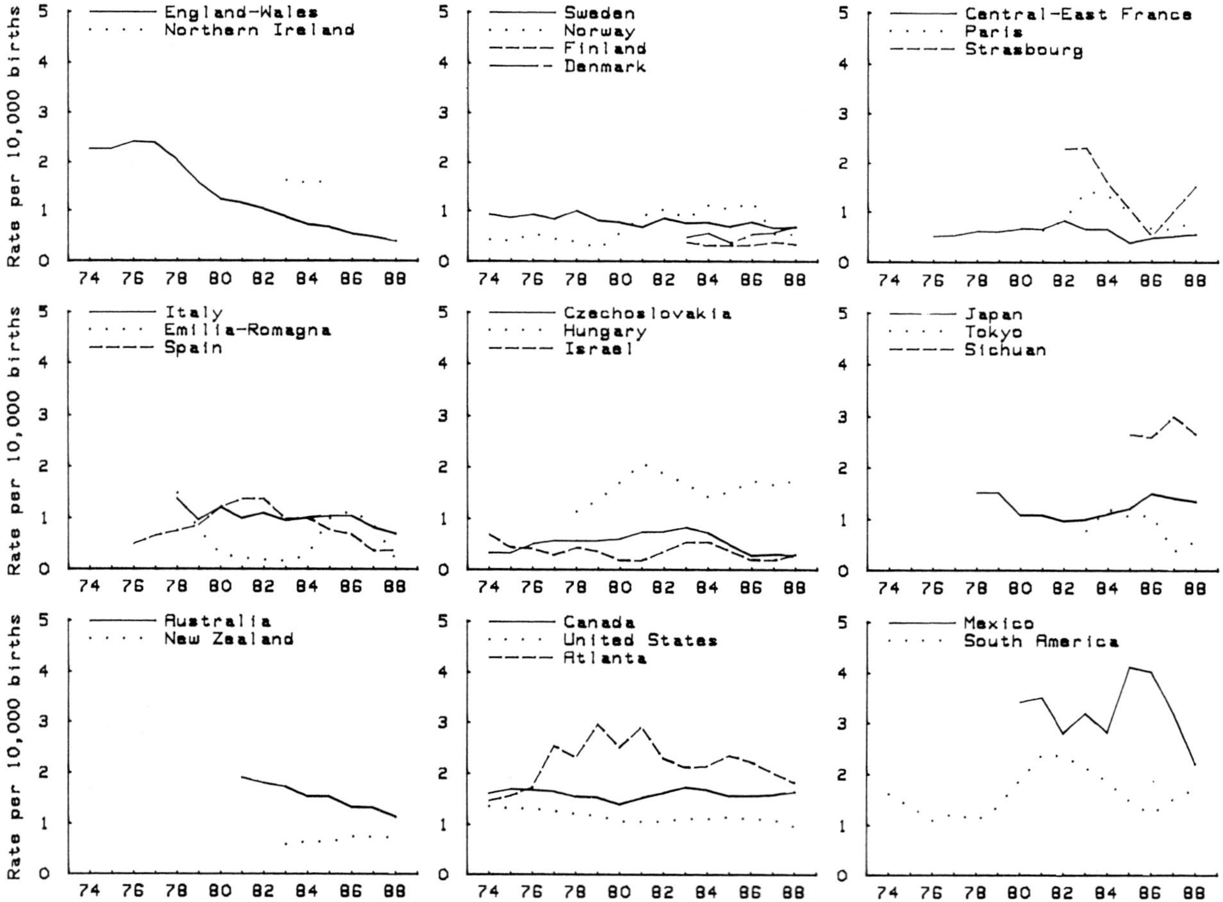

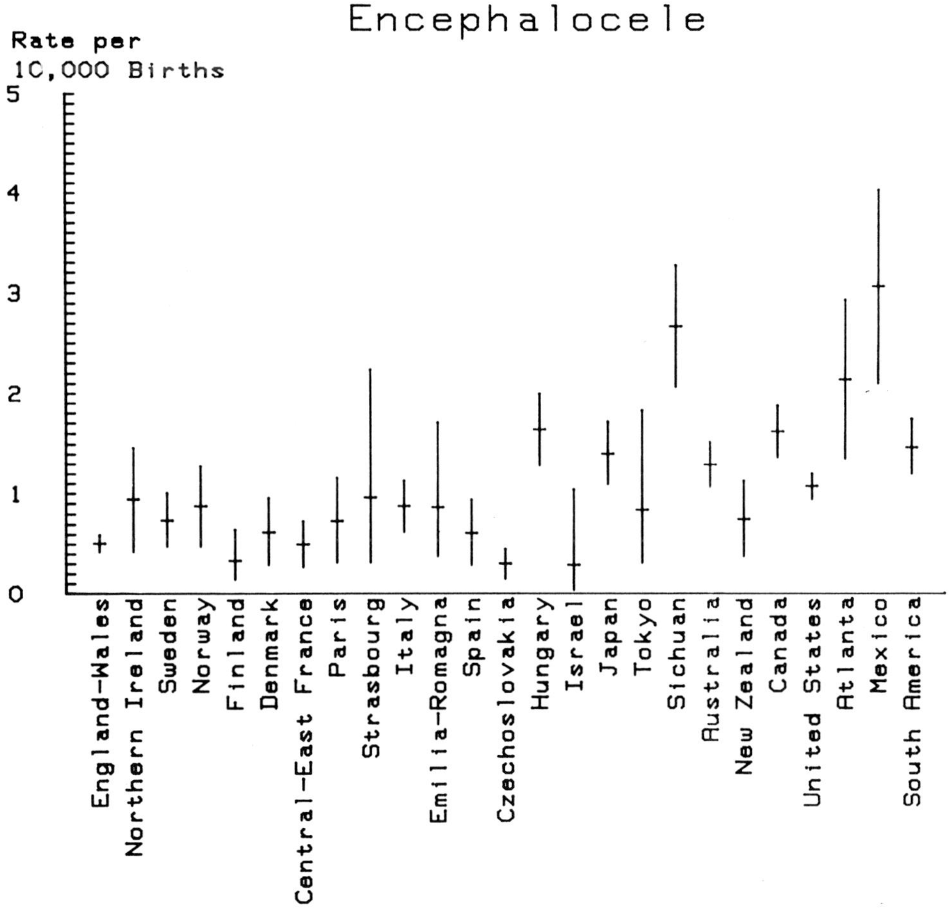

Diagram showing average rates of encephalocele in different programs for the years 1985-1988. Vertical lines indicate 95% confidence intervals of the recorded rates.

Comments

The comparative infrequency of this malformation results in random fluctuations in recorded rates. Relatively high rates are seen, however, in Sichuan, Atlanta, and Mexico.

The recorded rates decline markedly in England-Wales and to a lesser extent in Australia, while for most programs the rates remain relatively constant.

Around 1986, Mexico experienced an increased rate of encephalocele. The affected infants sometimes also had cataracts. A special investigation was made of this constellation of malformations in the *Clearinghouse*, but the finding could not be substantiated in other programs.

Hydrocephaly

Hydrocephaly is a condition characterized by an abnormal accumulation of cerebrospinal fluid, either within the brain ventricles or between the brain and skull. The head circumference may increase abnormally and, if untreated, brain development becomes impaired. Many different causes of hydrocephaly exist. Some are secondary to spina bifida or encephalocele and are not included in the tables given below. In other instances, brain malformations are the basis of hydrocephaly. Prenatal infections may cause hydrocephaly. There are genetic forms, either autosomal recessive or X-linked recessive, but generally the recurrence risk is moderate. Hydrocephaly may develop secondarily to birth trauma, notably after premature births.

Hydrocephaly may be present at birth or may develop even months after birth. Severe cases can be detected by ultrasound prenatal investigation and elective abortion can be made.

Hydrocephaly can be treated surgically by shunting, leading excess cerebrospinal fluid away from the skull. If brain development was not already impaired, neurological and mental development can be adequate.

Hydrocephaly

Definition: A congenital abnormality characterized by dilatation of the ventricular system, not associated with a primary brain atrophy, with or without enlargement of the head, and diagnosed before birth or during the first week of life. Not counted when present with encephalocele or open spina bifida.

A. Number of infants born with hydrocephaly

Monitoring program	1974	1975	1976	1977	1978	1979	1980	1981	1982	1983	1984	1985	1986	1987	1988	Total
Atlanta	24	15	15	29	25	26	44	26	18	15	28	28	27	22	13	355
Australia								57	107	96	95	96	67	82	93	693
Canada	76	79	121	92	150	147	143	125	127	151	150	146	154	139	110	1910
Central-East France			17	9	8	12	18	10	19	28	24	40	23	28	28	264
Czechoslovakia	26	45	46	48	38	54	35	46	49	34	32	48	35	30	31	597
Denmark										15	15	12	16	17	14	89
Emilia-Romagna					4	1	2	8	8	13	13	10	9	13	5	86
England-Wales	691	615	552	545	536	473	490	424	339	331	283	263	226	117	137	6022
Finland	5	18	13	14	10	10	20	18	9	17	20	17	10	10	11	202
Hungary	151	181	132	107	78	93	95	66	52	68	37	29	58	34	45	1226
Israel	3	5	1	5	6	5	8	5	8	6	6	10	4	2	5	79
Italy					14	26	33	31	43	56	50	49	54	43	58	457
Japan					27	50	49	47	57	50	41	75	83	67	78	624
Mexico							26	20	21	27	14	11	10	17	16	162
New Zealand							34	20	17	20	15	15	24	17	20	182
Northern Ireland							19	13	11	20	16	7				86
Norway	31	26	12	14	21	35	20	18	15	15	23	19	26	16	28	319
Paris								28	24	18	22	21	21	15	12	161
Sichuan												41	70	60	41	212
South America	14	21	16	24	28	24	25	25	43	64	66	73	91	88	117	719
Spain			3	0	5	8	18	15	11	15	8	18	12	11	21	145
Strasbourg									11	10	10	7	4	8	8	58
Sweden	35	34	33	21	27	30	30	40	30	34	24	37	36	25	24	460
Tokyo							1	3	1	3	5	6	7	7	4	37
United States	439	419	431	500	412	453	329	469	453	492	418	411	403	362	295	6286

B. Rate per 10,000 infants.

Monitoring program	1974	1975	1976	1977	1978	1979	1980	1981	1982	1983	1984	1985	1986	1987	1988	Average
Atlanta	9.7	6.5	6.6	12.3	10.2	10.2	16.1	9.7	6.5	5.4	9.6	9.0	8.2	6.3	3.5	8.5
Australia								5.0	4.5	4.0	4.0	4.0	2.8	3.4	3.8	3.9
Canada	3.4	3.4	5.3	4.0	6.1	5.8	6.0	5.1	5.0	6.2	6.0	5.6	5.9	5.6	5.1	5.3
Central-East France			2.6	1.3	1.2	1.7	2.4	1.3	2.5	3.3	2.8	4.4	2.5	3.1	3.1	2.5
Czechoslovakia	1.3	2.3	2.5	2.6	2.1	3.1	2.3	3.2	3.5	2.5	2.3	3.5	2.6	2.3	2.3	2.5
Denmark										2.9	2.9	2.2	2.9	3.0	2.4	2.7
Emilia-Romagna					5.7	1.6	1.6	5.6	4.4	6.0	5.6	4.2	3.9	5.7	2.2	4.4
England-Wales	10.7	10.1	9.4	9.5	8.9	7.4	7.4	6.6	5.4	5.2	4.4	4.0	3.4	1.7	2.0	6.3
Finland	0.8	2.8	2.0	2.1	1.6	1.6	3.2	2.8	1.4	2.5	3.1	2.7	1.6	1.7	1.8	2.1
Hungary	8.0	9.2	7.1	6.0	4.6	5.8	6.3	4.6	3.9	5.3	2.9	2.2	4.5	2.7	3.6	5.4
Israel	4.3	6.7	1.2	6.1	3.3	2.7	4.3	2.7	4.5	3.3	3.3	5.6	2.3	1.2	2.9	3.4
Italy					3.2	3.6	4.0	2.9	3.4	4.0	3.7	3.7	3.8	3.1	4.2	3.6
Japan						3.1	3.1	3.4	4.7	4.0	3.3	5.8	5.3	4.6	5.6	4.5
Mexico							6.2	5.8	6.1	7.1	4.2	4.6	4.1	4.2	3.9	5.2
New Zealand							7.4	4.0	3.5	4.0	3.0	2.9	4.6	3.1	3.6	4.0
Northern Ireland							6.6	4.7	4.0	7.3	5.7	2.5				5.2
Norway	5.1	4.6	2.2	2.7	4.0	6.7	3.9	3.5	2.9	3.0	4.5	3.7	4.9	2.9	4.8	4.0
Paris								7.2	6.2	4.5	5.5	5.1	5.2	3.7	2.9	5.0
Sichuan												6.5	8.8	7.1	6.3	7.3
South America	1.6	3.2	2.1	3.6	3.8	3.5	4.5	4.5	3.0	4.1	3.9	4.0	4.3	4.5	6.2	4.0
Spain			2.5	0	1.4	1.2	3.2	2.7	1.8	2.1	1.2	2.7	2.1	2.2	4.0	2.1
Strasbourg									8.1	8.0	7.9	5.4	3.1	6.2	6.0	6.4
Sweden	3.2	3.3	3.3	2.2	2.9	3.1	3.1	4.2	3.2	3.7	2.5	3.7	3.5	2.4	2.1	3.1
Tokyo							0.5	1.7	0.5	1.6	2.6	3.1	3.8	4.0	2.5	2.2
United States	4.0	3.9	4.1	4.6	4.2	4.4	4.3	5.4	5.5	6.0	5.6	5.7	5.9	6.0	5.8	4.9

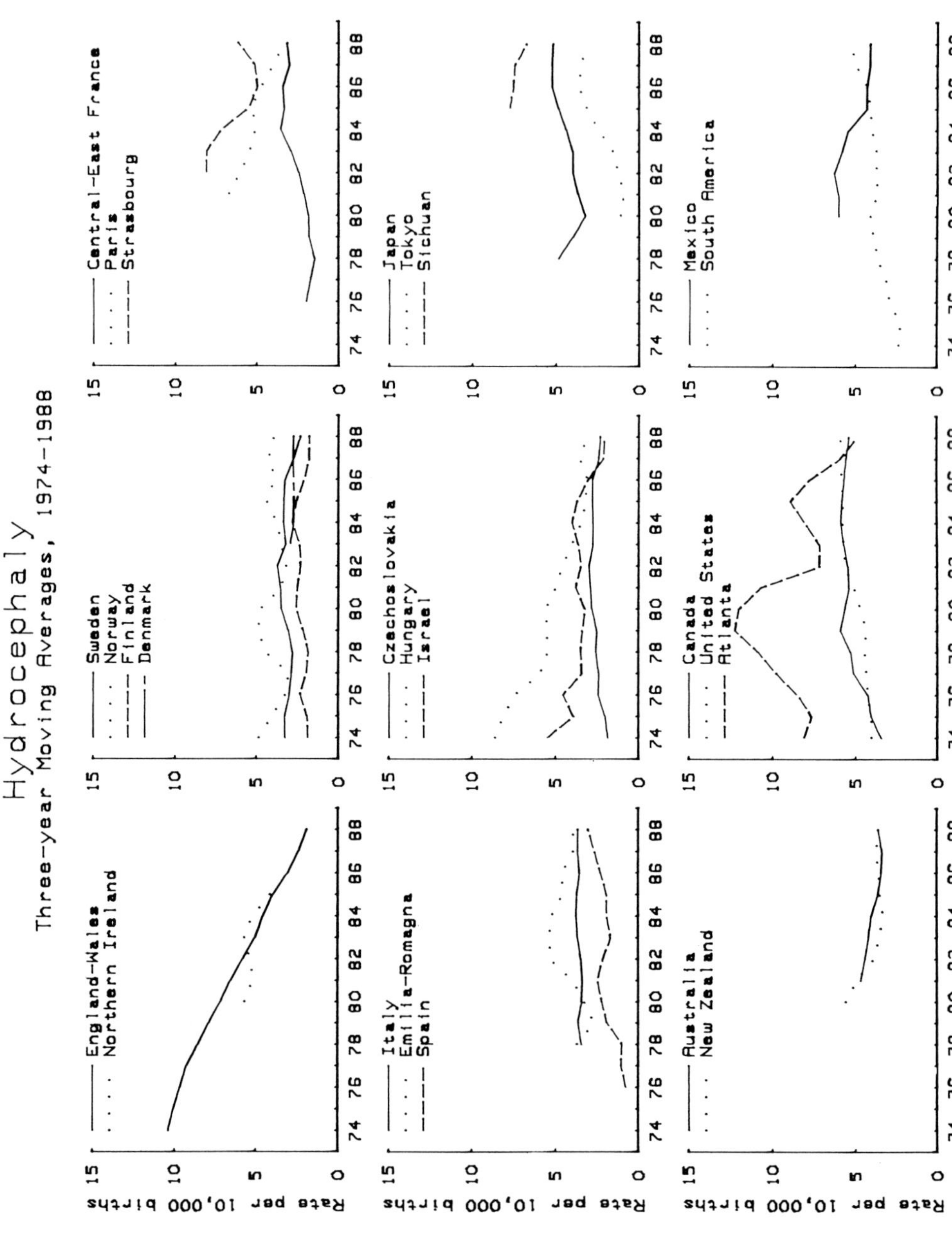
Hydrocephaly
Three-year Moving Averages, 1974-1988
England-Wales
Northern Ireland
Sweden
Norway
Finland
Denmark
Central-East France
Paris
Strasbourg
Italy
Emilia-Romagna
Spain
Czechoslovakia
Hungary
Israel
Japan
Tokyo
Sichuan
Australia
New Zealand
Canada
United States
Atlanta
Mexico
South America
Rate per 10,000 births
0
5
10
15
74
76
78
80
82
84
86
88

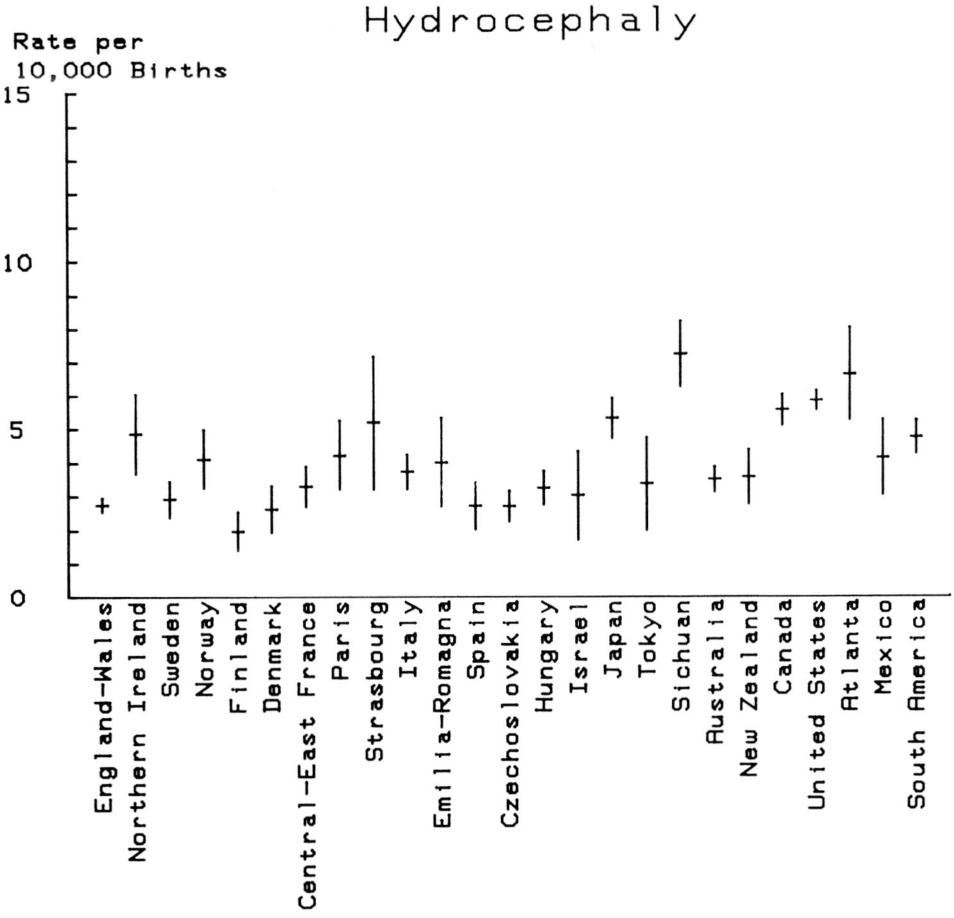

Diagram showing average rates of hydrocephaly in different programs for the years 1985-1988. Vertical lines indicate 95% confidence intervals of the recorded rates.

Comments

High rates are seen in Canada, United States and Atlanta, and also in Sichuan. Variations in rate are probably partly due to actual differences, but even more so to variability in the definition of hydrocephaly, the length of time the newborns are followed up, and the inclusion of perinatally originating conditions.

An increasing trend is seen in several programs - Spain, the two Japanese programs, Canada, United States, South America, and in Central-East France - while the two other French programs, Atlanta, and Mexico show, if anything, the opposite trend. A strongly declining trend is seen in England-Wales and Hungary.

Prenatal diagnosis and selective abortion may play a role, possibly explaining the declining trend in Paris, for example. However, no strong impact on the rate of hydrocephaly is seen in other countries with well-developed prenatal diagnostic services (like Denmark and Sweden).

Microtia

In microtia the ear is reduced in size and is abnormal in shape. The malformation is usually unilateral, most often on the right side. Different degrees of microtia occur, with the most severe form representing total or nearly total absence of the ear (anotia). The ear canal is often missing and hearing is usually impaired.

Microtia often occurs together with other malformations. As such, it does not threaten the infant's life, but reduced or absent hearing is a handicap to which should be added the cosmetic problem.

In many cases heredity is present, autosomal dominant or recessive. Little is known about exogenous causes of the malformation, but it is included in a complex seen after maternal use of a vitamin A analogue (isotretinoin) and was seen in infants damaged by thalidomide.

The malformation cannot be detected prenatally.

Microtia

Definition: A congenital malformation characterized by absent parts of the pinna, with or without atresia of the ear canal, commonly expressed in grades (I-IV) of which the extreme form (grade IV) is anotia.

A. Number of infants born with microtia

Monitoring program	1974	1975	1976	1977	1978	1979	1980	1981	1982	1983	1984	1985	1986	1987	1988	Total
Atlanta	6	4	5	2	3	4	4	2	5	4	2	4	4	8	4	61
Australia								6	20	18	22	23	26	19	19	153
Central-East France			2	0	2	3	2	4	6	5	4	7	2	14	9	60
Czechoslovakia	6	3	0	0	1	1	1	1	3	1	1	2	2	0	2	24
Denmark										3	3	2	2	1	1	12
Emilia-Romagna					0	0	1	2	2	5	1	5	4	4	4	28
England-Wales						126	148	234	175	192	225	177	175	215	158	1825
Finland										8	4	4	5	7	3	31
Hungary					39	25	25	29	38	39	39	35	27	24	27	346
Israel					2	1	1	2	2	2	3	1	3	2	1	20
Italy								14	25	18	23	22	33	17	15	167
Japan					5	18	18	19	10	18	11	12	16	20	9	156
Mexico							33	15	28	25	23	18	12	21	24	199
New Zealand										6	6	2	0	4	0	18
Northern Ireland										5	4	2				11
Norway												3	5	13	9	32
Paris								0	2	1	2	2	2	2	2	13
Sichuan												13	43	43	34	133
South America	46	22	56	40	51	41	23	27	55	43	63	85	95	78	92	817
Spain			4	3	3	10	15	10	7	13	15	19	10	6	6	121
Strasbourg									3	0	1	1	4	3	3	15
Sweden	23	21	28	28	14	21	15	20	22	24	21	23	21	22	18	321
Tokyo								2	1	3	2	3	2	5	5	23

B. Rate per 10,000 infants.

Monitoring program	1974	1975	1976	1977	1978	1979	1980	1981	1982	1983	1984	1985	1986	1987	1988	Average
Atlanta	2.4	1.7	2.2	0.9	1.2	1.6	1.5	0.7	1.8	1.4	0.7	1.3	1.2	2.3	1.1	1.5
Australia								0.5	0.8	0.7	0.9	1.0	1.1	0.8	0.8	0.9
Central-East France			0.3	0	0.3	0.4	0.3	0.5	0.8	0.6	0.5	0.8	0.2	1.6	1.0	0.6
Czechoslovakia	0.3	0.2	0	0	0.1	0.1	0.1	0.1	0.2	0.1	0.1	0.1	0.1	0	0.2	0.1
Denmark										0.6	0.6	0.4	0.4	0.2	0.2	0.4
Emilia-Romagna					0	0	0.8	1.4	1.1	2.3	0.4	2.1	1.7	1.8	1.8	1.4
England-Wales						2.0	2.2	3.7	2.8	3.0	3.5	2.7	2.6	3.1	2.3	2.8
Finland										1.2	0.6	0.6	0.8	1.2	0.5	0.8
Hungary					2.3	1.5	1.7	2.8	2.8	3.0	3.0	2.7	2.1	1.9	2.2	2.3
Israel					1.1	0.5	0.5	1.1	1.1	1.1	1.7	0.6	1.7	1.2	0.6	1.0
Italy								1.3	2.0	1.3	1.7	1.7	2.3	1.2	1.1	1.6
Japan						1.1	1.1	1.4	0.8	1.4	0.9	0.9	1.0	1.4	0.7	1.1
Mexico							7.9	4.3	8.1	6.6	6.8	7.5	4.9	5.2	5.9	6.4
New Zealand										1.2	1.2	0.4	0	0.7	0	0.6
Northern Ireland										1.8	1.4	0.7				1.3
Norway										0.4	0	0.6	0.9	2.4	1.6	1.0
Paris								0	0.5	0.3	0.5	0.5	0.5	0.5	0.5	0.4
Sichuan												2.1	5.4	5.1	5.2	4.6
South America	5.4	3.4	7.2	5.9	7.0	5.9	4.2	4.8	3.8	2.8	3.7	4.7	4.5	4.0	4.9	4.6
Spain			3.3	1.1	0.8	1.5	2.6	1.8	1.1	1.8	2.2	2.8	1.7	1.2	1.1	1.8
Strasbourg									2.2	0	0.8	0.8	3.1	2.3	2.2	1.7
Sweden	2.1	2.0	2.8	2.9	1.5	2.2	1.5	2.1	2.4	2.6	2.2	2.3	2.1	2.1	1.6	2.2
Tokyo								1.1	0.5	1.6	1.0	1.6	1.1	2.8	3.1	1.6

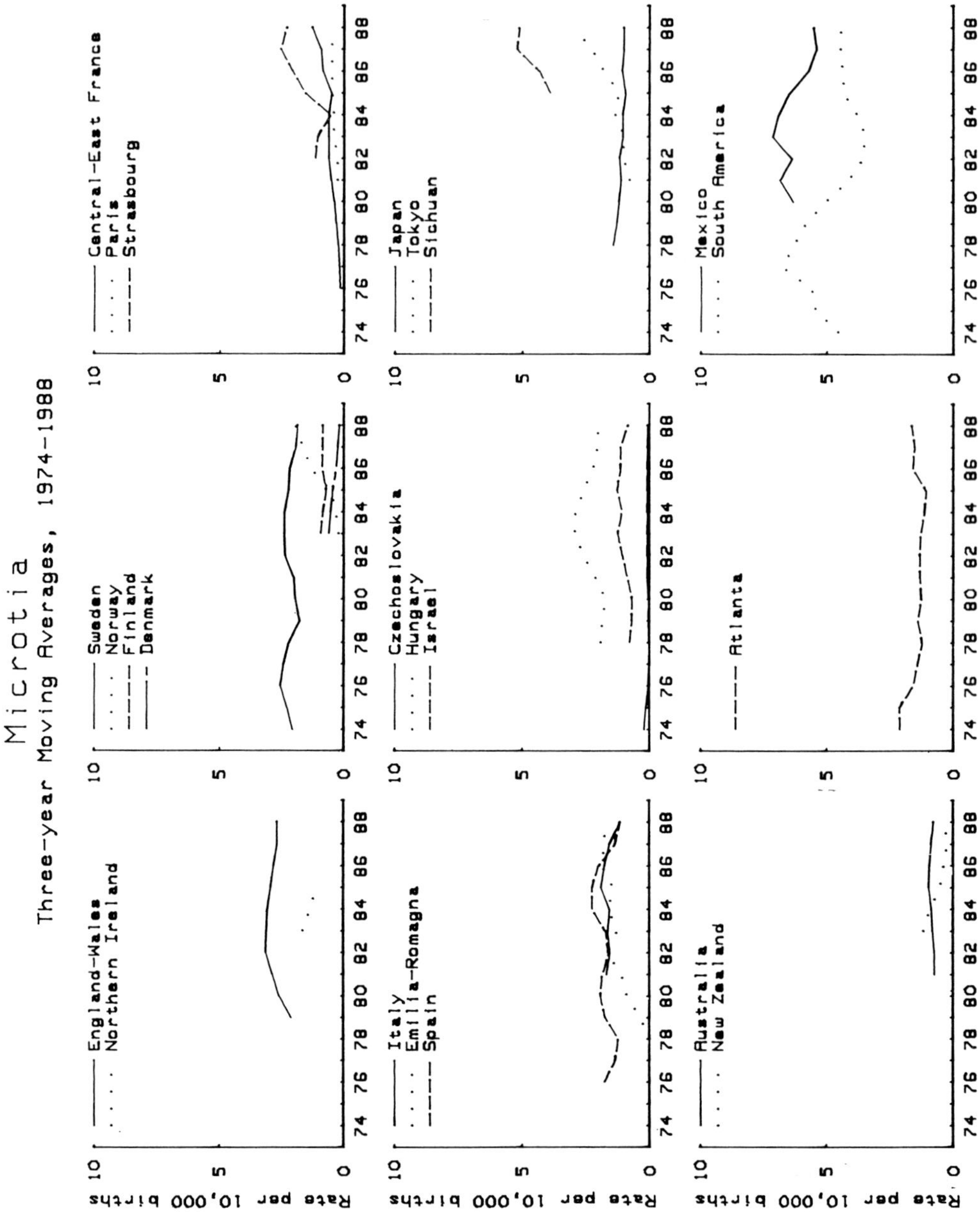
Microtia
Three-year Moving Averages, 1974-1988
England-Wales
Northern Ireland
Sweden
Norway
Finland
Denmark
Central-East France
Paris
Strasbourg
Italy
Emilia-Romagna
Spain
Czechoslovakia
Hungary
Israel
Japan
Tokyo
Sichuan
Australia
New Zealand
Atlanta
Mexico
South America
Rate per 10,000 births
10
5
0
74 76 78 80 82 84 86 88

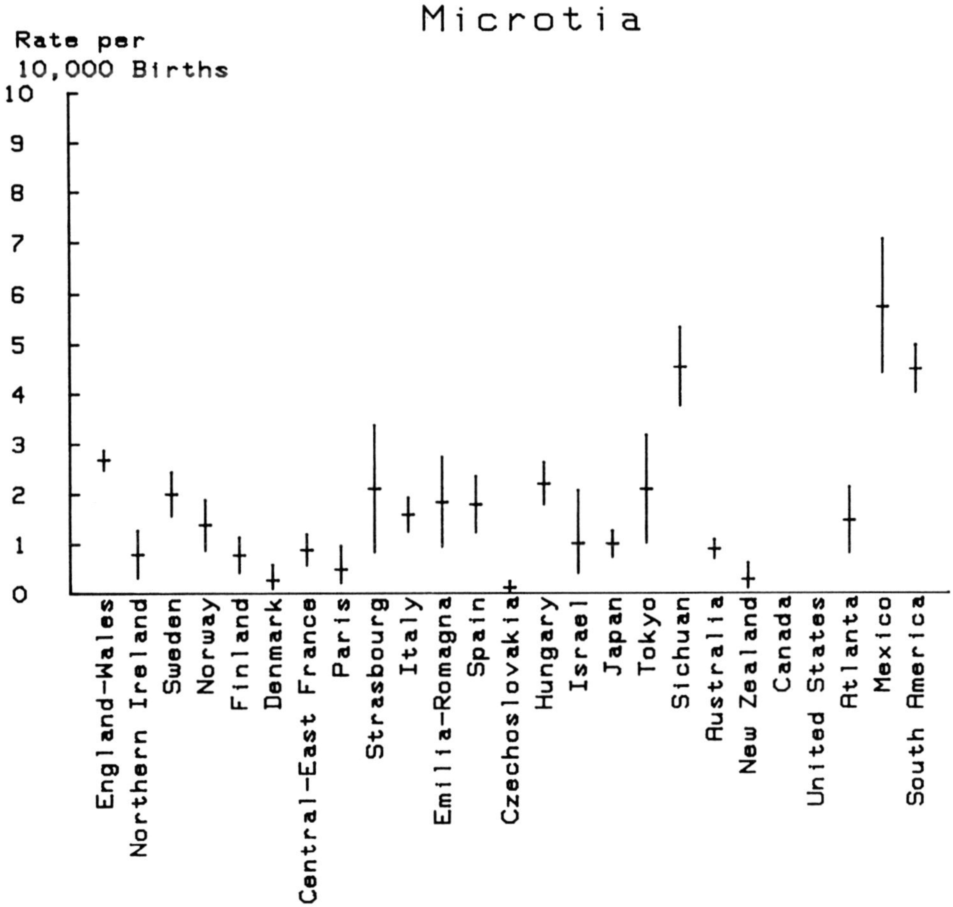

Diagram showing average rates of microtia in different programs for the years 1985-1988. Vertical lines indicate 95% confidence intervals of the recorded rates.

Comments

Rates are low, so random fluctuations of rates will occur. Relatively high rates are seen in Sichuan, Mexico, and South America.

In most programs the recorded rates are comparatively stable, but increases are seen in Central-East France, Tokyo, and at the end of the 1970s in South America.

Transposition of the great vessels (TGV)

This is a serious heart defect that arises through a maldivision of the arterial truncus which gives rise to the aorta and the pulmonary artery. The division occurs by a spiralized septum, and if the septum development is abnormal, the aorta will emerge from the right ventricle and the pulmonary truncus from the left ventricle.

The malformation results in serious effects on the circulation, and for long-term survival an operation has to be performed. If the infant survives the operation, prognosis is fair.

As in all congenital heart defects, a genetic component exists that causes a low but definite recurrence rate in sibs. Prenatal diagnosis can detect the condition in late pregnancy. Various exogenous causes have been suggested but not proved.

Transposition of the great vessels

Definition: A group of congenital malformations characterized by various degrees of transposition of the great vessels and inversion of the heart chambers.

A. Number of infants born with transposition of the great vessels

Monitoring program	1974	1975	1976	1977	1978	1979	1980	1981	1982	1983	1984	1985	1986	1987	1988	Total
Atlanta	9	11	9	10	16	9	14	7	16	16	18	14	12	16	17	194
Australia								34	74	76	72	91	80	96	114	637
Canada	44	55	52	58	113	94	94	114	118	118	126	162	127	143	100	1518
Central-East France			17	28	18	26	21	21	33	22	26	21	32	34	35	334
Czechoslovakia	79	66	86	57	58	58	49	35	30	40	28	36	24	25	21	692
Emilia-Romagna					1	0	3	4	4	11	5	4	9	4	5	50
England-Wales	21	23	30	16	23	28	24	32	31	41	36	38	50	35	33	461
Hungary					6	12	21	22	16	30	18	13	31	17	21	207
Israel													2	6	7	15
Italy								8	11	11	14	17	30	30	30	151
Japan					0	0	0	0	0	0	0	0	0	0	0	0
New Zealand														1	5	6
Norway	3	1	3	1	1	4	4	5	5	2	3	3	3	4	17	59
Paris								5	13	13	15	11	8	10	8	83
Sichuan														1	0	1
South America	0	1	2	0	0	2	0	1	9	9	5	10	16	15	5	75
Spain			0	1	1	1	5	2	0	8	6	3	5	4	8	44
Strasbourg									4	5	5	10	5	8	12	49
Sweden								26	31	41	34	36	28	29	34	259
Tokyo							1	1	0	1	1	0	2	0	0	6
United States	95	74	83	96	87	101	56	86	70	82	93	98	90	88	83	1282

B. Rate per 10,000 infants.																
Monitoring program	1974	1975	1976	1977	1978	1979	1980	1981	1982	1983	1984	1985	1986	1987	1988	Average
Atlanta	3.6	4.8	4.0	4.3	6.6	3.5	5.1	2.6	5.7	5.7	6.2	4.5	3.7	4.6	4.6	4.6
Australia								3.0	3.1	3.2	3.0	3.8	3.3	4.0	4.7	3.5
Canada	1.9	2.4	2.3	2.5	4.6	3.7	3.9	4.7	4.7	4.9	5.0	6.2	4.8	5.8	4.6	4.2
Central-East France			2.6	4.1	2.6	3.7	2.8	2.7	4.4	2.6	3.0	2.3	3.5	3.8	3.8	3.2
Czechoslovakia	4.1	3.4	4.6	3.1	3.2	3.4	3.2	2.4	2.1	2.9	2.0	2.6	1.8	1.9	1.6	2.9
Emilia-Romagna					1.4	0	2.4	2.8	2.2	5.1	2.2	1.7	3.9	1.8	2.2	2.6
England-Wales	0.3	0.4	0.5	0.3	0.4	0.4	0.4	0.5	0.5	0.6	0.6	0.6	0.8	0.5	0.5	0.5
Hungary					0.4	0.7	1.4	1.5	1.2	2.3	1.4	1.0	2.4	1.3	1.7	1.4
Israel													1.1	3.6	4.0	2.9
Italy								0.7	0.9	0.8	1.0	1.3	2.1	2.2	2.2	1.4
Japan						0	0	0	0	0	0	0	0	0	0	0
New Zealand														0.2	0.9	0.5
Norway	0.5	0.2	0.6	0.2	0.2	0.8	0.8	1.0	1.0	0.4	0.6	0.6	0.6	0.7	2.9	0.7
Paris								1.3	3.3	3.3	3.8	2.7	2.0	2.5	1.9	2.6
Sichuan														0.1	0	0.1
South America	0	0.2	0.3	0	0	0.3	0	0.2	0.6	0.6	0.3	0.5	0.8	0.8	0.3	0.4
Spain			0	0.4	0.3	0.1	0.9	0.4	0	1.1	0.9	0.4	0.9	0.8	1.5	0.6
Strasbourg									3.0	4.0	3.9	7.7	3.9	6.2	9.0	5.4
Sweden								2.8	3.3	4.5	3.6	3.6	2.7	2.8	3.0	3.3
Tokyo							0.5	0.6	0	0.5	0.5	0	1.1	0	0	0.4
United States	0.9	0.7	0.8	0.9	0.9	1.0	0.7	1.0	0.9	1.0	1.3	1.4	1.3	1.5	1.6	1.0

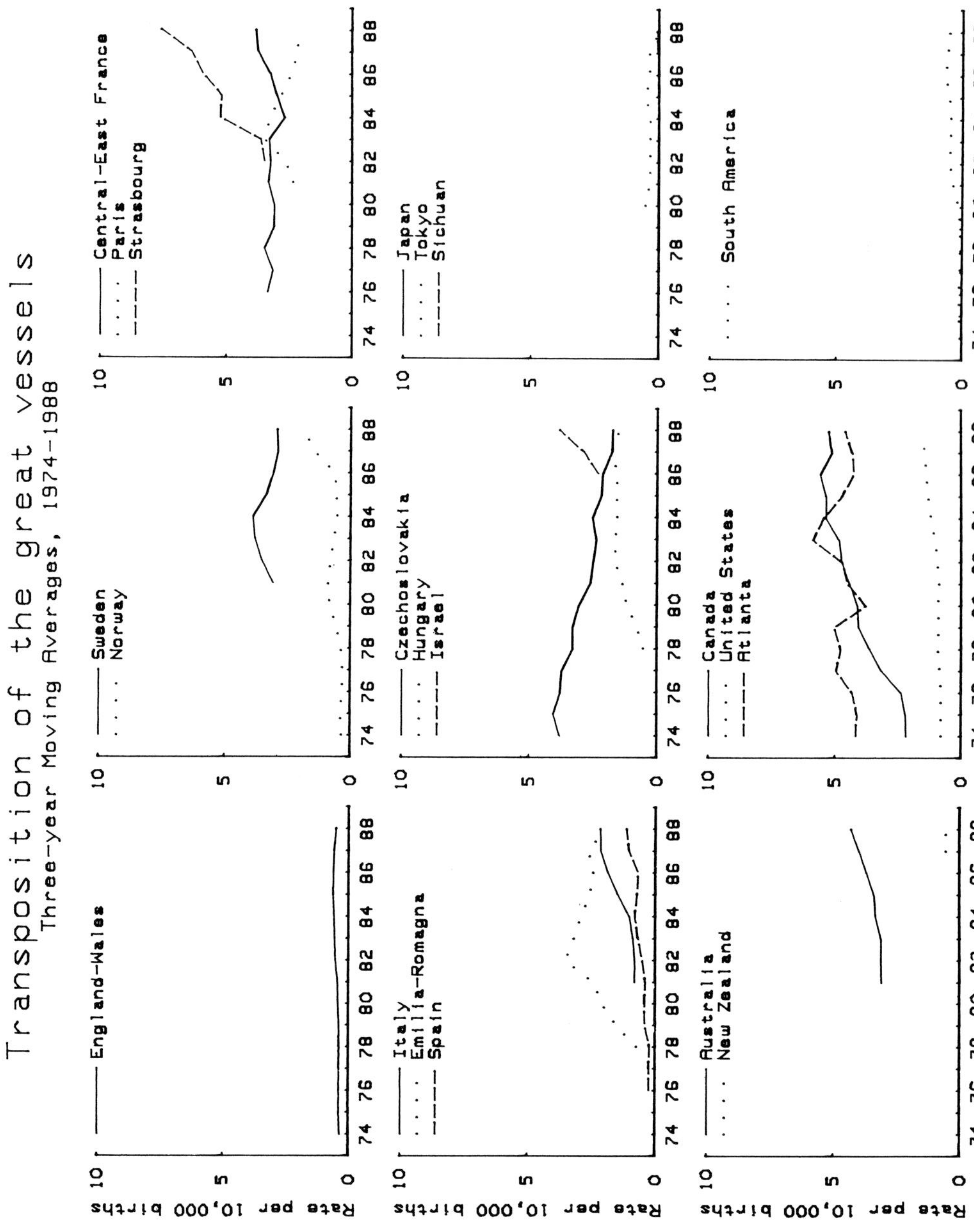
Transposition of the great vessels
Three-year Moving Averages, 1974-1988
Rate per 10,000 births
England-Wales
Sweden
Norway
Central-East France
Paris
Strasbourg
Italy
Emilia-Romagna
Spain
Czechoslovakia
Hungary
Israel
Japan
Tokyo
Sichuan
Australia
New Zealand
Canada
United States
Atlanta
South America
0
5
10
74
76
78
80
82
84
86
88

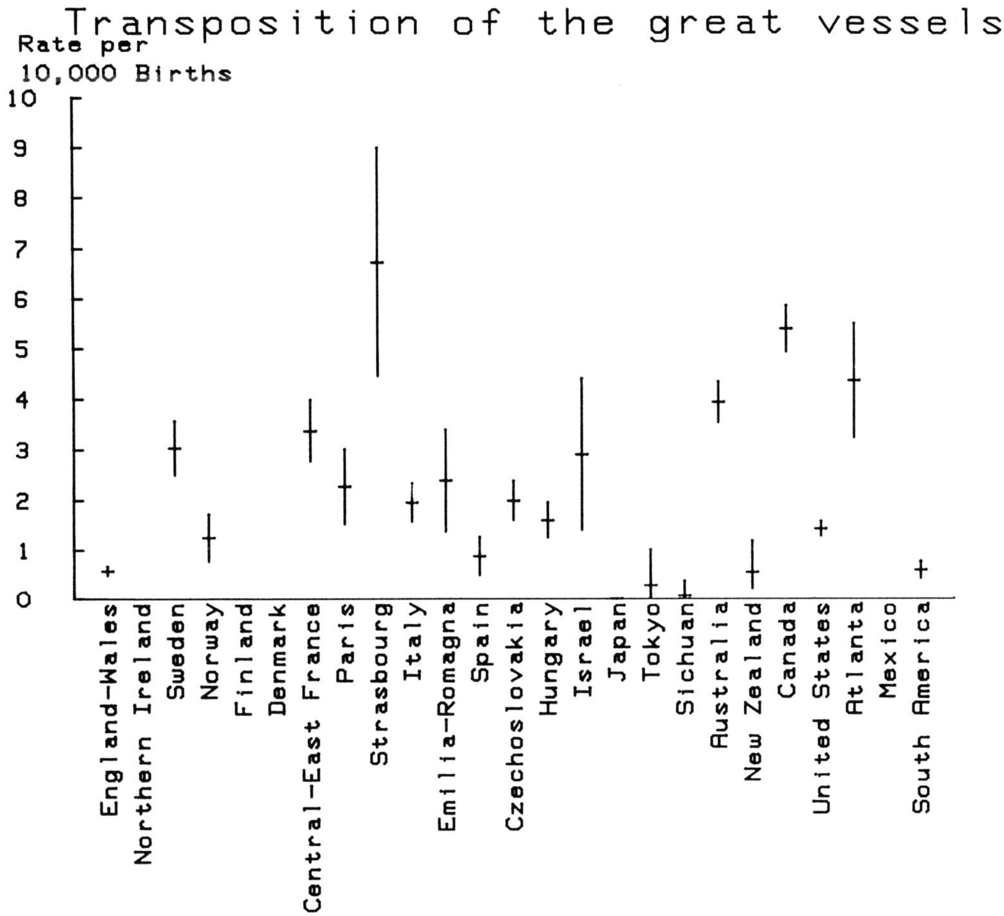

Diagram showing average rates of transpositions in different programs for the years 1985-1988. Vertical lines indicate 95% confidence intervals of the recorded rates.

Comments

The recorded rates of this cardiac malformation vary immensely - from very low rates around 1:20,000 in England-Wales, Sichuan, Tokyo, New Zealand, and South America to high rates around 1:2,500 in Sweden, Central-East France, Australia, Canada, and Atlanta, and even higher in Strasbourg. As this malformation is sometimes not diagnosed during the first few days of life, part of the variation can be explained by the length of the follow-up time.

New diagnostic possibilities, such as echocardiography, may increase ascertainment and may partly explain the increase in rates seen in some programs

(Strasbourg, Italy, Australia, Canada). On the other hand, a clear-cut decrease is seen in the Czechoslovakian rate.

The malformation is not routinely monitored in some programs.

Hypoplastic left heart syndrome (HLHS)

HLHS is a lethal cardiac defect consisting of a severely underdeveloped left heart ventricle as a result of aortic valve atresia, mitral valve atresia, or a combination of both. The right ventricle is enlarged and an intra-atrial septum defect is usually present. The ductus arteriosus is wide. The origin of the aortic atresia is probably found in a maldevelopment of the outflow portion of the left ventricle during the 5th-8th embryonic week. Extracardiac malformations may exist, but the HLHS is the dominant condition with respect to survival.

No adequate therapy is available, and death usually occurs within the first weeks of life. Heart transplantation has been tried.

Hypoplastic left heart syndrome

Definition: A congenital malformation resulting from an obstructive valvular or vascular lesion on the left side of the heart with varying degrees of hypoplasia of the left ventricle.

A. Number of infants born with hypoplastic left heart syndrome

Monitoring program	1974	1975	1976	1977	1978	1979	1980	1981	1982	1983	1984	1985	1986	1987	1988	Total
Atlanta	9	8	8	6	10	5	11	11	9	10	12	11	6	14	11	141
Australia								34	56	69	74	47	55	49	57	441
Canada							52	64	52	64	64	57	73	56	56	538
Central-East France			6	7	6	6	12	19	14	15	22	26	11	22	17	183
Czechoslovakia	16	29	40	25	31	50	33	24	30	21	24	36	18	29	33	439
Emilia-Romagna					0	0	1	3	0	3	5	6	4	3	3	28
England-Wales						6	10	8	13	18	21	25	16	18	10	145
Hungary					1	10	4	9	10	5	4	5	6	5	16	75
Israel													3	2	4	9
Italy								10	9	11	13	15	27	18	20	123
New Zealand														5	4	9
Norway													3	16	6	25
Paris								4	12	7	7	7	10	6	3	56
South America	0	0	0	0	0	0	0	0	1	0	0	0	0	0	4	5
Spain			0	1	1	1	0	2	3	5	2	3	4	4	2	28
Strasbourg									4	3	3	4	1	7	4	26
Sweden								24	22	26	25	17	16	18	25	173
Tokyo							0	0	0	1	0	0	0	1	0	2
United States						64	36	66	57	69	45	78	83	77	59	634

B. Rate per 10,000 infants.

Monitoring program	1974	1975	1976	1977	1978	1979	1980	1981	1982	1983	1984	1985	1986	1987	1988	Average
Atlanta	3.6	3.5	3.5	2.6	4.1	2.0	4.0	4.1	3.2	3.6	4.1	3.5	1.8	4.0	3.0	3.4
Australia								3.0	2.3	2.9	3.1	1.9	2.3	2.0	2.3	2.5
Canada							2.2	2.6	2.1	2.6	2.5	2.2	2.8	2.3	2.6	2.4
Central-East France			0.9	1.0	0.9	0.8	1.6	2.5	1.9	1.7	2.5	2.9	1.2	2.5	1.9	1.8
Czechoslovakia	0.8	1.5	2.1	1.4	1.7	2.9	2.1	1.7	2.1	1.5	1.8	2.6	1.3	2.2	2.5	1.9
Emilia-Romagna					0	0	0.8	2.1	0	1.4	2.2	2.5	1.7	1.3	1.3	1.4
England-Wales						0.1	0.2	0.1	0.2	0.3	0.3	0.4	0.2	0.3	0.1	0.2
Hungary					0.1	0.6	0.3	0.6	0.7	0.4	0.3	0.4	0.5	0.4	1.3	0.5
Israel													1.7	1.2	2.3	1.7
Italy								0.9	0.7	0.8	1.0	1.1	1.9	1.3	1.4	1.2
New Zealand														0.9	0.7	0.8
Norway													0.6	2.9	1.0	1.5
Paris								1.0	3.1	1.8	1.8	1.7	2.5	1.5	0.7	1.7
South America	0	0	0	0	0	0	0	0	0.1	0	0	0	0	0	0.2	0
Spain			0	0.4	0.3	0.1	0	0.4	0.5	0.7	0.3	0.4	0.7	0.8	0.4	0.4
Strasbourg									3.0	2.4	2.4	3.1	0.8	5.4	3.0	2.9
Sweden								2.5	2.4	2.8	2.7	1.7	1.6	1.7	2.2	2.2
Tokyo							0	0	0	0.5	0	0	0	0.6	0	0.1
United States						0.6	0.5	0.8	0.7	0.8	0.6	1.1	1.2	1.3	1.2	0.8

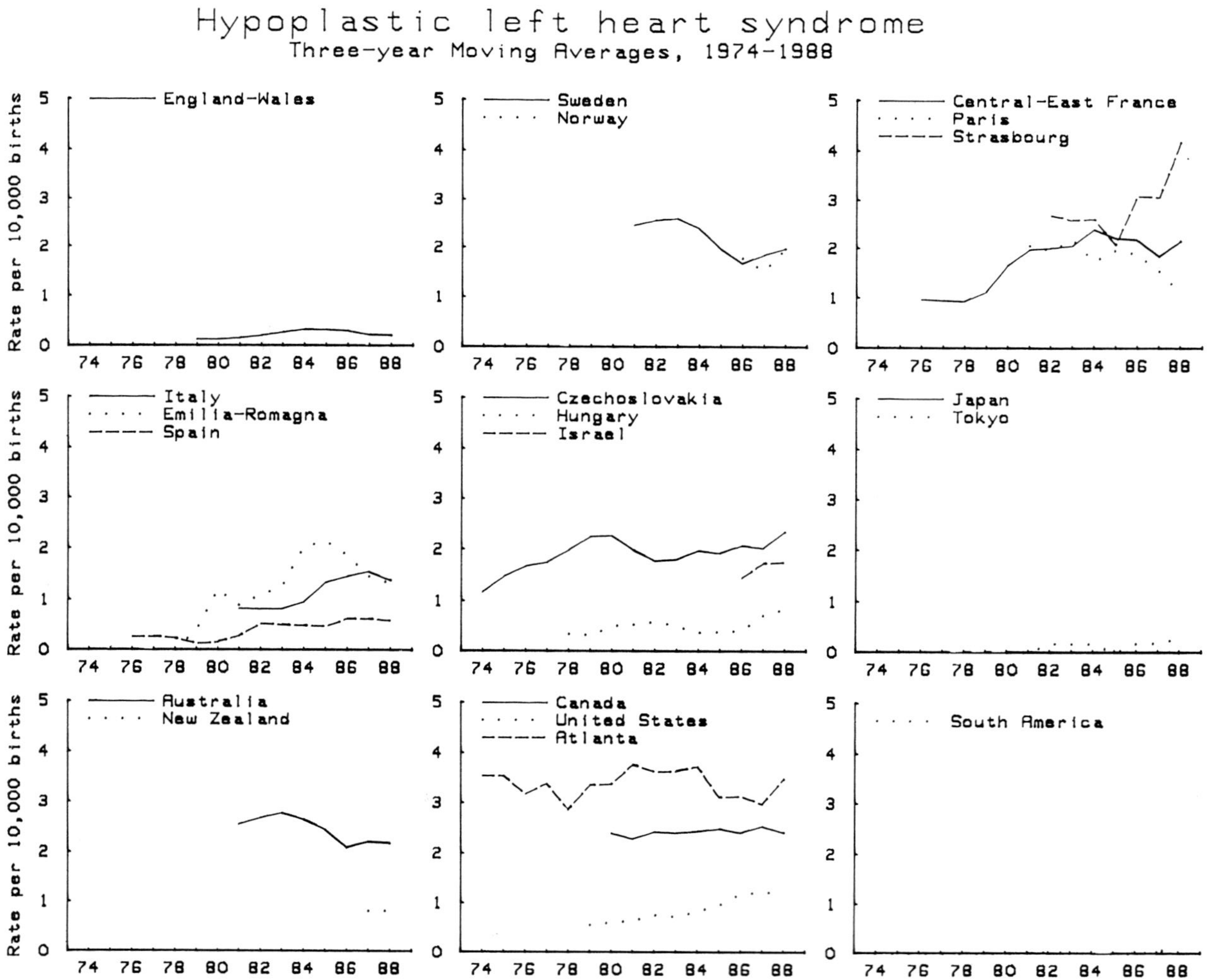

Hypoplastic left heart syndrome
Three-year Moving Averages, 1974-1988
Rate per 10,000 births
England-Wales
Sweden
Norway
Central-East France
Paris
Strasbourg
Italy
Emilia-Romagna
Spain
Czechoslovakia
Hungary
Israel
Japan
Tokyo
Australia
New Zealand
Canada
United States
Atlanta
South America
74 76 78 80 82 84 86 88
0 1 2 3 4 5

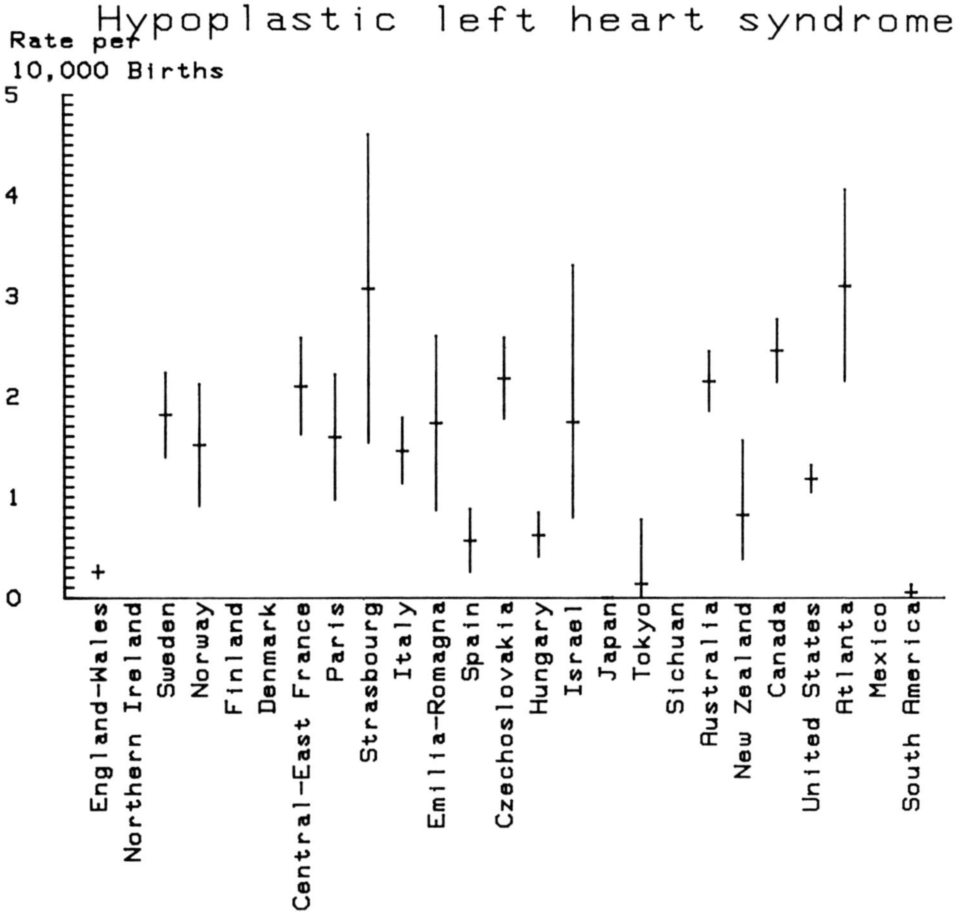

Diagram showing average rates of HLHS in different programs for the years 1985-1988. Vertical lines indicate 95% confidence intervals of the recorded rates.

Comments

The recorded rates of HLHS vary enormously. Most programs record rates of around 2 per 10,000, but lower rates are seen in Spain, Hungary, New Zealand, and the United States, while in England-Wales, Tokyo, and South America the diagnosis is only rarely recorded. The highest recorded rates are in Strasbourg and Atlanta, but in both instances the rates have large confidence intervals. The recording of the malformation is heavily influenced by factors such as access to echocardiography, length of follow-up time, and autopsy rate.

In some programs, like Central-East France, Strasbourg, and Czechoslovakia, the rates increased, in some instances followed by a more steady level. In other programs, like Australia and Atlanta, the rates are relatively steady during the whole observation period. In still other programs, like Sweden and Paris, a decreasing tendency can be seen. All these changes can probably be explained by changes in the diagnostic and recording procedures.

Some programs could not provide data on this malformation.

Cleft palate

This condition is characterized by a cleft through the soft and/or hard palate, usually positioned in the mid-line, but without clefting of lips or alveolar process. The cleft originates in the non-fusion of the maxillar palatal processes during the 10th week of embryonic development, but details of the pathogenesis are debated. The cleft may be submucous. Some clefts are associated with a small lower jaw (micrognathia) where the tongue may have mechanically prevented fusion of palatal processes (Pierre Robin sequence). Cleft palate is often associated with other malformations in various syndromes.

Genetic factors play a role in non-syndromic isolated cleft palate, and a recurrence risk exists in sibs. Environmental factors may increase the risk for an isolated cleft palate, e.g., certain drugs and possibly maternal smoking.

The palatal cleft impairs swallowing and later speech. Treatment usually starts with a prosthesis to cover the cleft, followed by surgical repair. If no serious malformations are associated, prognosis is excellent.

Cleft palate

Definition: A congenital malformation characterized by a fissure defect of the hard and/or soft palate behind the foramen incisivum without cleft lip.

A. Numbers of infants born with cleft palate

Monitoring program	1974	1975	1976	1977	1978	1979	1980	1981	1982	1983	1984	1985	1986	1987	1988	Total
Atlanta	19	22	14	15	17	23	10	8	11	12	16	11	20	20	17	235
Australia								76	132	128	141	113	135	124	132	981
Canada	125	122	153	132	146	165	170	164	154	199	184	175	189	205	115	2398
Central-East France			17	32	29	29	28	31	46	37	46	46	43	31	58	473
Czechoslovakia	107	94	98	126	105	104	94	96	100	103	89	73	85	85	81	1440
Denmark										30	27	36	32	28	41	194
Emilia-Romagna					2	3	4	4	11	14	9	14	15	15	15	106
England-Wales	706	638	635	621	612	625	683	628	640	618	656	601	637	251	274	8825
Finland	49	51	55	47	51	60	76	72	70	52	83	75	79	71	73	964
Hungary	72	63	80	47	71	81	60	85	64	41	60	62	52	42	39	919
Israel	4	3	6	3	3	6	10	8	8	9	6	7	13	13	4	103
Italy					28	33	40	62	72	70	59	59	66	57	69	615
Japan					126	198	209	190	76	74	57	57	82	71	82	1222
Mexico							16	11	9	17	7	2	14	20	9	105
New Zealand							28	27	34	30	37	33	40	50	40	319
Northern Ireland							18	26	24	27	26	20				141
Norway	26	27	25	21	27	25	29	21	28	21	31	32	31	27	30	401
Paris								11	26	18	15	8	13	11	14	116
Sichuan												25	29	16	7	77
South America	28	17	19	25	42	17	17	21	59	67	57	71	78	64	58	640
Spain			4	15	13	25	26	29	34	44	27	34	20	19	19	309
Strasbourg									6	13	13	10	9	13	15	79
Sweden	59	61	67	57	59	63	54	61	53	73	77	72	67	82	78	983
Tokyo							12	6	7	14	13	10	21	3	12	98
United States	570	495	509	586	468	533	376	449	385	468	419	429	381	316	270	6654

B. Rate per 10,000 infants.

Monitoring program	1974	1975	1976	1977	1978	1979	1980	1981	1982	1983	1984	1985	1986	1987	1988	Average
Atlanta	7.7	9.6	6.2	6.4	7.0	9.0	3.7	3.0	3.9	4.3	5.5	3.5	6.1	5.7	4.6	5.6
Australia								6.7	5.5	5.3	6.0	4.7	5.6	5.1	5.4	5.5
Canada	5.5	5.3	6.7	5.7	5.9	6.5	7.1	6.8	6.1	8.2	7.3	6.7	7.2	8.3	5.3	6.6
Central-East France			2.6	4.7	4.2	4.1	3.7	4.0	6.1	4.3	5.3	5.1	4.7	3.5	6.4	4.6
Czechoslovakia	5.5	4.9	5.2	6.9	5.9	6.0	6.1	6.6	7.1	7.5	6.5	5.4	6.4	6.5	6.1	6.1
Denmark										5.9	5.2	6.7	5.8	5.0	6.9	5.9
Emilia-Romagna					2.8	4.7	3.2	2.8	6.0	6.4	3.9	5.8	6.6	6.6	6.6	5.4
England-Wales	10.9	10.5	10.8	10.8	10.2	9.7	10.3	9.8	10.2	9.8	10.2	9.1	9.6	3.7	3.9	9.2
Finland	7.9	7.8	8.3	7.2	8.0	9.5	12.1	11.3	10.6	7.8	12.8	11.9	13.0	11.9	12.2	10.1
Hungary	3.8	3.2	4.7	2.6	4.2	5.0	4.0	5.9	4.8	3.2	4.8	4.7	4.0	3.3	3.1	4.0
Israel	5.7	4.0	7.1	3.7	1.6	3.2	5.4	4.4	4.5	4.9	3.3	3.9	7.4	7.8	2.3	4.5
Italy					6.3	4.6	4.9	5.8	5.7	5.0	4.3	4.5	4.7	4.2	5.0	4.9
Japan						12.5	13.3	13.6	6.3	5.9	4.5	4.4	5.2	4.9	5.9	8.7
Mexico							3.8	3.2	2.6	4.5	2.1	0.8	5.7	4.9	2.2	3.4
New Zealand							6.1	5.4	7.0	5.9	7.4	6.4	7.6	9.2	7.3	7.0
Northern Ireland							6.2	9.4	8.8	9.8	9.3	7.2				8.5
Norway	4.3	4.7	4.6	4.1	5.2	4.8	5.6	4.1	5.4	4.2	6.1	6.2	5.9	5.0	5.2	5.0
Paris								2.8	6.7	4.5	3.8	2.0	3.2	2.7	3.4	3.6
Sichuan												4.0	3.7	1.9	1.1	2.6
South America	3.3	2.6	2.4	3.7	5.8	2.4	3.1	3.8	4.1	4.3	3.4	3.9	3.7	3.3	3.1	3.6
Spain			3.3	5.5	3.7	3.6	4.6	5.2	5.5	6.1	3.9	5.1	3.4	3.7	3.6	4.5
Strasbourg									4.4	10.5	10.2	7.7	7.0	10.1	11.2	8.7
Sweden	5.3	5.9	6.8	5.9	6.3	6.5	5.5	6.5	5.7	7.9	8.2	7.3	6.5	7.8	6.9	6.6
Tokyo							6.4	3.3	3.6	7.4	6.7	5.2	11.5	1.7	7.4	5.9
United States	5.3	4.6	4.8	5.4	4.8	5.2	4.9	5.2	4.7	5.8	5.6	5.9	5.6	5.3	5.3	5.2

Cleft palate

Three-year Moving Averages, 1974-1988

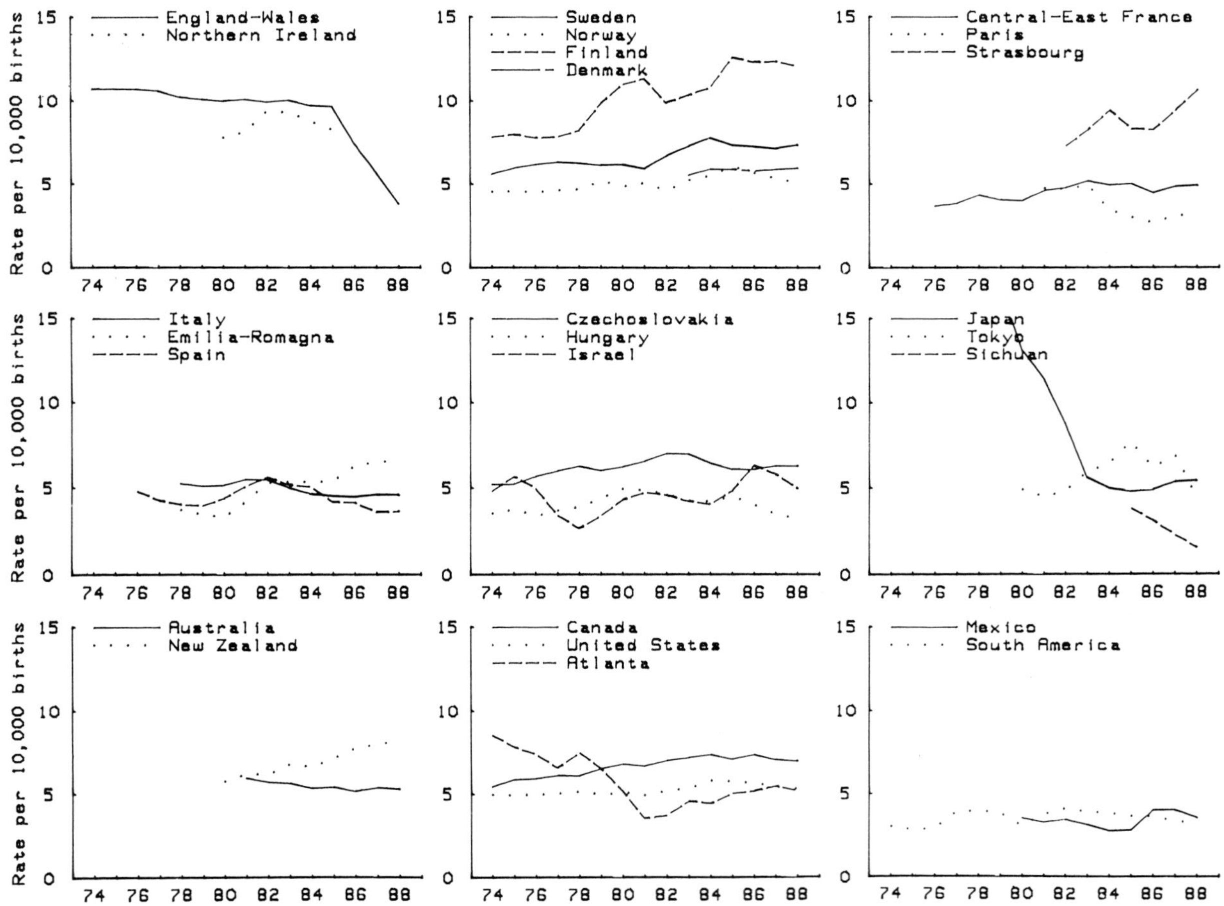

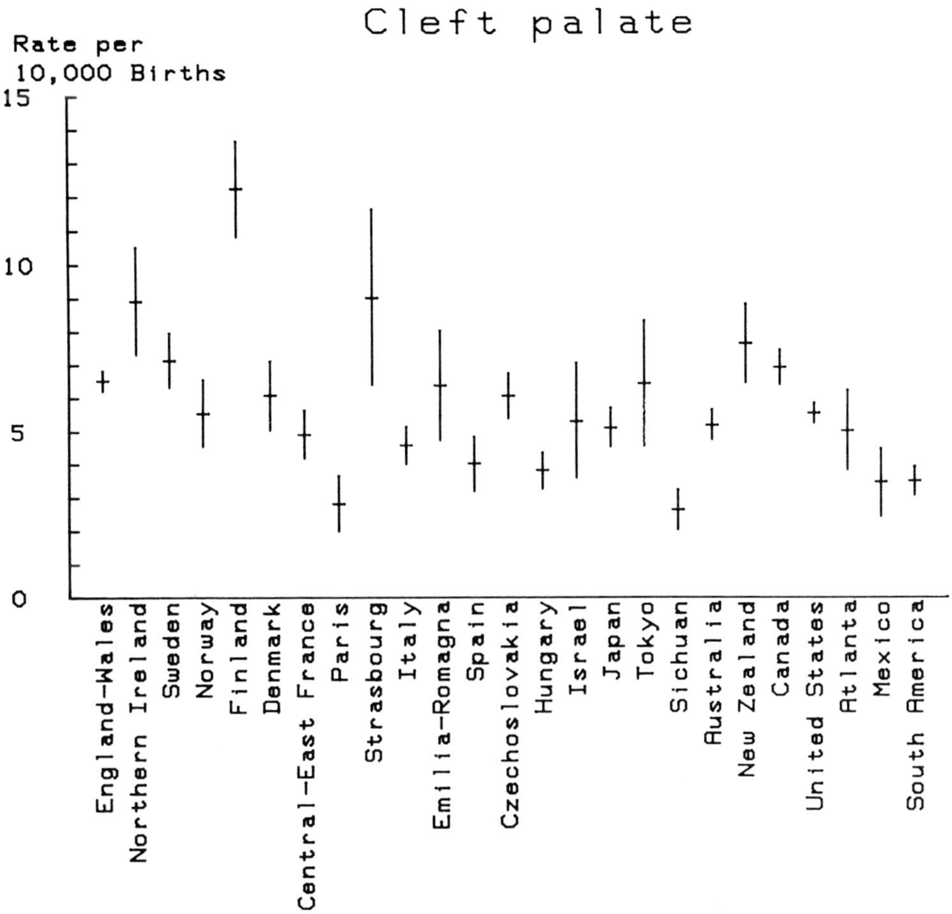

Diagram showing average rates of cleft palate in different programs for the years 1985-1988. Vertical lines indicate 95% confidence intervals of the recorded rates.

Comments

In most programs, the rate is around 5 per 10,000 births and remains reasonably constant during the observation period. Some remarkable exceptions can be seen.

In England-Wales, Japan, and Atlanta very high rates exist at the beginning of the observation period followed by a marked decrease down to the approximate level of most other programs.

High and increasing rates are seen in Finland. A tendency to an increase is seen in Sweden, Strasbourg, and perhaps to a lesser extent in some other programs. Although such changes might have arisen by an increased inclusion of mild cases, a special study made in the *Clearinghouse* on this problem yielded no convincing evidence that this was a major cause of the observed changes.

Total cleft lip

Clefts of the lip arise by non-fusion of various processes that build up the face. Clefting of the lip ("harelip") may also include the alveolar processes and the palate. Clefts may be unilateral, predominantly on the left side, or bilateral. Most infants with clefts of the lips have no associated malformations.

Clefts can be surgically repaired with complete functional and cosmetic restoration, but often a series of treatments are necessary until the child is of school age or more.

There is a genetic background to cleft lip and a recurrence risk exists for sibs. Exogenous factors probably play a role, e.g., certain drugs and maternal smoking.

Facial clefts may be detected prenatally by ultrasound, but usually not until late in pregnancy.

Total cleft lip

Definition: A congenital malformation characterized by clefting of the upper lip, with or without clefting of the alveolar ridge and palate.

A. Numbers of infants born with total cleft lip

Monitoring program	1974	1975	1976	1977	1978	1979	1980	1981	1982	1983	1984	1985	1986	1987	1988	Total
Atlanta	33	27	28	17	28	31	32	28	29	37	28	34	26	30	33	441
Australia								128	222	206	226	215	214	231	208	1650
Canada	237	260	227	257	271	267	275	280	274	313	382	325	331	291	274	4264
Central-East France			52	57	51	48	49	50	68	42	63	41	49	71	62	703
Czechoslovakia	206	143	195	173	179	179	181	156	134	119	149	168	151	135	147	2415
Denmark										70	82	71	90	75	94	482
Emilia-Romagna					4	4	9	7	18	10	25	22	14	17	12	142
England-Wales	700	583	586	566	558	592	629	605	565	568	579	556	611	588	529	8815
Finland	48	53	42	51	47	62	54	37	59	51	62	54	48	56	49	773
Hungary	195	205	213	180	215	164	166	227	121	151	120	126	140	110	108	2441
Israel	3	4	5	5	11	7	7	8	7	11	7	10	13	11	10	119
Italy					32	66	59	85	97	94	70	84	89	86	92	854
Japan					133	220	186	174	165	172	158	190	234	183	212	2027
Mexico							60	33	50	50	49	25	34	41	60	402
New Zealand							50	38	46	35	51	44	54	38	42	398
Northern Ireland							16	30	26	30	15	34				151
Norway	80	103	69	65	70	74	85	77	64	73	59	72	88	69	86	1134
Paris								27	44	24	28	29	16	22	25	215
Sichuan												107	144	127	98	476
South America	90	54	101	76	70	76	54	57	146	146	163	155	222	209	207	1826
Spain			2	12	17	34	30	37	33	39	46	35	33	30	25	373
Strasbourg									14	14	10	9	11	15	8	81
Sweden	153	149	139	116	115	139	120	145	131	155	115	136	125	121	130	1989
Tokyo							12	19	19	30	20	22	19	22	38	201
United States	1003	1020	930	966	839	782	615	758	724	750	664	642	650	561	436	11340

B. Rate per 10,000 infants.																
Monitoring program	1974	1975	1976	1977	1978	1979	1980	1981	1982	1983	1984	1985	1986	1987	1988	Average
Atlanta	13.3	11.7	12.3	7.2	11.5	12.1	11.7	10.4	10.4	13.2	9.6	11.0	7.9	8.6	9.0	10.5
Australia								11.3	9.3	8.5	9.5	8.9	8.9	9.6	8.5	9.2
Canada	10.5	11.3	10.0	11.1	10.9	10.6	11.5	11.5	10.8	12.9	15.2	12.4	12.6	11.7	12.7	11.7
Central-East France			7.8	8.3	7.4	6.8	6.6	6.5	9.1	4.9	7.3	4.5	5.4	7.9	6.8	6.8
Czechoslovakia	10.6	7.5	10.4	9.5	10.0	10.4	11.8	10.8	9.5	8.7	10.9	12.4	11.3	10.3	11.1	10.3
Denmark										13.7	15.8	13.2	16.2	13.3	15.9	14.7
Emilia-Romagna					5.7	6.3	7.2	4.9	9.8	4.6	10.8	9.2	6.1	7.5	5.3	7.2
England-Wales	10.8	9.6	9.9	9.8	9.3	9.2	9.5	9.5	9.0	9.0	9.0	8.4	9.2	8.6	7.6	9.2
Finland	7.7	8.1	6.3	7.8	7.4	9.8	8.6	5.8	8.9	7.6	9.5	8.6	7.9	9.4	8.2	8.1
Hungary	10.4	10.5	11.4	10.0	12.7	10.1	11.1	15.8	9.0	11.8	9.5	9.6	10.9	8.7	8.6	10.7
Israel	4.3	5.4	5.9	6.1	6.0	3.7	3.8	4.4	3.9	6.0	3.9	5.6	7.4	6.6	5.7	5.2
Italy					7.2	9.2	7.2	7.9	7.7	6.7	5.1	6.4	6.3	6.3	6.7	6.8
Japan						13.8	11.9	12.5	13.6	13.7	12.6	14.6	14.8	12.7	15.3	14.5
Mexico							14.4	9.6	14.4	13.1	14.6	10.4	13.8	10.1	14.7	12.8
New Zealand							10.8	7.6	9.5	6.9	10.2	8.6	10.3	7.0	7.6	8.7
Northern Ireland							5.5	10.9	9.6	10.9	5.4	12.2				9.1
Norway	13.3	18.1	12.7	12.6	13.4	14.2	16.5	15.1	12.4	14.5	11.7	14.0	16.7	12.7	14.9	14.2
Paris								6.9	11.3	6.0	7.0	7.1	3.9	5.5	6.0	6.7
Sichuan												17.0	18.1	15.0	15.1	16.3
South America	10.6	8.3	13.0	11.3	9.6	10.9	9.7	10.2	10.1	9.5	9.6	8.5	10.5	10.7	11.0	10.2
Spain			1.6	4.4	4.8	4.9	5.3	6.6	5.4	5.4	6.6	5.2	5.7	5.9	4.7	5.4
Strasbourg									10.3	11.3	7.9	6.9	8.6	11.6	6.0	8.9
Sweden	13.8	14.3	14.1	12.0	12.3	14.4	12.3	15.4	14.1	16.8	12.2	13.8	12.2	11.5	11.6	13.3
Tokyo							6.4	10.5	9.9	15.9	10.2	11.5	10.4	12.5	23.3	12.1
United States	9.2	9.5	8.9	9.0	8.6	7.6	8.0	8.8	8.8	9.2	8.9	8.9	9.5	9.3	8.6	8.8

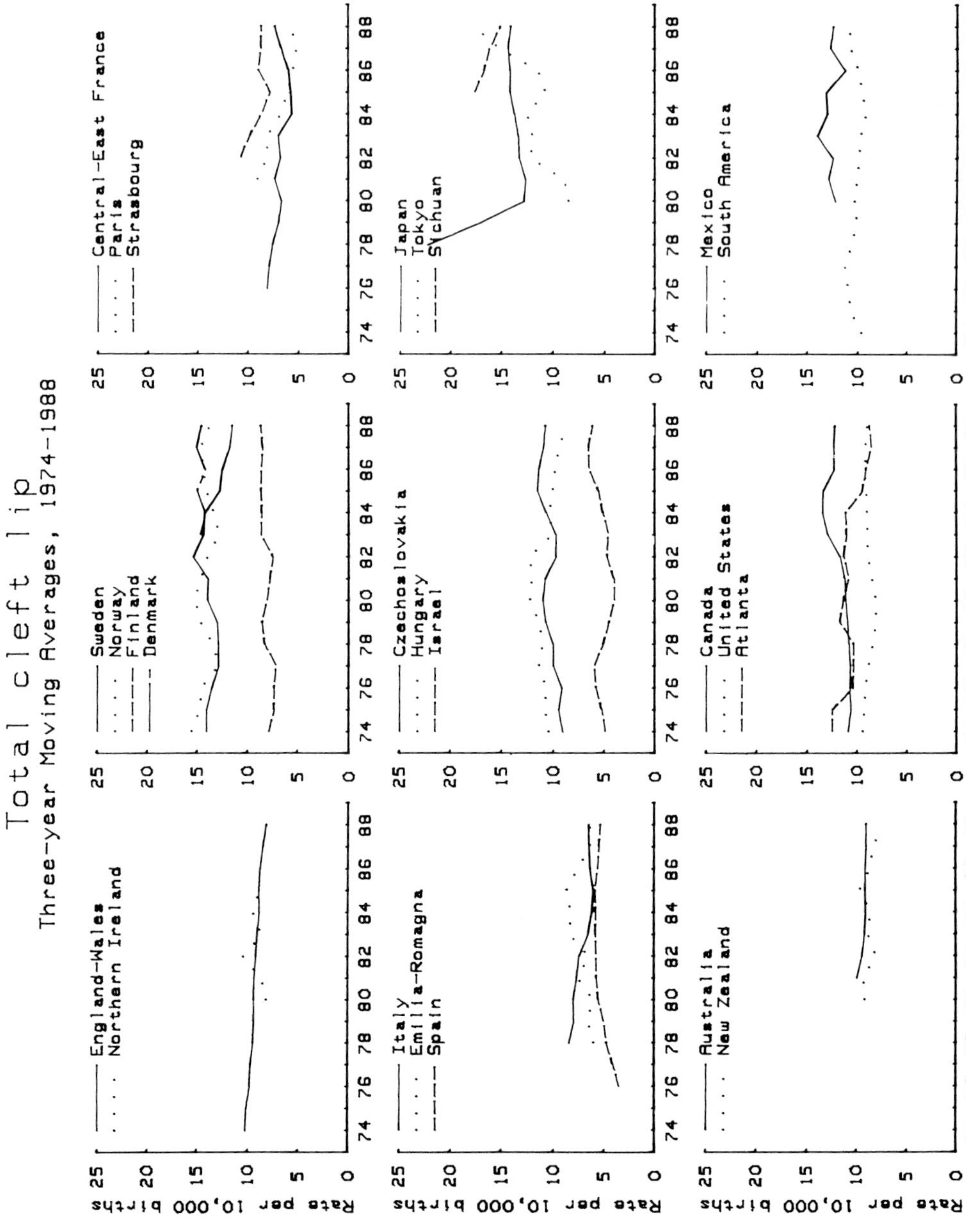
Total cleft lip
Three-year Moving Averages, 1974-1988
England-Wales
Northern Ireland
Sweden
Norway
Finland
Denmark
Central-East France
Paris
Strasbourg
Italy
Emilia-Romagna
Spain
Czechoslovakia
Hungary
Israel
Japan
Tokyo
Sichuan
Australia
New Zealand
Canada
United States
Atlanta
Mexico
South America
Rate per 10,000 births
0
5
10
15
20
25
74
76
78
80
82
84
86
88

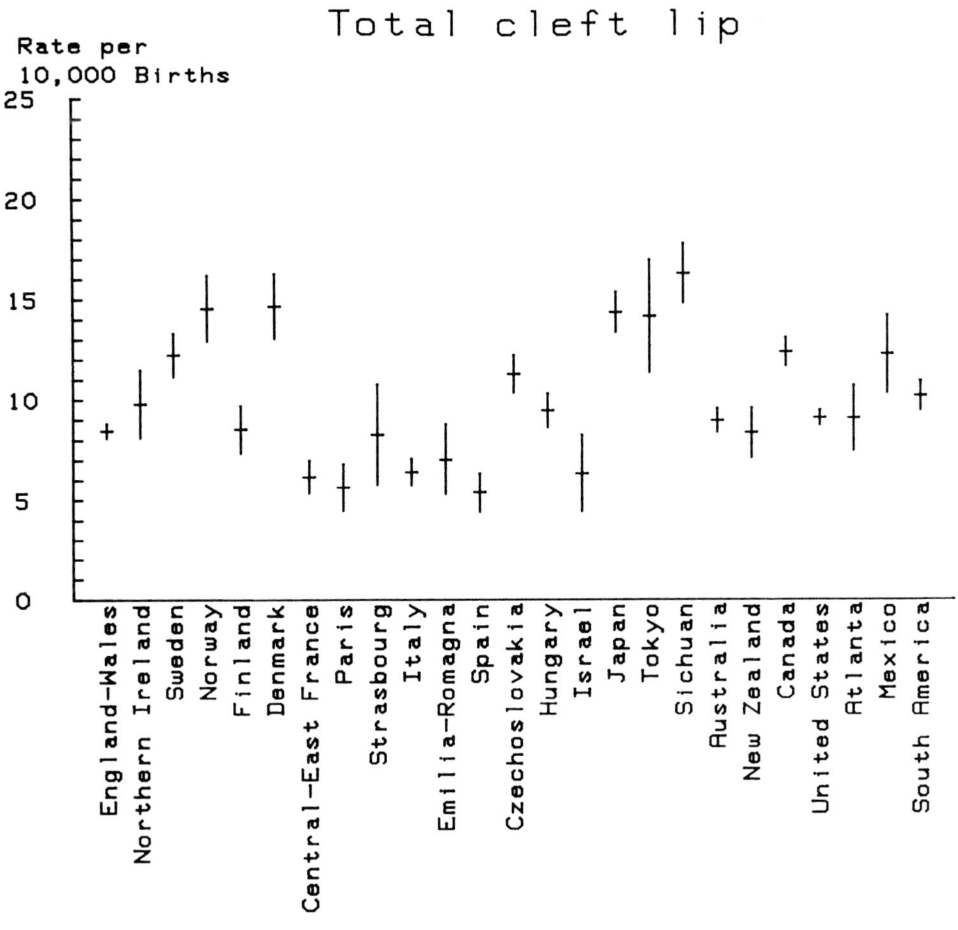

Diagram showing average rates of total cleft lip in different programs for the years 1985-1988. Vertical lines indicate 95% confidence intervals of the recorded rates.

Comments

This is one of the most stable malformations among those studied, probably because it is a condition easily observed and described. Some temporal changes can be noted, however. Up to about 1982, the rates in Canada and Atlanta were virtually identical, but since that time the Canadian rate increased and the Atlanta rate decreased slightly. A slightly increasing trend is seen in the Tokyo program.

More remarkable is the difference in actual recorded rates. All programs in southern Europe and Israel have rates around 6 per 10,000, while the Scandinavian programs, the Asian programs, and Canada have rates about twice as high.

The rate of total cleft lip apparently differs in different populations and it is likely that genetic factors play a decisive role for this difference in a way similar to that well known for neural tube defects.

Esophageal atresia

In esophageal atresia the passage through the esophagus is blocked because the lumen is obliterated. Various types exist, but in 90% the upper part of the esophagus ends blindly and the lower part has a fistula to the trachea. In a substantial percentage of the infants, other malformations exist.

The esophagus and the trachea are formed from the embryonic foregut and are separated by a septum, the maldevelopment of which causes esophageal atresia during the fourth week of embryonic development.

The malformation often causes hydramnios and can be suspected even before birth. It is usually diagnosed rapidly after birth, and a life-saving operation has to be performed. If the infant survives surgery and no other lethal malformations exist, life expectancy is good and no handicap should remain.

Although a genetic background is probable, the recurrence risk in sibs is low. Little is known about the cause of esophageal atresia, and although various exogenous factors have been suggested, none has been proved.

Esophageal atresia

Definition: A congenital malformation characterized by occlusion or narrowing of the esophagus, with or without tracheal fistula.

A. Numbers of infants born with esophageal atresia

Monitoring program	1974	1975	1976	1977	1978	1979	1980	1981	1982	1983	1984	1985	1986	1987	1988	Total
Atlanta	7	8	2	5	5	4	7	13	5	4	6	13	6	6	6	97
Australia								32	85	77	74	76	56	87	69	556
Canada	35	32	34	21	22	20										164
Central-East France			18	19	9	19	17	14	20	21	36	22	16	31	28	270
Czechoslovakia	21	16	18	16	20	25	16	28	22	19	26	32	21	26	21	327
Denmark										5	8	17	13	15	13	71
Emilia-Romagna					5	0	3	5	6	8	12	9	8	7	7	70
England-Wales	95	87	107	98	113	104	108	112	105	104	98	123	94	97	70	1515
Finland	8	2	14	9	7	2	5	12	9	7	21	19	11	10	6	142
Hungary			45	31	36	32	22	31	22	22	22	12	30	21	19	345
Israel	0	2	2	1	2	3	4	5	1	2	2	5	4	3	10	46
Italy					12	29	23	33	36	39	33	34	38	39	44	360
Japan					8	23	13	23	11	13	9	22	24	22	28	196
Mexico							7	2	3	8	3	2	3	6	9	43
New Zealand							8	4	12	10	7	14	11	6	13	85
Northern Ireland							8	13	11	5	9	8				54
Norway	17	12	12	11	8	7	8	9	9	10	8	10	9	12	15	157
Paris								9	11	10	16	13	8	11	3	81
Sichuan												3	1	3	4	11
South America	12	9	21	14	18	15	9	14	32	45	56	31	44	56	60	436
Spain			0	2	3	8	8	11	21	16	17	15	10	10	2	123
Strasbourg									6	2	1	6	0	3	3	21
Sweden	28	27	16	29	22	29	28	34	25	27	21	26	25	35	32	404
Tokyo							3	2	4	2	4	2	9	9	6	41
United States	175	190	174	154	141	183	152	177	148	147	144	206	172	141	121	2425

B. Rate per 10,000 infants.

Monitoring program	1974	1975	1976	1977	1978	1979	1980	1981	1982	1983	1984	1985	1986	1987	1988	Average
Atlanta	2.8	3.5	0.9	2.1	2.0	1.6	2.6	4.8	1.8	1.4	2.1	4.2	1.8	1.7	1.6	2.3
Australia								2.8	3.6	3.2	3.1	3.2	2.3	3.6	2.8	3.1
Canada	1.5	1.4	1.5	0.9	0.9	0.8										1.2
Central-East France			2.7	2.8	1.3	2.7	2.3	1.8	2.7	2.4	4.2	2.4	1.8	3.5	3.1	2.6
Czechoslovakia	1.1	0.8	1.0	0.9	1.1	1.5	1.0	1.9	1.6	1.4	1.9	2.4	1.6	2.0	1.6	1.4
Denmark										1.0	1.5	3.1	2.3	2.7	2.2	2.2
Emilia-Romagna					7.1	0	2.4	3.5	3.3	3.7	5.2	3.7	3.5	3.1	3.1	3.6
EnglandWales	1.5	1.4	1.8	1.7	1.9	1.6	1.6	1.8	1.7	1.6	1.5	1.9	1.4	1.4	1.0	1.6
Finland	1.3	0.3	2.1	1.4	1.1	0.3	0.8	1.9	1.4	1.0	3.2	3.0	1.8	1.7	1.0	1.5
Hungary			2.4	1.7	2.1	2.0	1.5	2.2	1.6	1.7	1.7	0.9	2.3	1.7	1.5	1.8
Israel	0	2.7	2.4	1.2	1.1	1.6	2.2	2.7	0.6	1.1	1.1	2.8	2.3	1.8	5.7	2.0
Italy					2.7	4.0	2.8	3.1	2.9	2.8	2.4	2.6	2.7	2.8	3.2	2.9
Japan						1.4	0.8	1.6	0.9	1.0	0.7	1.7	1.5	1.5	2.0	1.4
Mexico							1.7	0.6	0.9	2.1	0.9	0.8	1.2	1.5	2.2	1.4
New Zealand							1.7	0.8	2.5	2.0	1.4	2.7	2.1	1.1	2.4	1.9
Northern Ireland							2.8	4.7	4.0	1.8	3.2	2.9				3.2
Norway	2.8	2.1	2.2	2.1	1.5	1.3	1.6	1.8	1.7	2.0	1.6	1.9	1.7	2.2	2.6	2.0
Paris								2.3	2.8	2.5	4.0	3.2	2.0	2.7	0.7	2.5
Sichuan												0.5	0.1	0.4	0.6	0.4
South America	1.4	1.4	2.7	2.1	2.5	2.2	1.6	2.5	2.2	2.9	3.3	1.7	2.1	2.9	3.2	2.4
Spain			0	0.7	0.8	1.2	1.4	2.0	3.4	2.2	2.4	2.2	1.7	2.0	0.4	1.8
Strasbourg									4.4	1.6	0.8	4.6	0	2.3	2.2	2.3
Sweden	2.5	2.6	1.6	3.0	2.3	3.0	2.9	3.6	2.7	2.9	2.2	2.6	2.4	3.3	2.8	2.7
Tokyo							1.6	1.1	2.1	1.1	2.0	1.0	4.9	5.1	3.7	2.5
United States	1.6	1.8	1.7	1.4	1.4	1.8	2.0	2.0	1.8	1.8	1.9	2.9	2.5	2.3	2.4	1.9

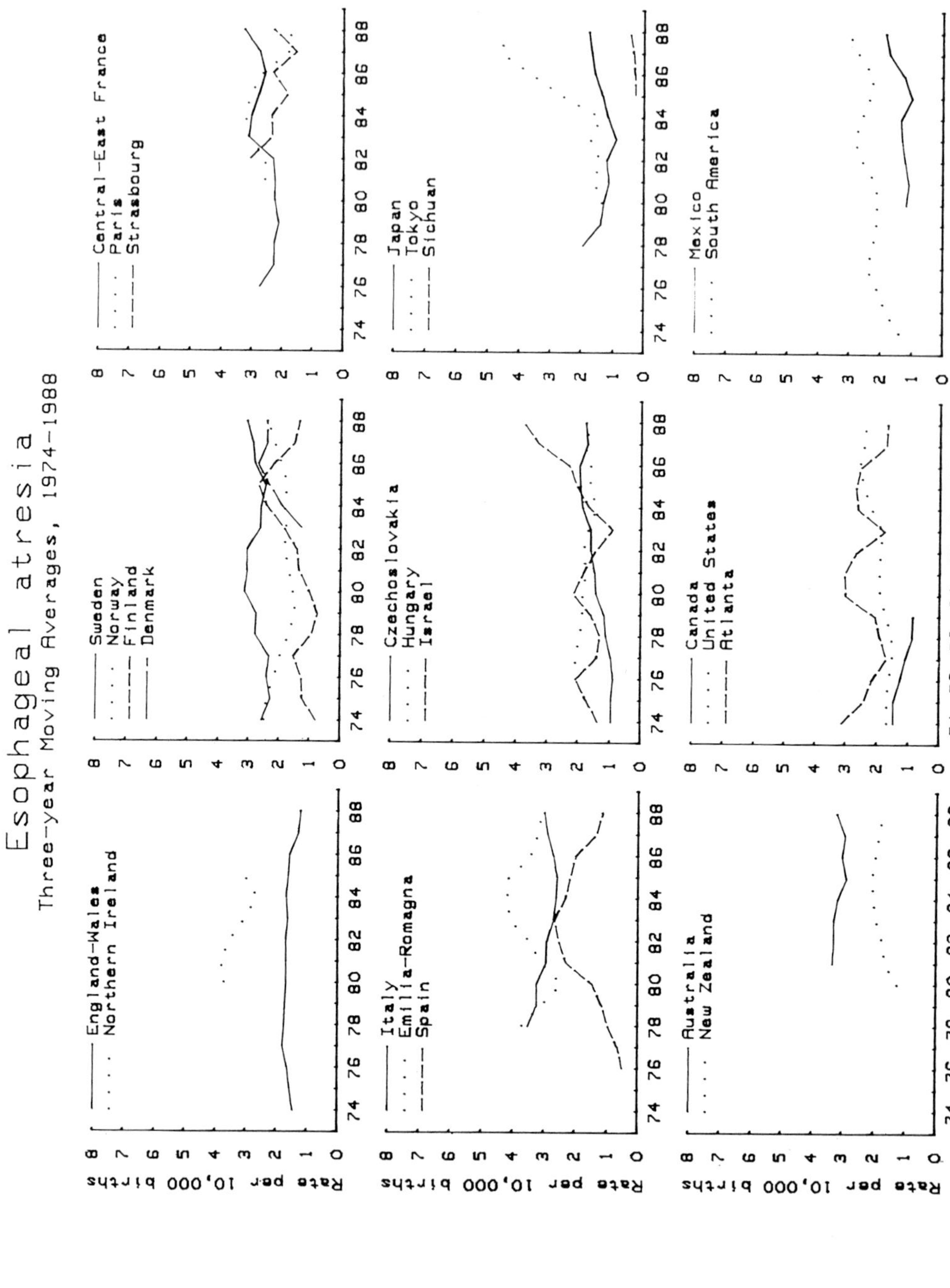
Esophageal atresia
Three-year Moving Averages, 1974-1988
England-Wales
Northern Ireland
Sweden
Norway
Finland
Denmark
Central-East France
Paris
Strasbourg
Italy
Emilia-Romagna
Spain
Czechoslovakia
Hungary
Israel
Japan
Tokyo
Sichuan
Australia
New Zealand
Canada
United States
Atlanta
Mexico
South America
Rate per 10,000 births

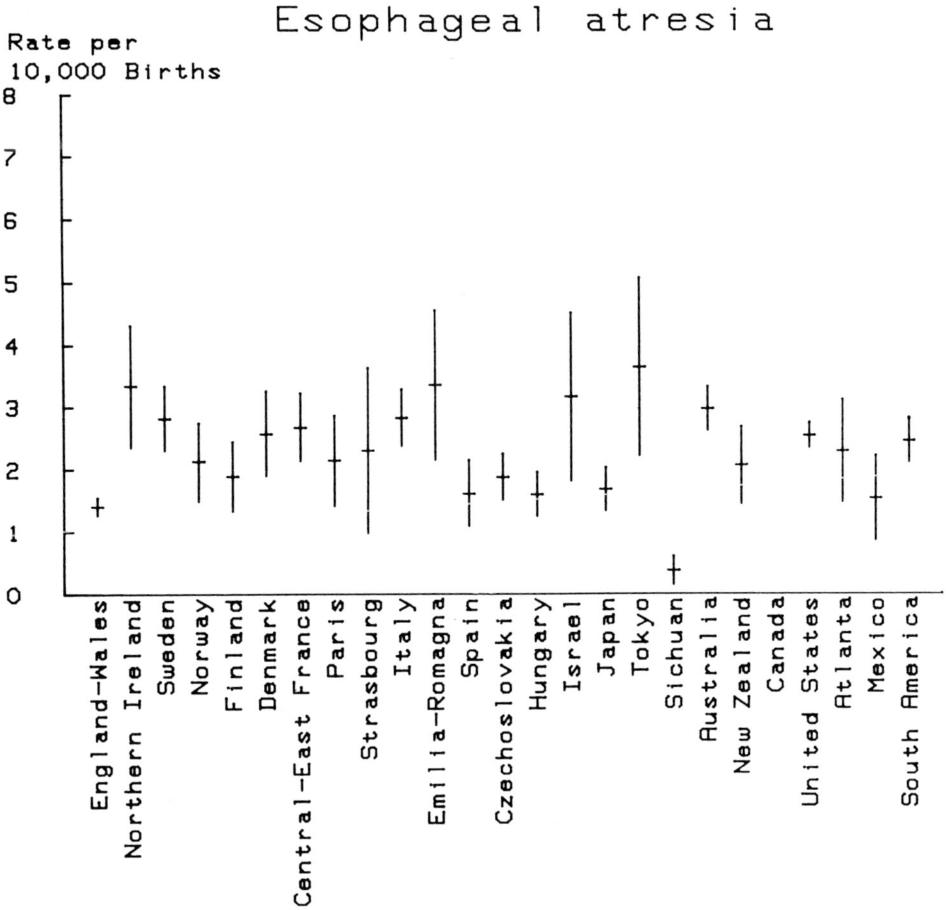

Diagram showing average rates of esophageal atresia in different programs for the years 1985-1988. Vertical lines indicate 95% confidence intervals of the recorded rates.

Comments

In most programs, the recorded rates have been relatively constant and around 2-3 per 10,000, though the rates in Sichuan have been consistently lower. An increasing trend is seen in Czechoslovakia, Finland, Israel, Tokyo, United States, and South America. A temporary increase noted in Central-East France in the mid-1980s was the subject of a special investigation, but no explanation could be found.

Similar temporary increases at about the same time may be seen in Paris, Emilia-Romagna, and Spain.

Anorectal atresia

Anorectal atresia consists of absence of an anus ("imperforate anus") or a lack of passage through the rectum or from the rectum to the anal canal. The anal atresia may be low or high; in the latter case, it is often associated with a fistula to urethra, bladder or vagina. The anal opening may also be dislocated from its normal site. In the majority of infants other malformations exist, often serious ones.

This group of malformations arise from the hindgut, which during development divides into a ventral urogenital sinus and a dorsal rectum rudiment. The latter fuses with a pouch from the ectoderm, the proctodeum. Non-development of proctodeum or absence of fusion results in atresia, and defective development of the septum causes a fistula.

The anorectal atresia is usually detected at the examination of the newborn or will be detected during the first few days of life. It can often be surgically repaired, although often a normal functional anus cannot be produced. The initial operation in the newborn is usually followed by supplementary repair at a later age.

Autosomal recessive heredity has been described in a few families. Usually, recurrence risk for sibs is low. Various exogenous causes have been discussed, but none is definite.

Anorectal atresia

Definition: A congenital malformation characterized by absence of anus or of communication between rectum and anus or narrowing of anal canal, with or without fistula to neighbouring organs.

A. Number of infants born with anorectal atresia

Monitoring program	1974	1975	1976	1977	1978	1979	1980	1981	1982	1983	1984	1985	1986	1987	1988	Total
Atlanta	13	12	8	9	11	10	11	10	8	10	10	16	13	18	8	167
Australia								49	88	75	68	79	67	97	69	592
Canada	94	111	100	105	101	93	120	101	105	145	136	150	128	131	125	1745
Central-East France			24	17	16	17	11	16	17	31	27	27	37	38	32	310
Czechoslovakia	28	33	40	40	37	50	40	40	46	28	35	36	36	31	36	556
Denmark										14	8	18	14	20	11	85
Emilia-Romagna					0	1	0	4	10	7	11	2	8	6	6	55
England-Wales	199	166	185	147	172	192	183	159	180	153	166	171	160	161	138	2532
Finland	5	10	8	9	11	7	5	6	3	4	11	20	11	14	10	134
Hungary					41	32	30	45	30	17	34	24	30	31	17	331
Israel	0	1	2	0	3	5	5	8	5	7	8	2	7	9	6	68
Italy					14	36	24	43	43	47	36	40	45	43	44	415
Japan					48	86	64	55	59	66	32	58	88	63	56	675
Mexico							20	9	12	18	13	10	19	11	16	128
New Zealand							8	11	16	15	7	14	14	17	12	114
Northern Ireland							8	22	10	12	8	6				66
Norway	10	15	4	9	6	5	12	11	8	10	12	15	12	10	8	147
Paris								13	13	16	18	12	9	8	4	93
Sichuan												29	26	17	15	87
South America	20	15	20	19	24	25	15	25	65	58	61	65	73	56	77	618
Spain			0	4	8	11	11	17	15	22	15	18	18	6	13	158
Strasbourg									5	8	5	5	8	9	3	43
Sweden	29	33	40	42	35	35	22	42	19	29	21	39	41	35	40	502
Tokyo							6	4	18	7	12	7	18	9	10	91
United States	367	344	336	346	307	321	260	302	250	261	266	296	268	216	181	4321

B. Rate per 10,000 infants.

Monitoring program	1974	1975	1976	1977	1978	1979	1980	1981	1982	1983	1984	1985	1986	1987	1988	Average
Atlanta	5.2	5.2	3.5	3.8	4.5	3.9	4.0	3.7	2.9	3.6	3.4	5.2	4.0	5.1	2.2	4.0
Australia								4.3	3.7	3.1	2.9	3.3	2.8	4.0	2.8	3.3
Canada	4.2	4.8	4.4	4.5	4.1	3.7	5.0	4.2	4.2	6.0	5.4	5.7	4.9	5.3	5.8	4.8
Central-East France			3.6	2.5	2.3	2.4	1.5	2.1	2.3	3.6	3.1	3.0	4.1	4.2	3.5	3.0
Czechoslovakia	1.4	1.7	2.1	2.2	2.1	2.9	2.6	2.8	3.2	2.0	2.6	2.6	2.7	2.4	2.7	2.4
Denmark										2.7	1.5	3.3	2.5	3.5	1.9	2.6
Emilia-Romagna					0	1.6	0	2.8	5.4	3.2	4.8	0.8	3.5	2.6	2.6	2.8
England-Wales	3.1	2.7	3.1	2.6	2.9	3.0	2.8	2.5	2.9	2.4	2.6	2.6	2.4	2.4	2.0	2.6
Finland	0.8	1.5	1.2	1.4	1.7	1.1	0.8	0.9	0.5	0.6	1.7	3.2	1.8	2.3	1.7	1.4
Hungary					2.4	2.0	2.0	3.1	2.2	1.3	2.7	1.8	2.3	2.4	1.4	2.2
Israel	0	1.3	2.4	0	1.6	2.7	2.7	4.4	2.8	3.8	4.4	1.1	4.0	5.4	3.4	3.0
Italy					3.2	5.0	2.9	4.0	3.4	3.4	2.6	3.1	3.2	3.1	3.2	3.3
Japan						5.4	4.1	3.9	4.9	5.3	2.6	4.5	5.6	4.4	4.0	4.8
Mexico							4.8	2.6	3.5	4.7	3.9	4.2	7.7	2.7	3.9	4.1
New Zealand							1.7	2.2	3.3	3.0	1.4	2.7	2.7	3.1	2.2	2.5
Northern Ireland							2.8	8.0	3.7	4.4	2.9	2.2				4.0
Norway	1.7	2.6	0.7	1.7	1.1	1.0	2.3	2.2	1.5	2.0	2.4	2.9	2.3	1.8	1.4	1.8
Paris								3.3	3.3	4.0	4.5	2.9	2.2	2.0	1.0	2.9
Sichuan												4.6	3.3	2.0	2.3	3.0
South America	2.4	2.3	2.6	2.8	3.3	3.6	2.7	4.5	4.5	3.8	3.6	3.6	3.5	2.9	4.1	3.4
Spain			0	1.5	2.3	1.6	1.9	3.0	2.4	3.1	2.2	2.7	3.1	1.2	2.5	2.3
Strasbourg									3.7	6.4	3.9	3.9	6.2	7.0	2.2	4.7
Sweden	2.6	3.2	4.0	4.4	3.7	3.6	2.3	4.4	2.0	3.1	2.2	3.9	4.0	3.3	3.6	3.4
Tokyo							3.2	2.2	9.4	3.7	6.1	3.7	9.8	5.1	6.1	5.5
United States	3.4	3.2	3.2	3.2	3.2	3.1	3.4	3.5	3.0	3.2	3.6	4.1	3.9	3.6	3.6	3.4

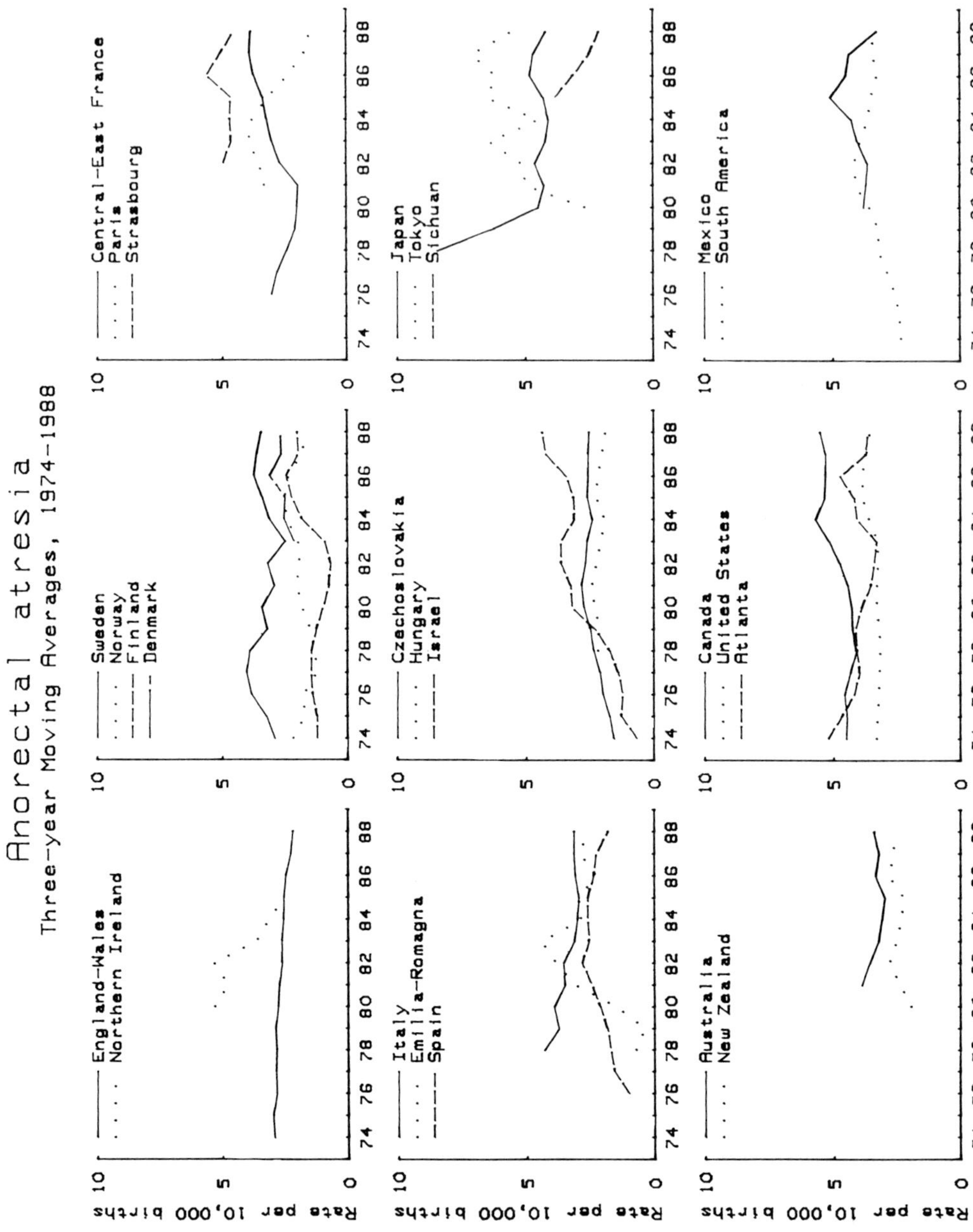
Anorectal atresia
Three-year Moving Averages, 1974-1988
Rate per 10,000 births
England-Wales
Northern Ireland
Sweden
Norway
Finland
Denmark
Central-East France
Paris
Strasbourg
Italy
Emilia-Romagna
Spain
Czechoslovakia
Hungary
Israel
Japan
Tokyo
Sichuan
Australia
New Zealand
Canada
United States
Atlanta
Mexico
South America
74 76 78 80 82 84 86 88
0 5 10

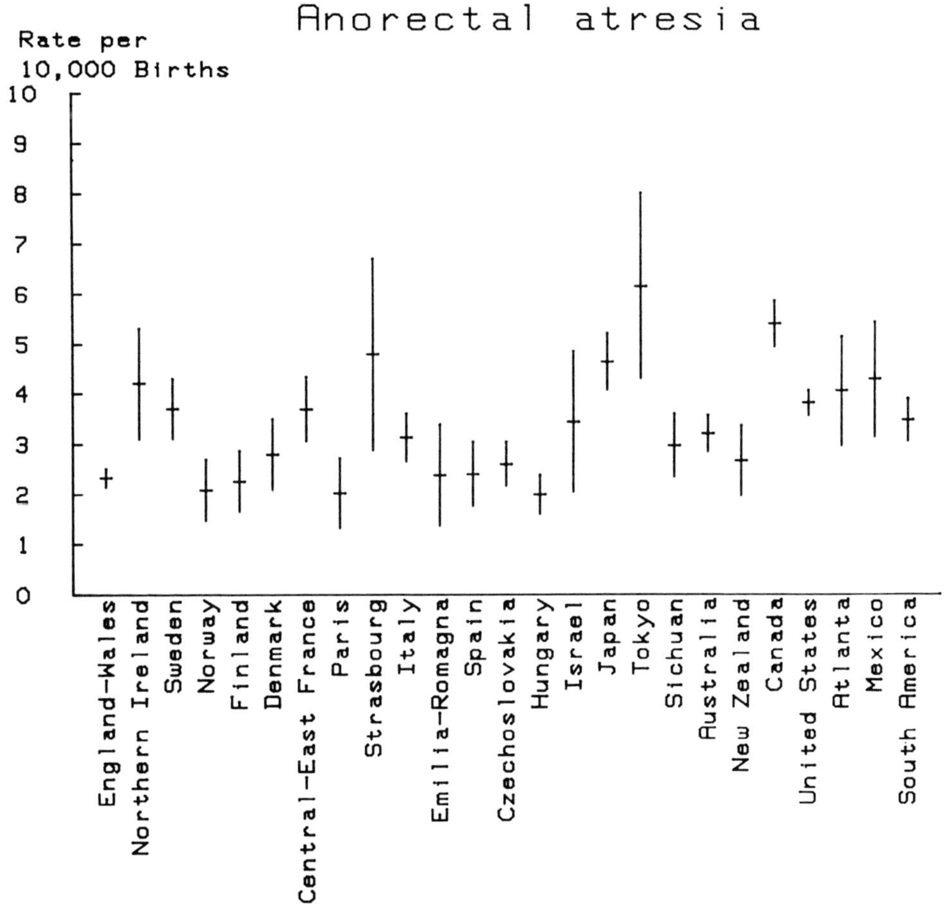

Diagram showing average rates of anorectal atresia in different programs for the years 1985-1988. Vertical lines indicate 95% confidence intervals of the recorded rates.

Comments

The rates vary somewhat among programs. High rates are seen in Strasbourg, Canada, Mexico, and the Japanese programs. In most programs the rate is similar to that of esophageal atresia, that is, around 3 per 10,000.

Most programs show a steady rate of anal atresia. An increase is noted in Canada and, during the early period, in Czechoslovakia, Israel, and South America. A decrease is noted in Australia and Northern Ireland.

Important sources of variation are probably inclusion or exclusion of cases of anorectal stenosis and the degree of detail in descriptions of multimalformed infants, as anal atresia often occurs together with other malformations.

Renal agenesis or dysgenesis

Complete absence of both kidneys or severe bilateral dysgenesis is not compatible with life. Other anomalies are usually also present in what is called the Potter sequence: lung hypoplasia, which is usually the direct cause of death, and abnormal facies with large floppy ears, epicanthic folds, a parrot-beak nose, and receding chin. These conditions are all thought to be secondary to the virtual absence of amniotic fluid and may also be found with bilateral polycystic kidneys. Positional foot defects, thought to be the result of crowding, are common. Esophageal and anorectal atresia and skeletal malformations are among the other malformations often found.

The infant usually expires within hours of birth, with a few surviving for a few days and then dying from renal failure.

No therapy is possible. The condition can often be identified by ultrasound investigation and an elective abortion can be made.

Families with autosomal recessive inheritance have been described, but in most instances the recurrence risk for sibs is low. No exogenous cause of these malformations has with certainty been demonstrated.

Renal agenesis/dysgenesis

Definition: A congenital malformation characterized by absence of kidneys or severely dysplastic kidneys. Polycystic kidneys not counted.

A. Number of infants born with renal a/dysgenesis

Monitoring program	1974	1975	1976	1977	1978	1979	1980	1981	1982	1983	1984	1985	1986	1987	1988	Total
Atlanta	9	12	8	9	9	10	8	6	8	12	10	10	10	10	11	142
Australia								36	71	66	58	69	47	56	38	441
Canada	60	58	67	72	81	85	79	70	107	91	106	118	141	111	81	1327
Central-East France			1	3	2	4	2	5	7	8	2	8	11	7	1	61
Czechoslovakia	34	24	44	24	32	22	22	27	17	24	18	17	13	14	8	340
Denmark										7	6	9	8	8	4	42
Emilia-Romagna					3	3	2	2	2	2	1	3	4	6	0	28
England-Wales	21	29	42	25	47	62	75	86	65	86	78	77	64	83	82	922
Finland											12	5	14	6	2	39
Hungary					18	24	26	17	15	10	3	10	11	22	11	167
Israel													1	2	2	5
Italy					6	16	13	8	12	24	23	10	17	11	6	146
New Zealand											2	0	0	3	4	9
Northern Ireland											6	7				13
Norway	2	0	0	0	2	0	1	4	2	10	4	8	5	15	12	65
Paris								6	11	12	22	12	17	21	16	117
Sichuan												4	5	1	1	11
South America	2	6	2	2	4	3	2	3	9	13	11	13	15	18	15	118
Spain			0	3	0	2	4	6	10	6	9	11	9	5	8	73
Strasbourg									4	7	5	4	6	2	9	37
Sweden	19	23	22	17	24	42	22	21	24	24	28	24	27	28	23	368
Tokyo							0	0	0	0	0	0	0	2	1	3
United States	109	120	152	111	129	126	95	123	140	146	120	143	157	133	120	1924

B. Rate per 10,000 infants.																
Monitoring program	1974	1975	1976	1977	1978	1979	1980	1981	1982	1983	1984	1985	1986	1987	1988	Average
Atlanta	3.6	5.2	3.5	3.8	3.7	3.9	2.9	2.2	2.9	4.3	3.4	3.2	3.0	2.9	3.0	3.4
Australia								3.2	3.0	2.7	2.4	2.9	1.9	2.3	1.6	2.5
Canada	2.7	2.5	2.9	3.1	3.3	3.4	3.3	2.9	4.2	3.8	4.2	4.5	5.4	4.5	3.8	3.7
Central-East France			0.2	0.4	0.3	0.6	0.3	0.6	0.9	0.9	0.2	0.9	1.2	0.8	0.1	0.6
Czechoslovakia	1.8	1.3	2.3	1.3	1.8	1.3	1.4	1.9	1.2	1.7	1.3	1.3	1.0	1.1	0.6	1.4
Denmark										1.4	1.2	1.7	1.4	1.4	0.7	1.3
Emilia-Romagna					4.3	4.7	1.6	1.4	1.1	0.9	0.4	1.2	1.7	2.6	0	1.4
England-Wales	0.3	0.5	0.7	0.4	0.8	1.0	1.1	1.3	1.0	1.4	1.2	1.2	1.0	1.2	1.2	1.0
Finland											1.8	0.8	2.3	1.0	0.3	1.3
Hungary					1.1	1.5	1.7	1.2	1.1	0.8	0.2	0.8	0.9	1.7	0.9	1.1
Israel													0.6	1.2	1.1	1.0
Italy					1.4	2.2	1.6	0.7	1.0	1.7	1.7	0.8	1.2	0.8	0.4	1.2
New Zealand											0.4	0	0	0.5	0	0.2
Northern Ireland											2.2	2.5				2.3
Norway	0.3	0	0	0	0.4	0	0.2	0.8	0.4	2.0	0.8	1.6	0.9	2.8	2.1	0.8
Paris								1.5	2.8	3.0	5.5	2.9	4.2	5.2	3.9	3.6
Sichuan												0.6	0.6	0.1	0.2	0.4
South America	0.2	0.9	0.3	0.3	0.5	0.4	0.4	0.5	0.6	0.8	0.6	0.7	0.7	0.9	0.8	0.7
Spain			0	1.1	0	0.3	0.7	1.1	1.6	0.8	1.3	1.6	1.5	1.0	1.5	1.1
Strasbourg									3.0	5.6	3.9	3.1	4.7	1.5	6.7	4.1
Sweden	1.7	2.2	2.2	1.8	2.6	4.3	2.3	2.2	2.6	2.6	3.0	2.4	2.6	2.7	2.0	2.5
Tokyo														1.1	0.6	0.2
United States	1.0	1.1	1.4	1.0	1.3	1.2	1.2	1.4	1.7	1.8	1.6	2.0	2.3	2.2	2.4	1.5

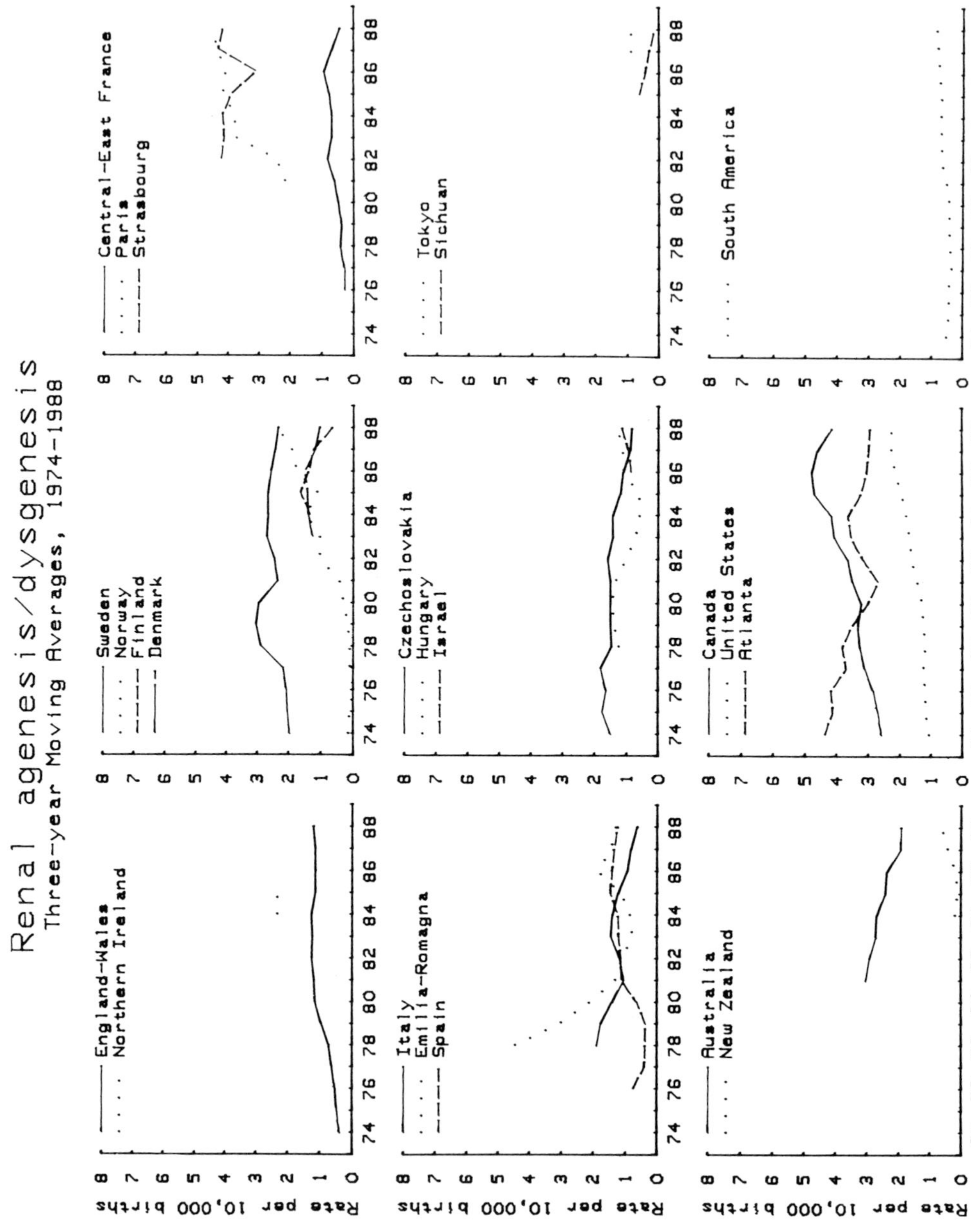
Renal agenesis/dysgenesis
Three-year Moving Averages, 1974-1988
Rate per 10,000 births
England-Wales
Northern Ireland
Sweden
Norway
Finland
Denmark
Central-East France
Paris
Strasbourg
Italy
Emilia-Romagna
Spain
Czechoslovakia
Hungary
Israel
Tokyo
Sichuan
Australia
New Zealand
Canada
United States
Atlanta
South America
74 76 78 80 82 84 86 88
0 1 2 3 4 5 6 7 8

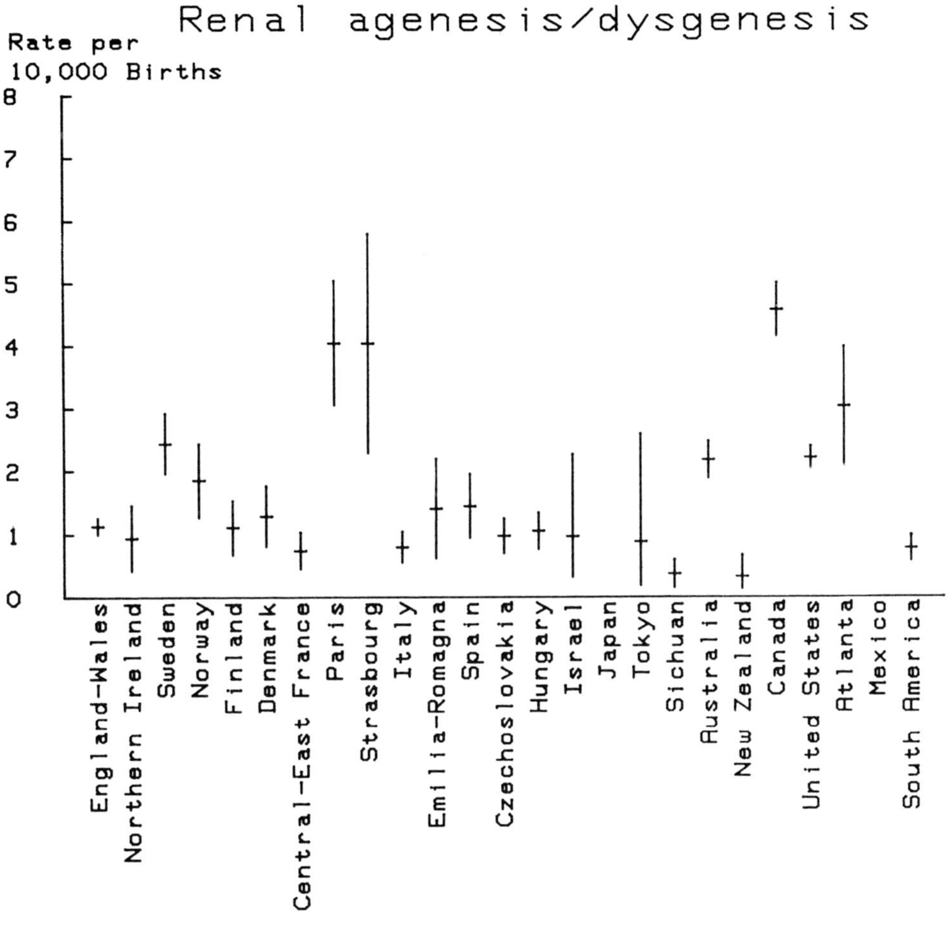

Diagram showing average rates of renal agenesis or dysgenesis in different programs for the years 1985-1988. Vertical lines indicate 95% confidence intervals of the recorded rates.

Comments

Some programs show high rates (e.g., Paris, Strasbourg, Canada, and Atlanta) while others show very low rates (e.g., Sichuan and New Zealand). The inclusion or exclusion of renal dysgenesis of various degrees and the frequency of autopsy will affect the recorded rates and their trends in different programs.

Increasing rates are seen in England-Wales, Norway, Canada, and the United States. A recently published analysis of the changing rate in the latter country found it to be caused by increased reporting of renal dysgenesis.

Hypospadias

Hypospadias means a malposition of the urethral opening on the underside of the penis. Rare cases of a similar malformation in females have been described. Various forms exist, from the most severe ones with the urethral opening at the base of the penis or even on the perineum to less severe forms with the opening on the shaft of the penis to the most common and least severe form with the opening in the coronal sulcus or on the underside of the glans. The penis is often severely curved and the urethral opening may be stenosed. Other genital anomalies are common (e.g., undescended testis) and in some infants also non-genital malformations occur. Hypospadias may also be a component of certain syndromes, including chromosome anomalies.

Hypospadias arises between weeks 6-14 of embryonic development at a time when the penis is formed from the genital folds and tubercle. This process is driven by androgens, and hypospadias can be regarded as a mild form of incomplete masculinization of the male embryo. It has been suggested that exogenous hormones may cause hypospadias, but this is uncertain. No definite non-genetic cause has been identified.

The malformation can be successfully treated surgically, usually before school age, but the mildest forms do not need an operation.

Hypospadias

Definition: A congenital malformation characterized by the opening of the urethra on the ventral side of the penis, irrespective of degree of severity.

A. Number of infants born with hypospadias

Monitoring program	1974	1975	1976	1977	1978	1979	1980	1981	1982	1983	1984	1985	1986	1987	1988	Total
Atlanta	65	80	68	70	76	87	62	75	67	79	79	101	113	105	116	1243
Australia								254	476	432	361	365	431	449	480	3248
Canada	361	367	405	341	554	554	584	557	624	672	699	660	652	625	472	8127
Central-East France			43	52	39	41	52	45	50	58	40	59	92	80	95	746
Czechoslovakia	381	399	349	289	328	290	321	289	273	260	285	321	274	317	291	4667
Denmark										61	65	73	90	84	88	461
Emilia-Romagna					7	10	37	32	21	46	46	47	47	52	52	397
England-Wales	900	869	881	899	944	1065	990	1010	1050	1150	1139	1062	1029	1109	1092	15189
Finland	26	24	19	27	23	15	25	33	42	30	30	35	37	29	44	439
Hungary	262	339	377	344	405	307	329	310	322	298	290	301	290	239	285	4698
Israel	33	20	26	33	45	42	48	53	42	62	39	44	57	64	44	652
Italy								193	239	275	271	323	401	362	363	2427
Japan					21	34	34	34	21	31	28	37	41	29	29	339
Mexico							19	8	17	20	13	7	7	22	15	128
New Zealand							56	49	59	87	71	75	72	86	59	614
Northern Ireland							31	23	19	25	29	22				149
Norway	63	59	65	75	79	76	79	59	70	62	81	85	72	88	120	1133
Paris								40	52	51	36	28	49	43	41	340
Sichuan												28	15	25	15	83
South America	68	52	46	50	51	42	35	44	76	142	155	162	173	147	149	1392
Spain			26	39	73	124	97	93	112	121	147	121	97	82	97	1229
Strasbourg									24	24	22	36	35	34	40	215
Sweden	212	217	204	202	191	211	206	188	141	183	200	195	174	210	194	2928
Tokyo							6	4	3	2	3	5	5	4	6	38
United States	2467	2509	2509	2551	2328	2567	2017	2349	2206	2411	2377	2323	2250	1989	1717	34570

B. Rate per 10,000 infants.																
Monitoring program	1974	1975	1976	1977	1978	1979	1980	1981	1982	1983	1984	1985	1986	1987	1988	Average
Atlanta	26.2	34.7	30.0	29.8	31.2	34.1	22.7	27.9	24.0	28.3	27.0	32.6	34.5	30.0	31.7	29.7
Australia								22.4	19.9	17.9	15.2	15.1	17.8	18.6	19.7	18.1
Canada	16.0	15.9	17.8	14.7	22.4	22.0	24.4	22.9	24.7	27.7	27.8	25.2	24.8	25.2	21.9	22.4
Central-East France			6.5	7.6	5.7	5.8	7.0	5.8	6.7	6.8	4.6	6.5	10.1	8.9	10.4	7.2
Czechoslovakia	19.6	20.8	18.6	15.9	18.3	16.8	20.9	20.0	19.3	18.9	20.8	23.6	20.5	24.2	21.9	19.8
Denmark										11.9	12.5	13.5	16.2	14.9	14.9	14.0
Emilia-Romagna					9.9	15.7	29.7	22.3	11.4	21.1	19.9	19.6	20.6	22.9	22.8	20.3
England-Wales	13.9	14.3	14.9	15.6	15.7	16.6	15.0	15.8	16.7	18.2	17.8	16.1	15.5	16.2	15.7	15.9
Finland	4.2	3.7	2.9	4.1	3.6	2.4	4.0	5.2	6.4	4.5	4.6	5.6	6.1	4.8	7.3	4.6
Hungary	13.9	17.3	20.2	19.2	23.9	19.0	22.0	21.5	23.9	23.3	23.0	23.0	22.5	18.9	22.8	20.6
Israel	46.9	26.8	30.7	40.5	24.5	22.3	25.8	29.1	23.4	33.8	21.5	24.7	32.5	38.5	25.2	28.5
Italy								18.0	19.0	19.7	19.8	24.6	28.3	26.4	26.3	23.0
Japan						2.1	2.2	2.4	1.7	2.5	2.2	2.8	2.6	2.0	2.1	2.4
Mexico							4.6	2.3	4.9	5.2	3.9	2.9	2.8	5.4	3.7	4.1
New Zealand							12.1	9.8	12.2	17.2	14.2	14.6	13.7	15.8	10.7	13.4
Northern Ireland							10.8	8.4	7.0	9.1	10.4	7.9				8.9
Norway	10.4	10.3	12.0	14.6	15.1	14.6	15.3	11.6	13.5	12.3	16.0	16.5	13.6	16.2	20.7	14.2
Paris								10.3	13.4	12.8	9.0	6.8	12.0	10.7	9.9	10.6
Sichuan												4.4	1.9	3.0	2.3	2.8
South America	8.0	8.0	5.9	7.4	7.0	6.1	6.3	7.9	5.3	9.2	9.2	8.9	8.2	7.5	7.9	7.8
Spain			21.3	14.2	20.5	18.0	17.0	16.6	18.3	16.8	21.1	18.1	16.7	16.1	18.4	17.9
Strasbourg									17.7	19.3	17.3	27.7	27.2	26.3	30.0	23.7
Sweden	19.2	20.8	20.6	20.9	20.4	21.8	21.1	19.9	15.1	19.9	21.2	19.7	17.0	20.0	17.2	19.6
Tokyo							3.2	2.2	1.6	1.1	1.5	2.6	2.7	2.3	3.7	2.3
United States	22.7	23.5	23.9	23.7	23.9	24.9	26.2	27.2	26.8	29.6	32.0	32.1	32.9	33.1	33.7	27.0

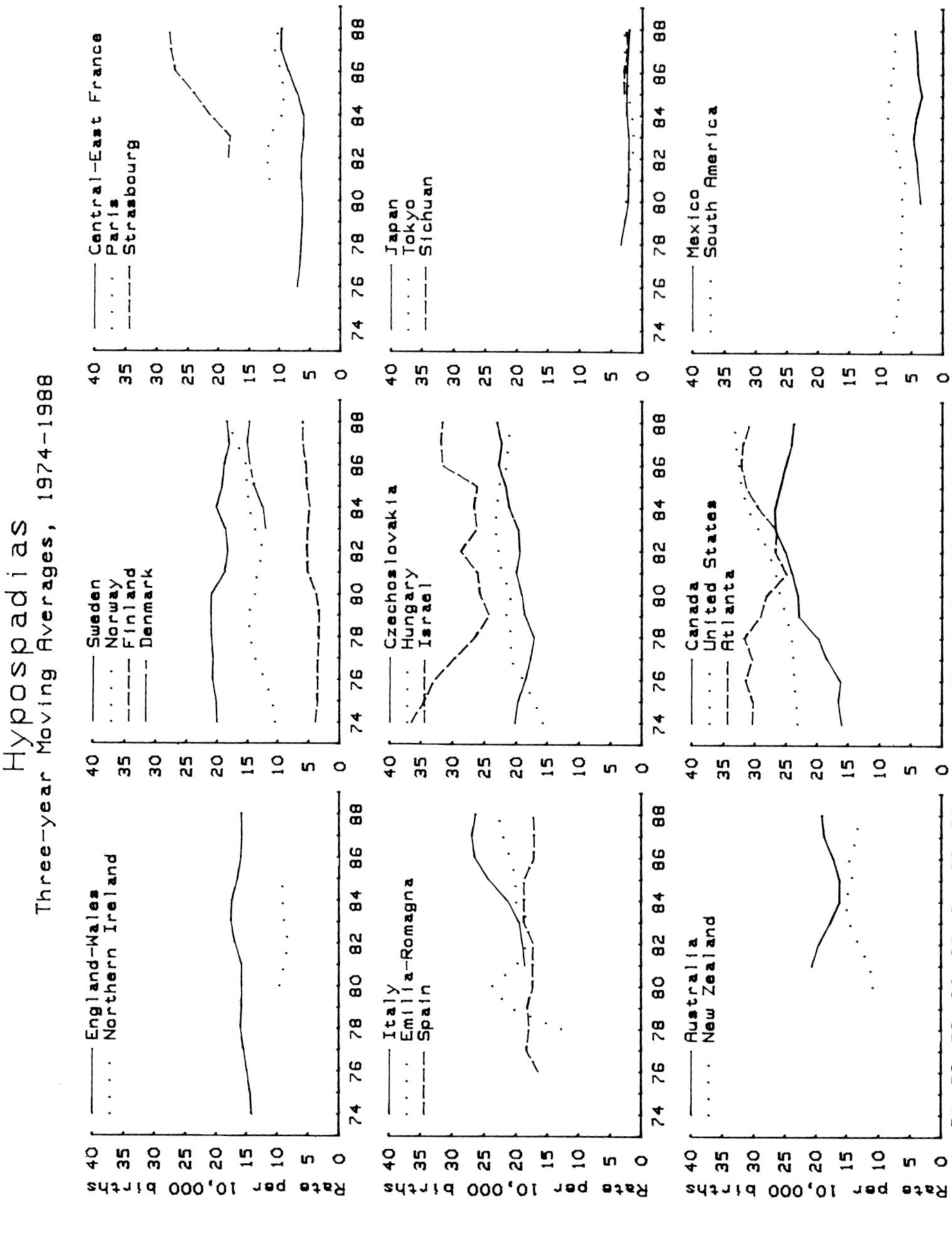
Hypospadias
Three-year Moving Averages, 1974-1988
England-Wales
Northern Ireland
Sweden
Norway
Finland
Denmark
Central-East France
Paris
Strasbourg
Italy
Emilia-Romagna
Spain
Czechoslovakia
Hungary
Israel
Japan
Tokyo
Sichuan
Australia
New Zealand
Canada
United States
Atlanta
Mexico
South America
Rate per 10,000 births

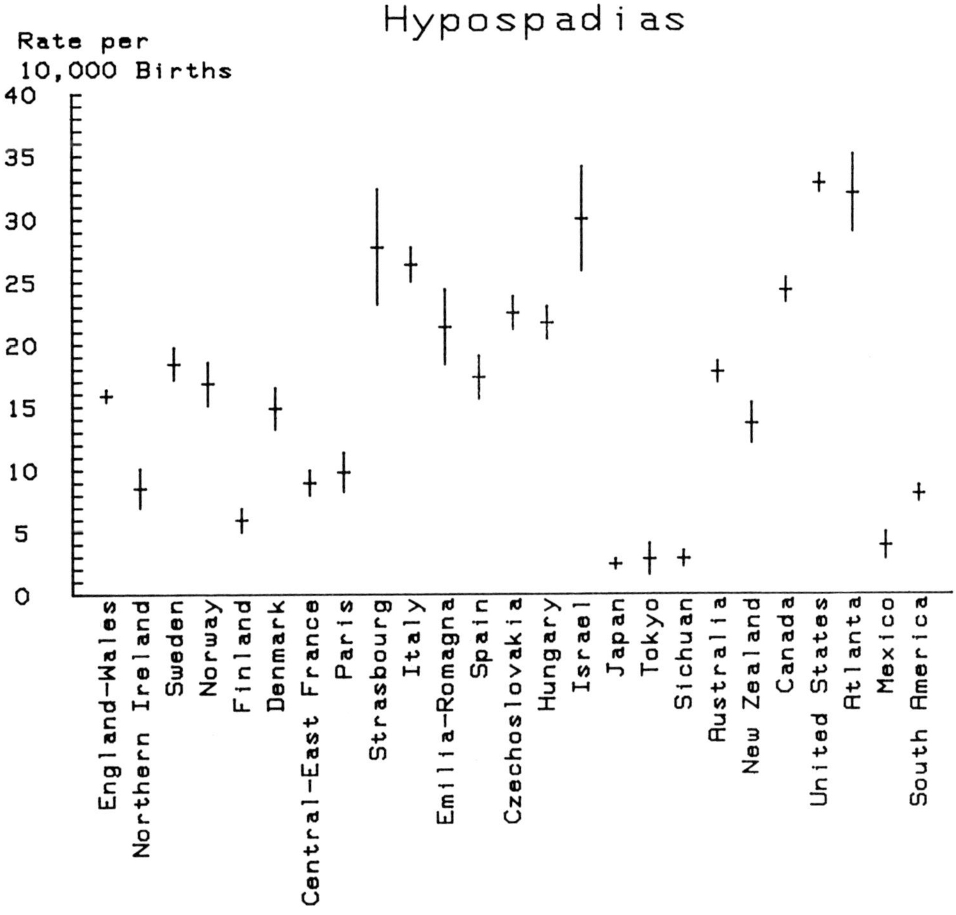

Diagram showing average rates of hypospadias in different programs for the years 1985-1988. Vertical lines indicate 95% confidence intervals of the recorded rates.

Comments

This is a rather common malformation and even in small programs the number of recorded cases is usually large. On the other hand, it occurs with very different degrees of severeness and rates are therefore difficult to compare.

There are very marked differences in the recorded rates. Low rates are seen in Finland, Northern Ireland, Central-East France, Paris, the Asian programs, Mexico, and South America. High rates are found in Strasbourg, Italy, Israel, and the two US programs. Detailed comparisons between some programs with markedly different rates have shown that the differences are probably not totally explained by different criteria or ascertainment.

A marked increase can be seen in the rates recorded in the United States as well as in Strasbourg and Italy. Some of these increases are certainly artifacts. In Italy the increase occurred simultaneously with a special case-control study of hypospadias and in Strasbourg it was due to a change in inclusion criteria.

Epispadias

In male epispadias the urethra opens on the dorsal side of the penis, which is usually small and often curved. In the female the urethra may open into or above the clitoris, which may be bifid. A defect may exist in the symphysis. The extent of the epispadias varies considerably. Epispadias often occurs with bladder exstrophy, but the tables are restricted to epispadias without that malformation. Usually no extragenital malformations exist.

Mild forms can be successfully repaired surgically.

An autosomal recessive heredity may exist, but most forms are sporadic. Nothing is known about exogenous factors that might cause epispadias.

Epispadias

Definition: A congenital malformation characterized by the opening of the urethra on the dorsal side of the penis or above the clitoris. Epispadias together with bladder exstrophy is not counted.

A. Number of infants born with epispadias

Monitoring program	1974	1975	1976	1977	1978	1979	1980	1981	1982	1983	1984	1985	1986	1987	1988	Total
Atlanta	5	2	0	3	1	3	3	3	4	3	0	5	2	3	0	37
Australia								2	5	5	3	6	7	7	6	41
Central-East France			0	3	2	0	0	1	0	2	1	3	1	1	2	16
Czechoslovakia	1	0	1	0	0	1	1	0	0	1	1	0	0	1	0	7
Denmark										3	0	3	1	3	2	12
Emilia-Romagna					0	0	0	0	1	1	1	0	0	1	1	5
Israel	1	0	0	0	0	0	0	0	0	0	0	1	0	0	0	2
Italy								3	3	4	1	4	0	4	1	20
Mexico							0	0	0	0	0	3	0	1	2	6
Norway	1	1	2	2	1	2	1	0	1	4	3	4	2	1	2	27
Paris								0	0	0	1	2	3	1	5	12
Sichuan															0	0
South America	0	3	1	0	2	0	0	0	3	6	9	4	2	5	2	37
Spain			0	0	0	1	1	4	0	2	0	1	2	1	0	12
Strasbourg									0	0	0	0	0	0	0	0
Sweden	2	1	2	0	1	1	1	1	2	1	3	1	2	4	5	27

Epispadias
Three-year Moving Averages, 1974-1988

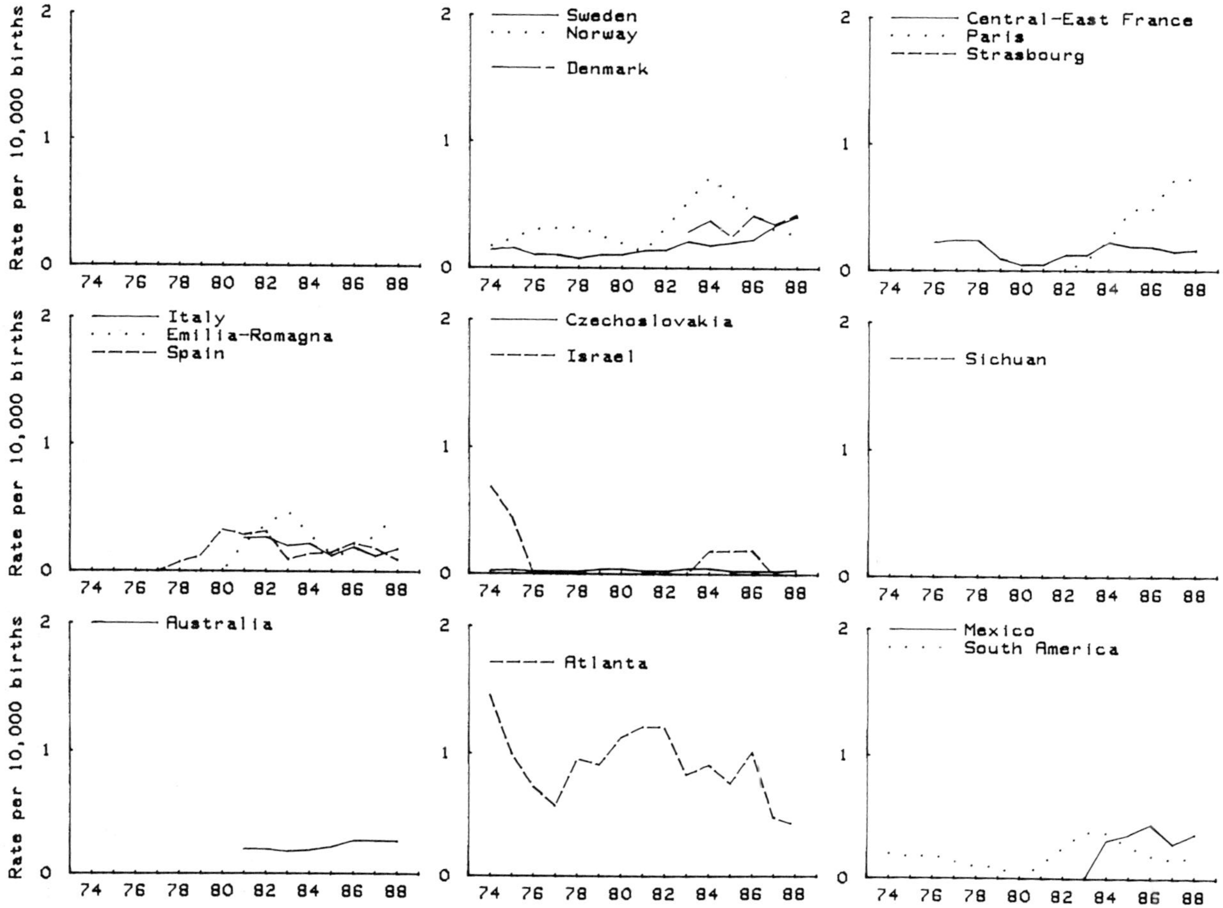

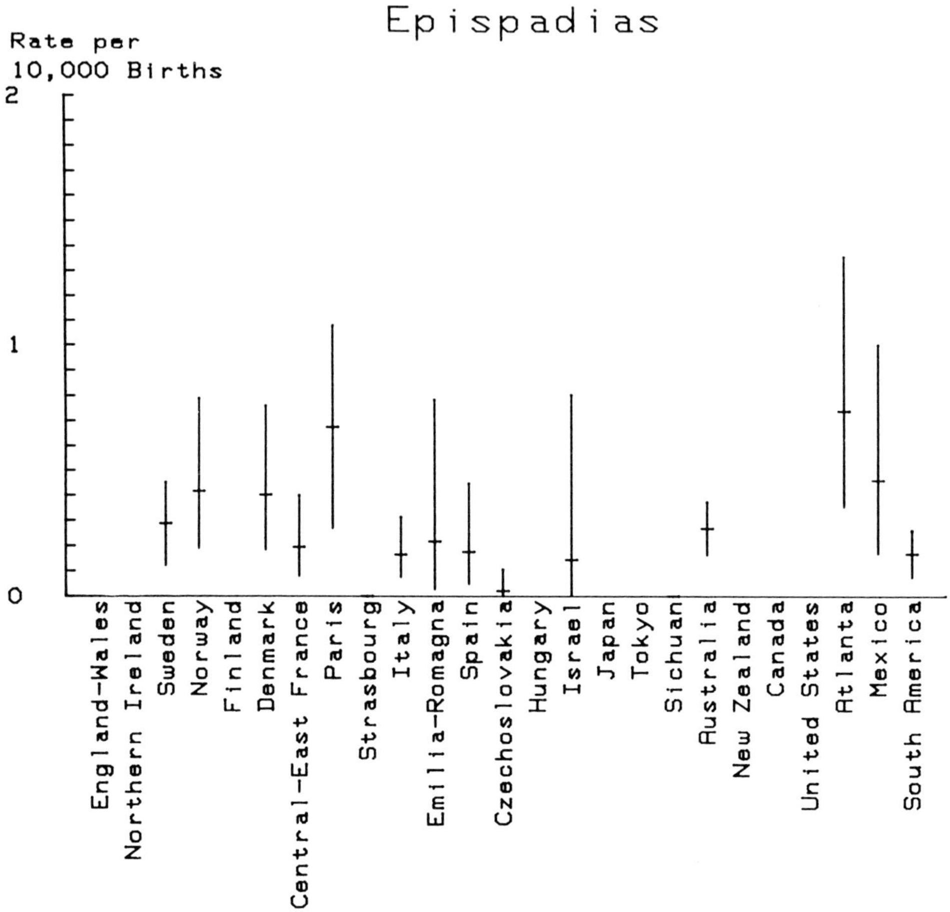

Diagram showing average rates of epispadias in different programs for the years 1985-1988. Vertical lines indicate 95% confidence intervals of the recorded rates.

Comments

Epispadias is a rare malformation, probably underdiagnosed at birth in girls. Data were reported from only some of the programs. The rates do not vary much between programs except for Atlanta, where the rate is markedly higher until the last few years when it goes down to a level similar to that of other programs. No other clear-cut time trends are seen except for Paris and possibly Mexico, but there are few cases and the trends may be random. Czechoslovakia has a very low rate.

Bladder exstrophy

Bladder exstrophy, or ectopia vesica, consists of the absence of the lower abdominal wall with the bladder exposed on the body surface. The pubic arch is open and the penis or clitoris is usually malformed. The malformation originates in a defect in the early mesoderm in the subumbilical region. Other malformations are often present and the bladder exstrophy may be part of a cloacal exstrophy sequence, where the rectum and the bladder are joined in an embryonic cloaca, exposed as described above.

Surgical treatment is moderately successful with respect to normal function, but it permits survival. Untreated cases may also survive.

Usually the cases are sporadic and nothing is known about possible exogenous factors causing this condition.

Prenatal diagnosis can identify this condition by ultrasound or alphafetoprotein determination.

Bladder exstrophy

Definition: A congenital malformation characterized by the broad exposure of the urinary bladder on the abdomen above the symphysis. Cloacal exstrophy is included.

A. Number of infants born with bladder exstrophy

Monitoring program	1974	1975	1976	1977	1978	1979	1980	1981	1982	1983	1984	1985	1986	1987	1988	Total
Atlanta	0	1	3	1	1	1	1	1	0	0	0	1	0	1	1	12
Australia								4	9	12	10	11	10	6	8	70
Canada	9	4	5	8	4	18	6	11	15	14	5	19	18	13	10	159
Central-East France			3	3	2	2	1	0	0	2	0	5	3	4	3	28
Czechoslovakia	1	3	3	7	0	2	1	4	1	2	3	1	2	2	2	34
Emilia-Romagna					1	0	1	1	1	0	0	1	5	1	2	13
England-Wales	19	26	20	19	9	13	13	17	16	11	16	14	12	15	13	233
Hungary					3	5	4	2	9	6	4	7	7	7	6	60
Israel	0	0	0	0	1	0	0	1	0	1	0	0	1	4	0	8
Italy					1	1	0	2	3	6	10	7	4	5	6	45
Japan						5	3	2	2	2	0	2	3	4	1	25
Mexico							2	0	1	2	4	1	2	1	2	15
Norway	2	2	2	0	0	1	1	3	3	1	6	1	0	1	3	26
Paris								0	4	0	0	3	2	2	1	12
Sichuan															0	0
South America	0	1	0	1	3	1	0	1	2	5	4	8	3	7	5	41
Spain			0	2	1	3	3	2	2	2	3	6	2	1	2	29
Strasbourg									0	1	1	1	0	2	0	5
Sweden	6	1	3	3	6	2	6	4	2	1	6	3	5	1	0	49
Tokyo							0	0	0	0	0	0	0	0	1	1
United States	30	22	33	36	26	34	19	24	21	26	26	16	23	20	19	375

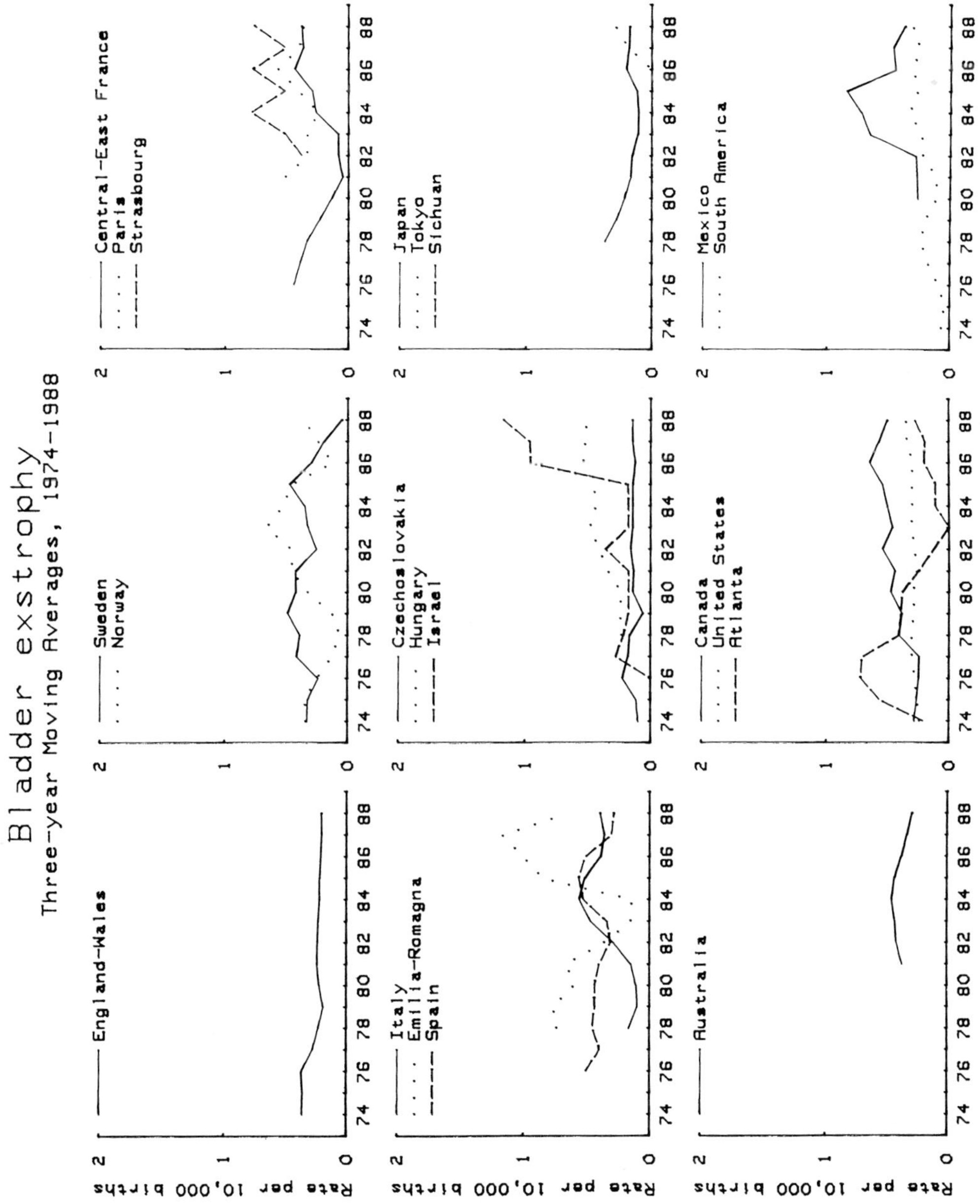
Bladder exstrophy
Three-year Moving Averages, 1974-1988
Rate per 10,000 births
England-Wales
Sweden
Norway
Central-East France
Paris
Strasbourg
Italy
Emilia-Romagna
Spain
Czechoslovakia
Hungary
Israel
Japan
Tokyo
Sichuan
Australia
Canada
United States
Atlanta
Mexico
South America
74 76 78 80 82 84 86 88
0 1 2

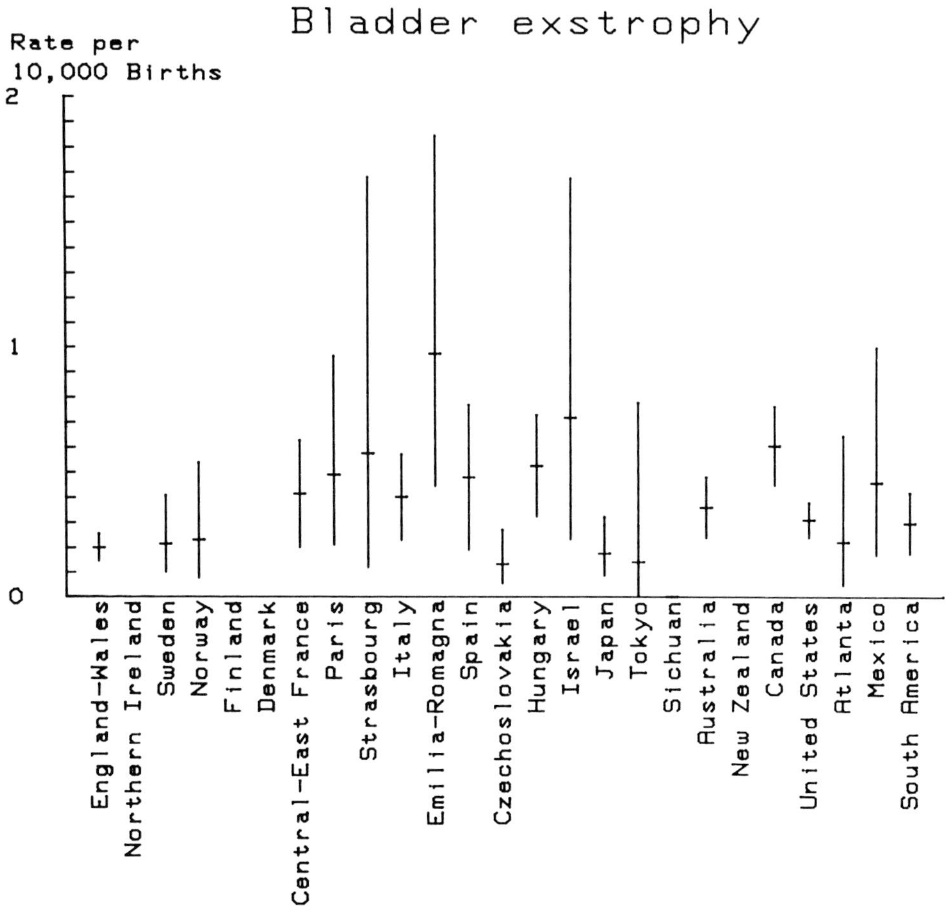

Diagram showing average rates of bladder exstrophy in different programs for the years 1985-1988. Vertical lines indicate 95% confidence intervals of the recorded rates.

Comments

Bladder exstrophy is a rare malformation and the recorded rates from small programs will show large confidence intervals. No major interprogram variation is seen. Changes in rate with time can be observed, but they are based on few cases and may well be random. A detailed analysis made by the *Clearinghouse* gave no evidence of any change in rate with time among the participating programs.

Limb reduction defects

This group of malformations spans a large range of severity, from a missing phalanx of a finger or toe to complete absence (amelia) of an entire limb. At least three main categories are discerned. In *transverse* reductions ("amputations"), the part of the limb distal to a specific level is missing. In *longitudinal* reductions, the radial (tibial) or ulnar (fibular) part of the limb is reduced or missing; the most common form is radial aplasia, often with absence of thumb. In *intercalary* reductions, the distal and proximal parts of a limb are reasonably normal, but the long bones of the middle part are shortened or absent. The latter form is sometimes called phocomelia, but this concept is ill defined. Transverse reductions are usually unilateral; longitudinal and intercalary forms are often bilateral. Non-limb malformations may concurrently exist. Some types are part of specific syndromes and are sometimes associated with chromosomal anomalies.

Survival depends on the severity of associated malformations. Surgical repair is usually not possible, but prosthesis may help.

Isolated reduction defects are usually not hereditary, but some syndromes may be, for example the autosomal dominant Holt-Oram syndrome having a cardiac defect and a radial longitudinal or an intercalary defect. Thalidomide is a well known exogenous cause of longitudinal or intercalary reductions. Other exogenous causes have been suggested, but none has been proved.

Limb reduction defects

Definition: A congenital malformation characterized by total or partial absence or severe hypoplasia of skeletal structures of the limbs.

A. Number of infants born with limb reduction

Monitoring program	1974	1975	1976	1977	1978	1979	1980	1981	1982	1983	1984	1985	1986	1987	1988	Total
Atlanta	14	15	18	18	16	14	14	10	17	13	14	12	17	15	14	221
Australia								73	117	109	97	93	107	99	119	814
Canada	105	112	118	102	143	118	134	101	141	156	143	135	169	115	103	1895
Central-East France			18	21	23	27	47	36	30	42	41	39	48	50	39	461
Czechoslovakia	55	79	85	92	103	69	66	67	70	80	81	64	72	49	55	1087
Denmark										19	30	26	24	50		149
Emilia-Romagna					3	2	3	9	7	9	12	13	9	12	15	94
England-Wales	415	343	311	275	308	277	325	283	288	328	364	359	303	311	301	4791
Finland	29	31	26	24	25	35	23	31	31	23	25	27	25	22	24	401
Hungary	58	80	78	74	59	44	42	54	57	40	42	65	62	41	53	849
Israel	4	2	3	3	7	5	3	8	3	5	7	5	6	4	5	70
Italy					22	48	66	66	76	93	89	76	97	82	70	785
Japan					48	60	62	41	37	47	26	40	55	61	35	512
Mexico							28	22	23	25	12	13	20	19	32	194
New Zealand							14	19	19	26	13	23	15	13	16	158
Northern Ireland							25	21	22	26	20	20				134
Norway	26	20	14	21	12	13	29	43	28	26	30	19	20	17	32	350
Paris								15	15	12	21	14	15	13	18	123
Sichuan												31	46	30	31	138
South America	32	28	39	27	51	35	32	33	95	110	108	126	119	126	105	1066
Spain			6	10	20	26	34	51	55	53	52	41	37	31	37	453
Strasbourg									7	8	10	7	7	11	8	58
Sweden	55	60	58	66	45	68	58	62	49	51	54	64	61	74	63	888
Tokyo							17	11	12	11	8	8	15	7	7	96
United States	401	340	349	362	319	365	293	311	275	326	270	284	251	235	180	4561

B. Rate per 10,000 infants.

Monitoring program	1974	1975	1976	1977	1978	1979	1980	1981	1982	1983	1984	1985	1986	1987	1988	Average
Atlanta	5.7	6.5	7.9	7.7	6.6	5.5	5.1	3.7	6.1	4.7	4.8	3.9	5.2	4.3	3.8	5.3
Australia								6.4	4.9	4.5	4.1	3.9	4.4	4.1	4.9	4.5
Canada	4.6	4.9	5.2	4.4	5.8	4.7	5.6	4.2	5.6	6.4	5.7	5.2	6.4	4.6	4.8	5.2
Central-East France			2.7	3.1	3.4	3.8	6.3	4.7	4.0	4.9	4.8	4.3	5.3	5.6	4.3	4.5
Czechoslovakia	2.8	4.1	4.5	5.1	5.8	4.0	4.3	4.6	4.9	5.8	5.9	4.7	5.4	3.7	4.1	4.6
Denmark										3.7	5.8	4.8	4.3	8.8		5.5
Emilia-Romagna					4.3	3.1	2.4	6.3	3.8	4.1	5.2	5.4	3.9	5.3	6.6	4.8
England-Wales	6.4	5.6	5.3	4.8	5.1	4.3	4.9	4.4	4.6	5.2	5.7	5.4	4.6	4.5	4.3	5.0
Finland	4.7	4.7	3.9	3.7	3.9	5.6	3.6	4.9	4.7	3.4	3.8	4.3	4.1	3.7	4.0	4.2
Hungary	3.1	4.1	4.2	4.1	3.5	2.7	2.8	3.7	4.2	3.1	3.3	5.0	4.8	3.2	4.2	3.7
Israel	5.7	2.7	3.5	3.7	3.8	2.7	1.6	4.4	1.7	2.7	3.9	2.8	3.4	2.4	2.9	3.1
Italy					5.0	6.7	8.0	6.2	6.0	6.7	6.5	5.8	6.8	6.0	5.1	6.3
Japan						3.8	4.0	2.9	3.0	3.7	2.1	3.1	3.5	4.2	2.5	3.7
Mexico							6.7	6.4	6.6	6.6	3.6	5.4	8.1	4.7	7.8	6.2
New Zealand							3.0	3.8	3.9	5.1	2.6	4.5	2.9	2.4	2.9	3.4
Northern Ireland							8.7	7.6	8.1	9.5	7.2	7.2				8.0
Norway	4.3	3.5	2.6	4.1	2.3	2.5	5.6	8.4	5.4	5.2	5.9	3.7	3.8	3.1	5.5	4.4
Paris								3.8	3.9	3.0	5.3	3.4	3.7	3.2	4.4	3.8
Sichuan												4.9	5.8	3.5	4.8	4.7
South America	3.8	4.3	5.0	4.0	7.0	5.0	5.8	5.9	6.6	7.1	6.4	6.9	5.6	6.5	5.6	5.9
Spain			4.9	3.6	5.6	3.8	6.0	9.1	9.0	7.4	7.5	6.1	6.4	6.1	7.0	6.6
Strasbourg									5.2	6.4	7.9	5.4	5.4	8.5	6.0	6.4
Sweden	5.0	5.8	5.9	6.8	4.8	7.0	5.9	6.6	5.3	5.5	5.7	6.5	6.0	7.0	5.6	6.0
Tokyo							9.0	6.1	6.2	5.8	4.1	4.2	8.2	4.0	4.3	5.8
United States	3.7	3.2	3.3	3.4	3.3	3.5	3.8	3.6	3.3	4.0	3.6	3.9	3.7	3.9	3.5	3.6

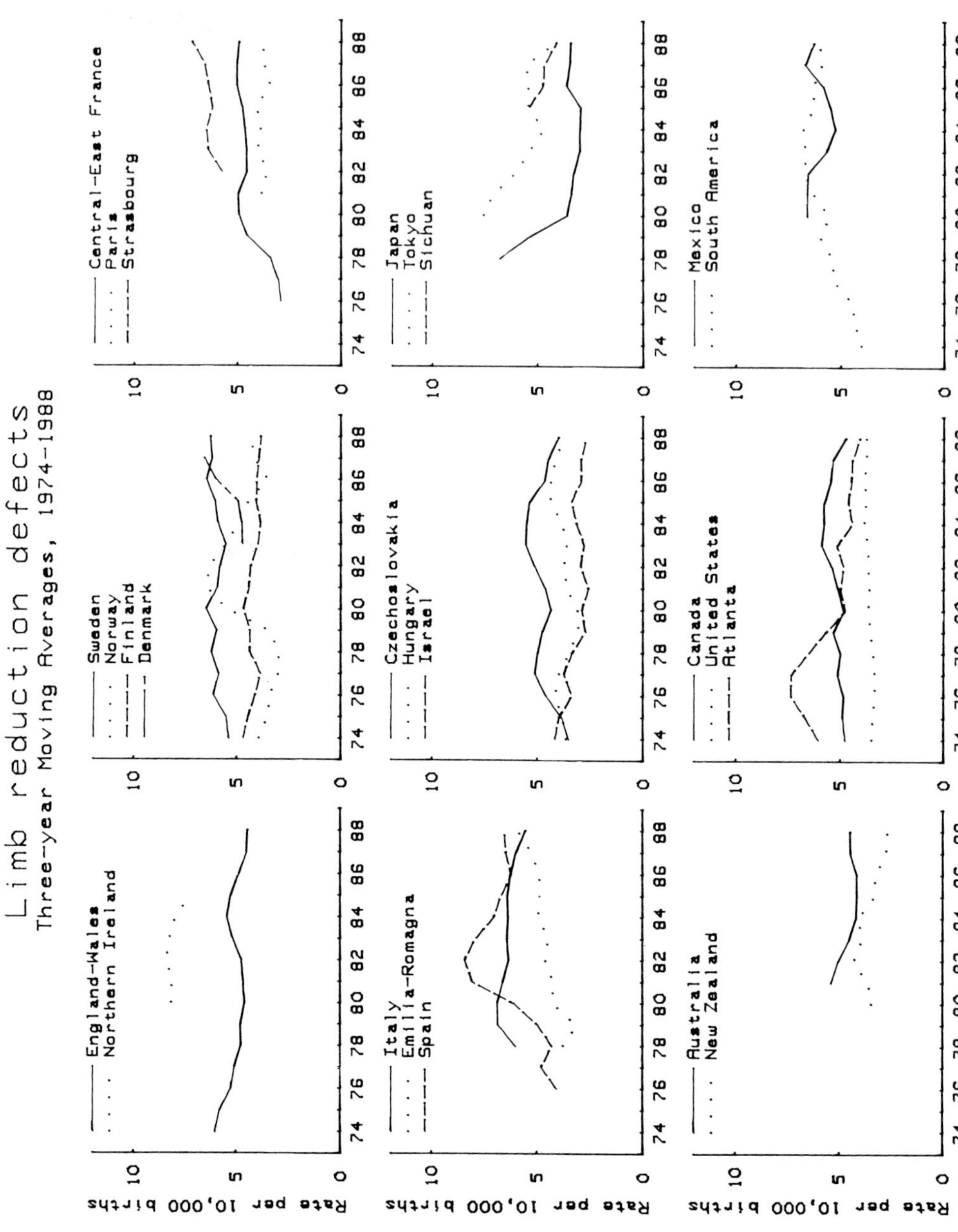

Limb reduction defects
Three-year Moving Averages, 1974-1988
Rate per 10,000 births
England-Wales
Northern Ireland
Sweden
Norway
Finland
Denmark
Central-East France
Paris
Strasbourg
Italy
Emilia-Romagna
Spain
Czechoslovakia
Hungary
Israel
Japan
Tokyo
Sichuan
Australia
New Zealand
Canada
United States
Atlanta
Mexico
South America
0
5
10
74 76 78 80 82 84 86 88

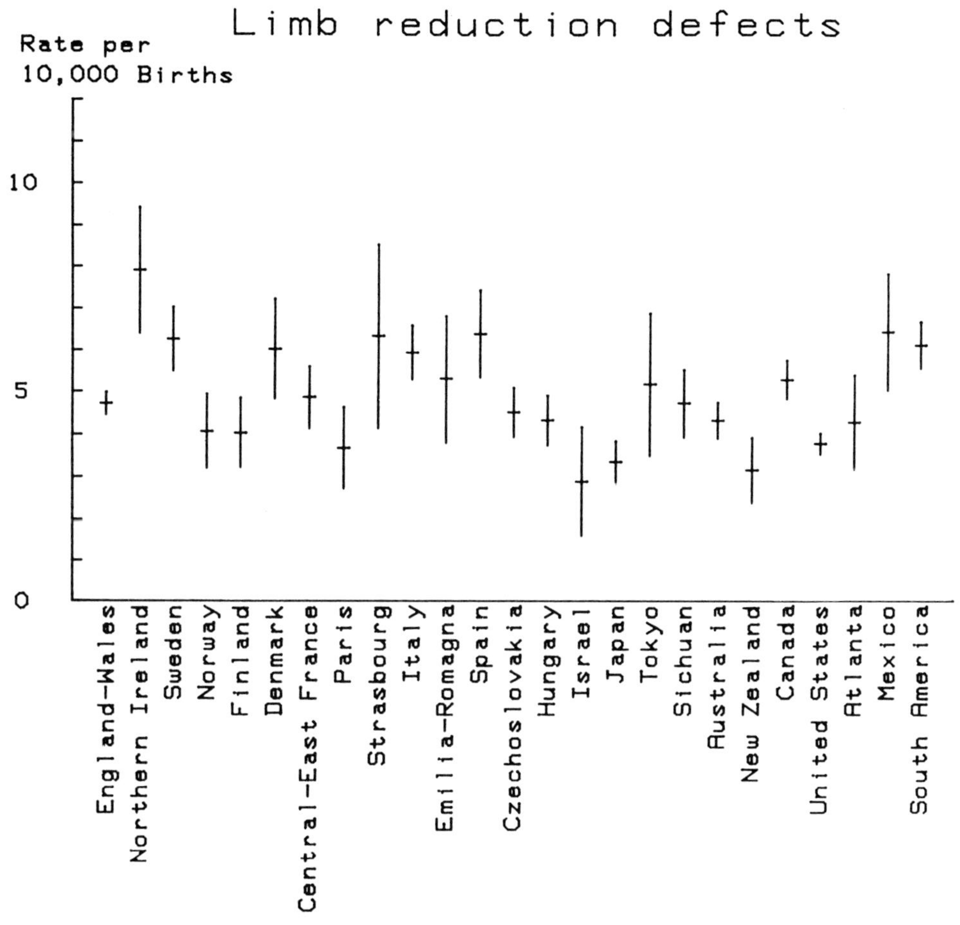

Diagram showing average rates of limb reduction defects in different programs for the years 1985-1988. Vertical lines indicate 95% confidence intervals of the recorded rates.

Comments

Most programs report rates around 4 to 6 per 10,000 births, with a higher rate in Northern Ireland. The inclusion or exclusion of minor phalangeal reductions may explain some variability.

With a few exceptions no marked time trends are seen. The rate in Atlanta seems to decrease with time (notably before 1980), and there is a marked increase in the rate in Norway in the early 1980s and in Spain a few years later. Without a detailed investigation of specific types of reduction defects, such changes are difficult to evaluate.

Diaphragmatic hernia

In diaphragmatic hernia a defect exists in the diaphragm, which permits abdominal organs to herniate into the thorax. Most cases diagnosed in the newborn consist of posterolateral defects (Bochdalek type) which originate during the 8th to 12th week of embryonic life when the diaphragm is formed and consist of an open passage through the diaphragm. Another type is the retrosternal hernia, in which a hernial sac almost always exists. The latter usually does not present symptoms in the newborn period. The main sign of the posterolateral diaphragmatic hernia is dyspnea and cyanosis due to the displacement and hypoplasia of lungs. Other malformations are common.

The defect can be repaired surgically, but survival depends on the degree of pulmonary hypoplasia and on associated malformations.

The condition is usually not hereditary and no markedly increased risk exists for sibs, but families with autosomal recessive inheritance are known. Nothing is known about exogenous factors that may cause the malformation.

Diaphragmatic hernia can be detected prenatally by ultrasound investigation, but usually only late in pregnancy.

Diaphragmatic hernia

Definition: A congenital malformation characterized by herniation into the thorax of abdominal contents through a defect of the diaphragm.

A. Number of infants born with diaphragmatic hernia

Monitoring program	1974	1975	1976	1977	1978	1979	1980	1981	1982	1983	1984	1985	1986	1987	1988	Total
Atlanta	6	8	6	8	2	3	7	3	9	4	7	2	11	10	12	98
Australia								46	60	69	69	76	79	74	54	527
Canada							92	95	92	96	105	116	97	122	88	903
Central-East France			16	13	17	9	11	18	32	26	23	24	19	24	33	265
Czechoslovakia	54	55	37	42	57	35	31	35	35	35	37	38	28	29	29	577
Denmark										14	16	11	6	8	17	72
Emilia-Romagna					0	0	3	0	4	2	6	5	2	8	4	34
England-Wales						75	103	86	88	81	128	83	111	96	92	943
Finland	0	0	0	0	0	0	0	0	0	5	9	3	8	0	2	27
Hungary	66	44	47	29	5	5	45	41	36	29	28	22	34	23	25	479
Israel					4	4	4	3	6	5	5	5	3	2	3	44
Italy								30	32	44	26	31	41	42	48	294
Mexico							4	0	2	2	2	1	0	6	2	19
New Zealand										5	9	9	8	8	8	47
Northern Ireland										10	8	3				21
Norway	10	7	4	13	15	14	13	14	10	10	14	17	7	20	9	177
Paris								9	9	13	12	24	17	18	23	125
Sichuan												8	5	5	5	23
South America	5	4	7	2	2	11	6	7	16	26	18	21	34	34	37	230
Strasbourg									10	3	5	7	6	5	4	40
Spain			3	1	7	19	11	17	22	16	23	16	8	11	11	165
Sweden	39	29	23	20	25	19	19	17	16	16	9	14	22	18	10	296
Tokyo							1	2	0	1	3	3	1	2	0	13

B. Rate per 10,000 infants.																
Monitoring program	1974	1975	1976	1977	1978	1979	1980	1981	1982	1983	1984	1985	1986	1987	1988	Average
Atlanta	2.4	3.5	2.6	3.4	0.8	1.2	2.6	1.1	3.2	1.4	2.4	0.6	3.4	2.9	3.3	2.3
Australia								4.1	2.5	2.9	2.9	3.2	3.3	3.1	2.2	2.9
Canada							3.8	3.9	3.6	4.0	4.2	4.4	3.7	4.9	4.1	4.1
Central-East France			2.4	1.9	2.5	1.3	1.5	2.3	4.3	3.0	2.7	2.7	2.1	2.7	3.6	2.6
Czechoslovakia	2.8	2.9	2.0	2.3	3.2	2.0	2.0	2.4	2.5	2.5	2.7	2.8	2.1	2.2	2.2	2.5
Denmark										2.7	3.1	2.0	1.1	1.4	2.9	2.2
Emilia-Romagna					0	0	2.4	0	2.2	0.9	2.6	2.1	0.9	3.5	1.8	1.7
England-Wales						1.2	1.6	1.3	1.4	1.3	2.0	1.3	1.7	1.4	1.3	1.4
Finland	0	0	0	0	0	0	0	0	0	0.7	1.4	0.5	1.3	0	0.3	0.3
Hungary	3.5	2.2	2.5	1.6	0.3	0.3	3.0	2.8	2.7	2.3	2.2	1.7	2.6	1.8	2.0	2.1
Israel					2.2	2.1	2.2	1.6	3.3	2.7	2.8	2.8	1.7	1.2	1.7	2.2
Italy								2.8	2.5	3.2	1.9	2.4	2.9	3.1	3.5	2.8
Mexico							1.0	0	0.6	0.5	0.6	0.4	0	1.5	0.5	0.6
New Zealand										1.0	1.8	1.8	1.5	1.5	1.5	1.5
Northern Ireland										3.6	2.9	1.1				2.5
Norway	1.7	1.2	0.7	2.5	2.9	2.7	2.5	2.7	1.9	2.0	2.8	3.3	1.3	3.7	1.6	2.2
Paris								2.3	2.3	3.3	3.0	5.9	4.2	4.5	5.6	3.9
Sichuan												1.3	0.6	0.6	0.8	0.8
South America	0.6	0.6	0.9	0.3	0.3	1.6	1.1	1.3	1.1	1.7	1.1	1.2	1.6	1.7	2.0	1.3
Spain			2.5	0.4	2.0	2.8	1.9	3.0	3.6	2.2	3.3	2.4	1.4	2.2	2.1	2.4
Strasbourg									7.4	2.4	3.9	5.4	4.7	3.9	3.0	4.4
Sweden	3.5	2.8	2.3	2.1	2.7	2.0	1.9	1.8	1.7	1.7	1.0	1.4	2.1	1.7	0.9	2.0
Tokyo							0.5	1.1	0	0.5	1.5	1.6	0.5	1.1	0	0.8

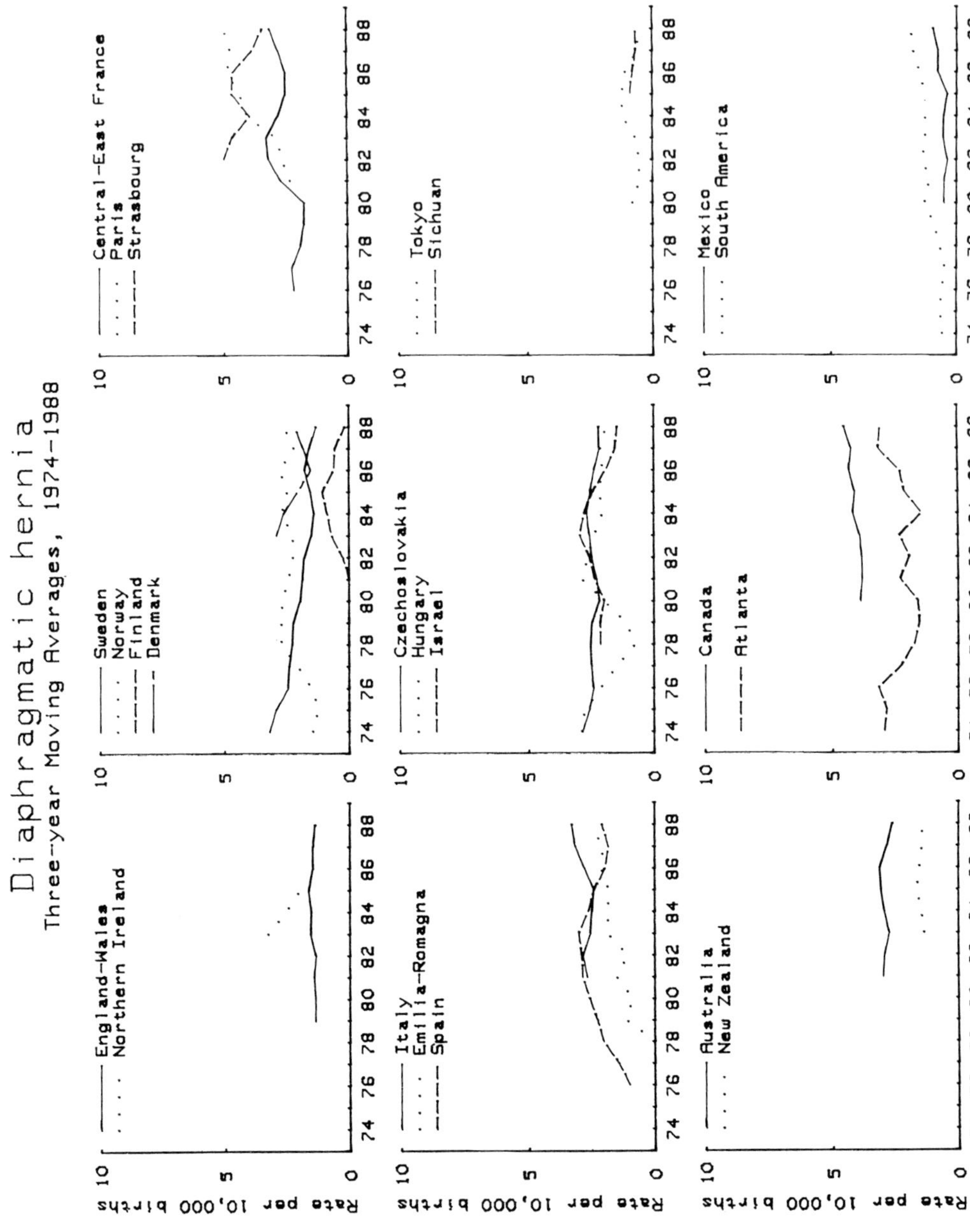
Diaphragmatic hernia
Three-year Moving Averages, 1974-1988
England-Wales
Northern Ireland
Sweden
Norway
Finland
Denmark
Central-East France
Paris
Strasbourg
Italy
Emilia-Romagna
Spain
Czechoslovakia
Hungary
Israel
Tokyo
Sichuan
Australia
New Zealand
Canada
Atlanta
Mexico
South America
Rate per 10,000 births
74 76 78 80 82 84 86 88

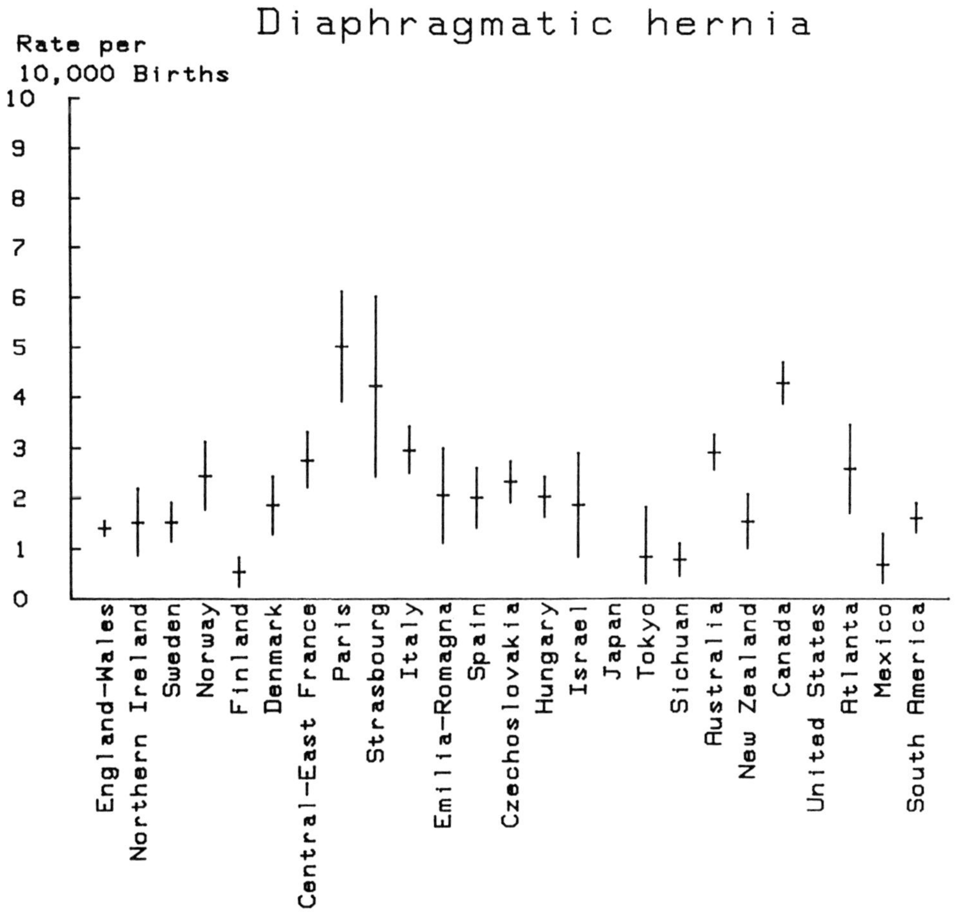

Diagram showing average rates of diaphragmatic hernia in different programs for the years 1985-1988. Vertical lines indicate 95% confidence intervals of the recorded rates.

Comments

The recording of diaphragmatic hernia may be partly dependent on the autopsy rate. Some variation may occur by inclusion or exclusion of hernias other than those of the Bochdalek type. The rates are high in Paris, Strasbourg, and Canada and low in Finland, Sichuan, Tokyo, and Mexico.

An increasing trend can be seen in some programs, e.g., Norway during the early part of the observation period, Central-East France, Paris, Italy, and South America.

Abdominal wall defects

Abdominal wall defects are a heterogenous group. The two main types are omphalocele and gastroschisis, both originating early in development. In *omphalocele* a sac is seen which - if unbroken - consists of amnion, herniated intestines, and perhaps other internal organs. The size may vary considerably. In a large percentage of infants with omphalocele, other malformations are present, often severe ones. *Gastroschisis* is a defect in the abdominal wall lateral to the intact navel and through which the intestines herniate. A gut atresia may be present; otherwise, the infant with gastroschisis usually has no further malformation.

Small or moderate omphaloceles can be repaired, but a large percentage of the infants have associated malformations that cause a high mortality. Gastroschisis can usually be surgically repaired to complete normality, and mortality is comparatively low.

Omphalocele may be part of a genetic or chromosomal syndrome. Most other cases are sporadic and no exogenous cause is known. Gastroschisis is not hereditary. Possible exogenous causes have been described, but none is proved.

Abdominal wall defects can be detected prenatally by ultrasound or from alphafetoprotein investigations. In most cases, a differential diagnosis between the two conditions can be made by ultrasound.

Abdominal wall defects

Definition: Contains omphalocele and gastroschisis (see later tables) and other rare types of abdominal wall defects.

A. Number of infants born with abdominal wall defects

Monitoring program	1974	1975	1976	1977	1978	1979	1980	1981	1982	1983	1984	1985	1986	1987	1988	Total
Atlanta	12	12	12	11	18	15	14	14	18	16	7	17	22	6	22	216
Australia								50	81	69	95	99	96	91	92	673
Canada							130	110	142	131	119	107	124	141	138	1142
Central-East France			12	11	8	9	14	15	11	18	22	17	14	16	30	197
Czechoslovakia	39	39	25	28	27	42	35	36	20	27	35	28	21	32	25	459
Denmark										14	18	20	21	28	16	117
Emilia-Romagna					2	1	4	5	2	7	6	11	8	10	4	60
England-Wales	453	417	362	383	417	489	515	489	458	505	413	390	398	411	449	6549
Finland											14	15	13	8	9	59
Hungary					48	45	45	41	40	46	21	25	42	28	23	404
Israel					2	4	1	8	3	7	8	4	3	3	1	44
Italy					5	10	22	34	35	30	32	27	35	35	24	289
Japan					27	26	40	26	35	27	20	35	66	57	58	417
Mexico							20	14	13	22	7	9	15	11	17	128
New Zealand							16	13	11	13	18	9	19	14	15	128
Northern Ireland							14	11	14	12	11	6				68
Norway							17	15	32	34	51	16	26	24	26	241
Paris								3	15	16	19	31	21	22	18	145
Sichuan												16	21	17	19	73
South America	14	10	9	5	11	15	5	23	35	40	41	63	72	60	57	460
Spain			0	5	3	9	19	17	18	18	16	14	11	19	7	156
Strasbourg									2	5	4	6	6	11	5	39
Sweden	35	24	30	32	15	24	19	20	16	26	23	20	22	14	11	331
Tokyo							10	9	16	7	7	3	9	6	3	70
United States						707	459	509	578	587	549	388	359	265	216	4617

B. Rate per 10,000 infants.

Monitoring program	1974	1975	1976	1977	1978	1979	1980	1981	1982	1983	1984	1985	1986	1987	1988	Average
Atlanta	4.8	5.2	5.3	4.7	7.4	5.9	5.1	5.2	6.5	5.7	2.4	5.5	6.7	1.7	6.0	5.2
Australia								4.4	3.4	2.9	4.0	4.1	4.0	3.8	3.8	3.7
Canada							5.4	4.5	5.6	5.4	4.7	4.1	4.7	5.7	6.4	5.2
Central-East France			1.8	1.6	1.2	1.3	1.9	1.9	1.5	2.1	2.5	1.9	1.5	1.8	3.3	1.9
Czechoslovakia	2.0	2.0	1.3	1.5	1.5	2.4	2.3	2.5	1.4	2.0	2.6	2.1	1.6	2.4	1.9	2.0
Denmark										2.7	3.5	3.7	3.8	5.0	2.7	3.6
Emilia-Romagna					2.8	1.6	3.2	3.5	1.1	3.2	2.6	4.6	3.5	4.4	1.8	3.1
England-Wales	7.0	6.8	6.1	6.7	6.9	7.6	7.8	7.7	7.3	8.0	6.5	5.9	6.0	6.0	6.4	6.8
Finland											2.2	2.4	2.1	1.3	1.5	1.9
Hungary					2.8	2.8	3.0	2.8	3.0	3.6	1.7	1.9	3.3	2.2	1.8	2.6
Israel					1.1	2.1	0.5	4.4	1.7	3.8	4.4	2.2	1.7	1.8	0.6	2.2
Italy					1.1	1.4	2.7	3.2	2.8	2.1	2.3	2.1	2.5	2.6	1.7	2.3
Japan						1.6	2.6	1.9	2.9	2.2	1.6	2.7	4.2	4.0	4.2	3.0
Mexico							4.8	4.1	3.8	5.8	2.1	3.7	6.1	2.7	4.2	4.1
New Zealand							3.5	2.6	2.3	2.6	3.6	1.8	3.6	2.6	2.7	2.8
Northern Ireland							4.9	4.8	5.1	4.4	3.9	2.2				4.1
Norway							3.3	2.9	6.2	6.8	10.1	3.1	4.9	4.4	4.5	5.1
Paris								0.8	3.9	4.0	4.8	7.6	5.2	5.5	4.4	4.5
Sichuan												2.5	2.6	2.0	2.9	2.5
South America	1.6	1.5	1.2	0.7	1.5	2.2	0.9	4.1	2.4	2.6	2.4	3.5	3.4	3.1	3.0	2.6
Spain			0	1.8	0.8	1.3	3.3	3.0	2.9	2.5	2.3	2.1	1.9	3.7	1.3	2.3
Strasbourg									1.5	4.0	3.2	4.6	4.7	8.5	3.7	4.3
Sweden	3.2	2.3	3.0	3.3	1.6	2.5	1.9	2.1	1.7	2.8	2.4	2.0	2.1	1.3	1.0	2.2
Tokyo							5.3	5.0	8.3	3.7	3.6	1.6	4.9	3.4	1.8	4.2
United States						6.9	6.0	5.9	7.0	7.2	7.4	5.4	5.3	4.4	4.2	6.1

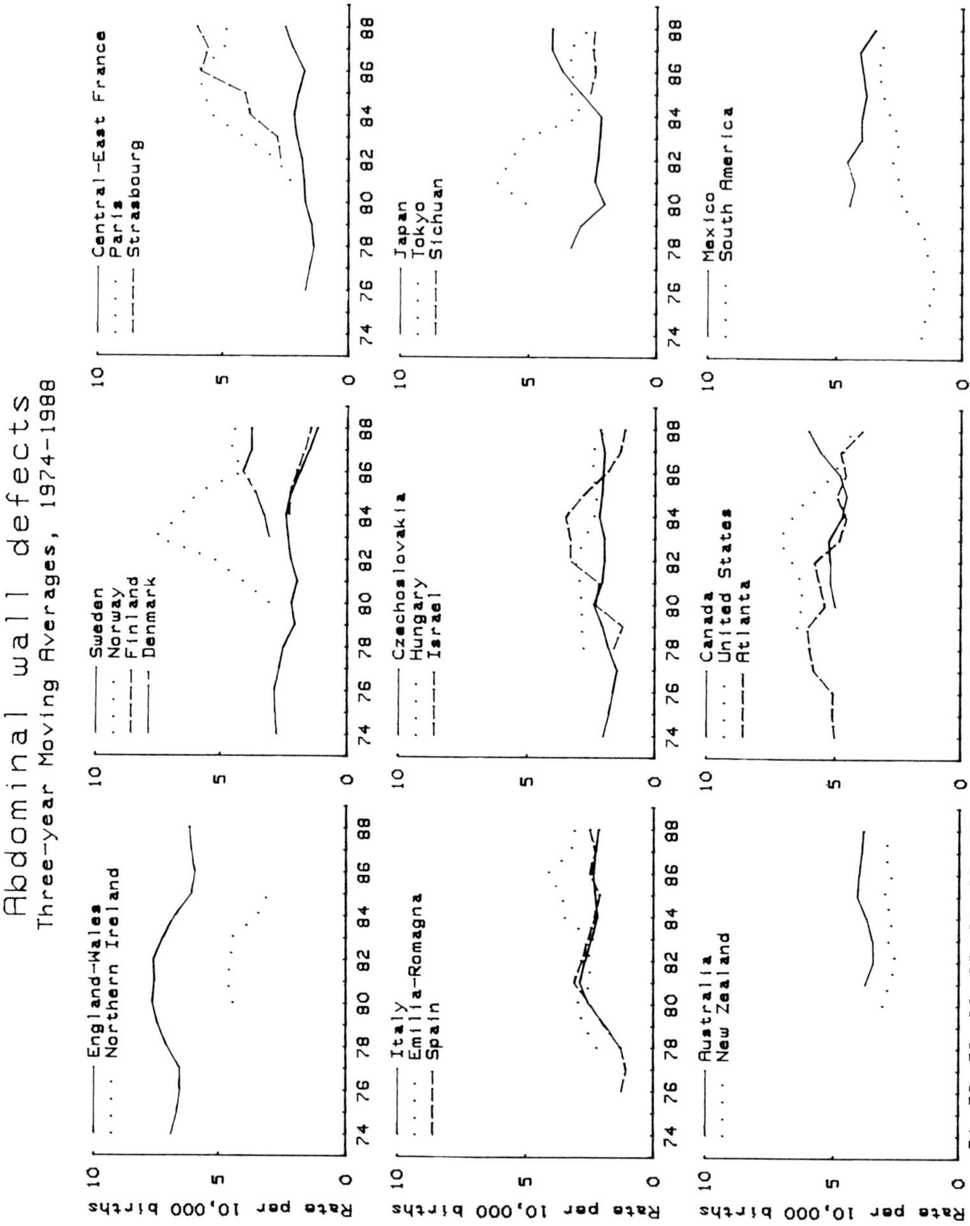
Abdominal wall defects
Three-year Moving Averages, 1974-1988
Rate per 10,000 births
England-Wales
Northern Ireland
Sweden
Norway
Finland
Denmark
Central-East France
Paris
Strasbourg
Italy
Emilia-Romagna
Spain
Czechoslovakia
Hungary
Israel
Japan
Tokyo
Sichuan
Australia
New Zealand
Canada
United States
Atlanta
Mexico
South America
0
5
10
74 76 78 80 82 84 86 88

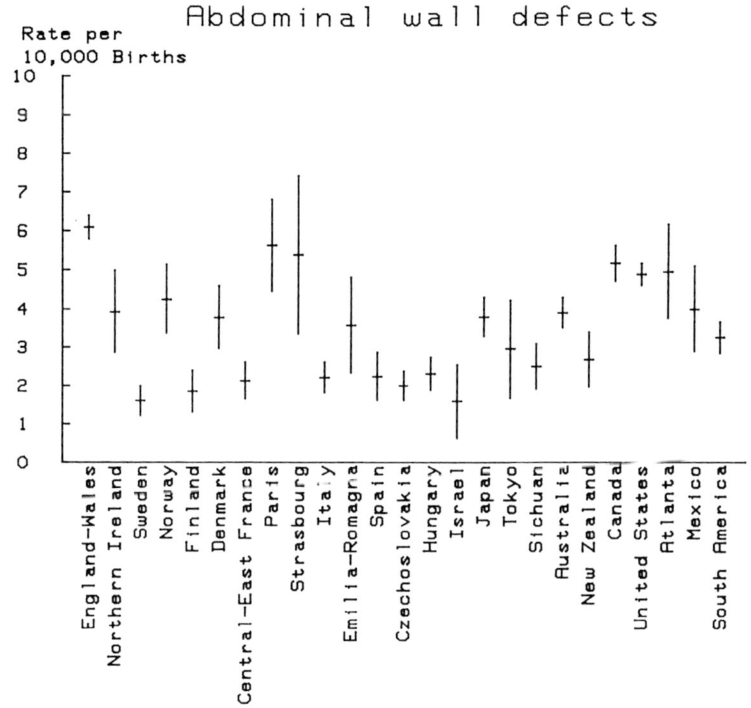

Diagram showing average rates of abdominal wall defects in different programs for the years 1985-1988. Vertical lines indicate 95% confidence intervals of the recorded rates.

Comments

This is a combination of three groups of malformations: omphalocele, gastroschisis and other rare types of abdominal wall defects. Not all programs have included the last group, but quantitatively it is probably too small to contribute much to the variation. A more significant source of variation might be the inclusion of umbilical hernias, which should not be included but which could be difficult to differentiate from true abdominal wall defects if an unspecific coding system is used.

Most programs record rates of 2-4 per 10,000 births, but a few have higher rates: England-Wales, Paris, Strasbourg, Canada, and the two United States programs. In Norway a remarkable peak is seen around 1984, followed by a decline.

During the last few years, a decreasing rate is seen in several programs, possibly as a result of prenatal diagnosis and selective abortion. In South America, the rate has increased steadily during the observation period, probably indicating an improved ascertainment. Increasing rates are also seen in the French programs.

Omphalocele

Definition: A congenital malformation characterized by herniation of abdominal contents through the umbilical insertion and covered by membrane which may or may not remain intact.

A. Number of infants born with omphalocele

Monitoring program	1974	1975	1976	1977	1978	1979	1980	1981	1982	1983	1984	1985	1986	1987	1988	Total
Atlanta	10	11	9	6	12	8	10	10	11	8	4	12	15	4	6	136
Australia								31	49	39	60	62	65	49	49	404
Central-East France			5	7	7	5	10	8	6	11	14	9	10	9	18	119
Denmark										9	12	14	19	21	8	83
Emilia-Romagna					2	1	3	1	1	5	2	7	5	5	4	36
England-Wales						78	109	119	93	118	122	94	111	104	106	1054
Finland					5	8	12	2	7	9	8	11	10	7	6	85
Israel	1	2	3	1	2	4	1	7	3	6	6	1	2	2	1	42
Italy					4	8	18	30	30	25	23	20	30	28	20	236
Japan						15	25	17	22	18	10	21	45	43	43	270
Mexico							11	4	4	6	4	5	6	4	5	49
New Zealand								13	11	13	17	3	11	12	7	87
Northern Ireland											5	2				7
Norway							10	12	25	30	41	13	24	16	12	183
Paris								3	9	13	9	14	13	12	12	85
Sichuan												6	5	7	4	22
South America	13	9	9	5	6	11	4	13	25	32	28	49	52	37	42	335
Spain			0	5	3	6	15	9	11	14	11	9	8	12	3	106
Strasbourg									2	4	3	1	5	7	3	25
Sweden	22	14	19	22	7	18	11	13	11	20	16	12	15	12	6	218
Tokyo							8	9	16	7	3	2	4	3	2	54

B. Rate per 10,000 infants.

Monitoring program	1974	1975	1976	1977	1978	1979	1980	1981	1982	1983	1984	1985	1986	1987	1988	Average
Atlanta	4.0	4.8	4.0	2.6	4.9	3.1	3.7	3.7	3.9	2.9	1.4	3.9	4.6	1.1	1.6	3.2
Australia								2.7	2.1	1.6	2.5	2.6	2.7	2.0	2.0	2.2
Central-East France			0.8	1.0	1.0	0.7	1.3	1.0	0.8	1.3	1.6	1.0	1.1	1.0	2.0	1.1
Denmark										1.8	2.3	2.6	3.4	3.7	1.4	2.5
Emilia-Romagna					2.8	1.6	2.4	0.7	0.5	2.3	0.9	2.9	2.2	2.2	1.8	1.8
England-Wales						1.2	1.6	1.9	1.5	1.9	1.9	1.4	1.7	1.5	1.5	1.6
Finland					0.8	1.3	1.9	0.3	1.1	1.3	1.2	1.8	1.6	1.2	1.0	1.2
Israel	1.4	2.7	3.5	1.2	1.1	2.1	0.5	3.8	1.7	3.3	3.3	0.6	1.1	1.2	0.6	1.8
Italy					0.9	1.1	2.2	2.8	2.4	1.3	1.7	1.5	2.1	2.0	1.4	1.9
Japan						0.9	1.6	1.2	1.8	1.4	0.8	1.6	2.9	3.0	3.1	1.9
Mexico							2.6	1.2	1.2	1.6	1.2	2.1	2.4	1.0	1.2	1.6
New Zealand											3.4	0.6	2.1	2.2	1.3	1.9
Northern Ireland											1.8	0.7				1.3
Norway							1.9	2.4	4.8	6.0	8.1	2.5	4.5	2.9	2.1	3.9
Paris								0.8	2.3	3.3	2.3	3.4	3.2	3.0	2.9	2.6
Sichuan												1.0	0.6	0.8	0.6	0.8
South America	1.5	1.4	1.2	0.7	0.8	1.6	0.7	2.3	1.7	2.1	1.7	2.7	2.5	1.9	2.2	1.9
Spain			0	1.8	0.8	0.9	2.6	1.6	1.8	1.9	1.6	1.3	1.4	2.4	0.6	1.5
Strasbourg									1.5	3.2	2.4	0.8	3.9	5.4	2.2	2.8
Sweden	2.0	1.3	1.9	2.3	0.7	1.9	1.1	1.4	1.2	2.2	1.7	1.2	1.5	1.1	0.5	1.5
Tokyo							4.2	5.0	8.3	3.7	1.5	1.0	2.2	1.7	1.2	3.3

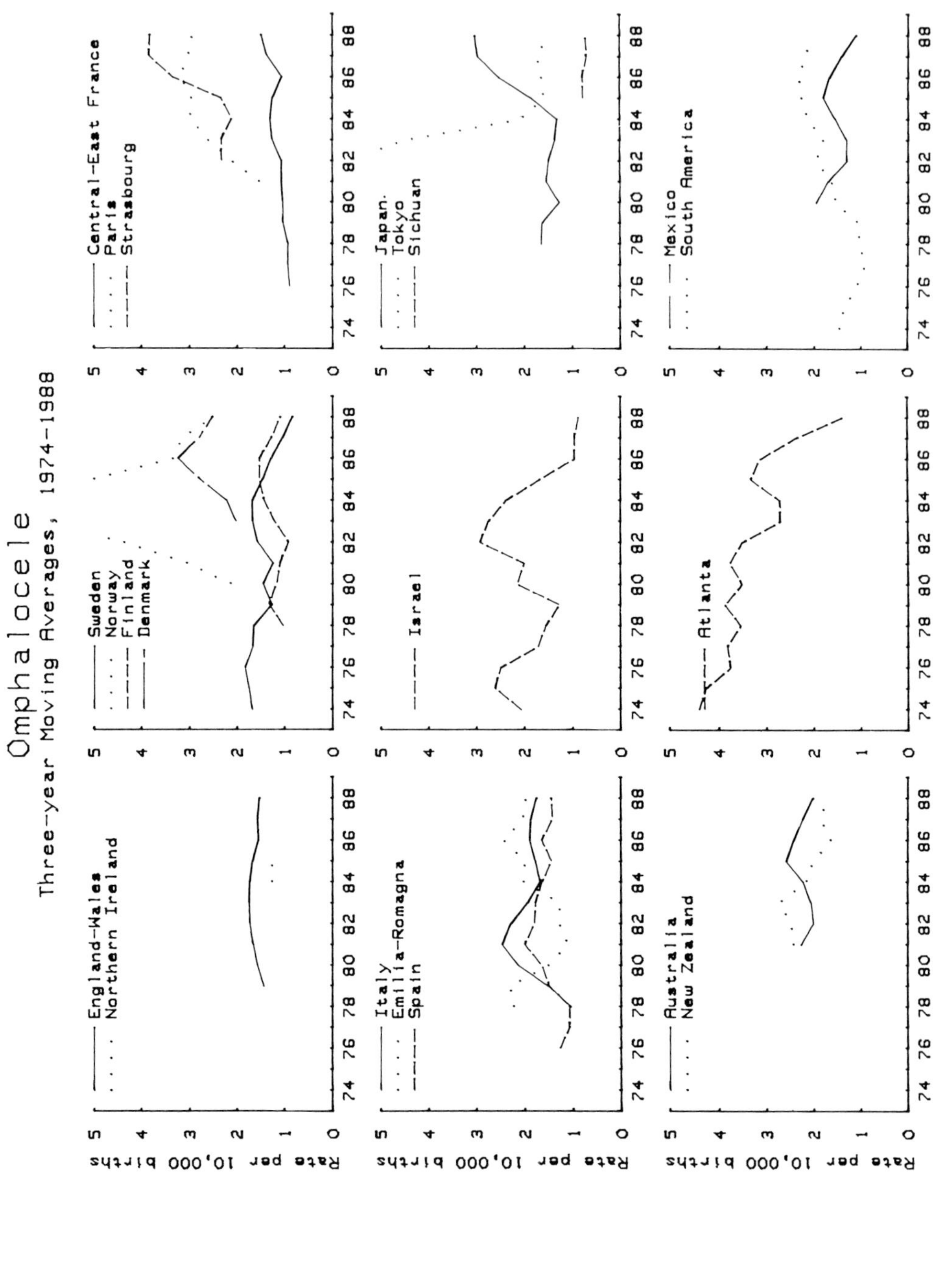
Omphalocele
Three-year Moving Averages, 1974-1988
England-Wales
Northern Ireland
Sweden
Norway
Finland
Denmark
Central-East France
Paris
Strasbourg
Italy
Emilia-Romagna
Spain
Israel
Japan
Tokyo
Sichuan
Australia
New Zealand
Atlanta
Mexico
South America
Rate per 10,000 births
74 76 78 80 82 84 86 88

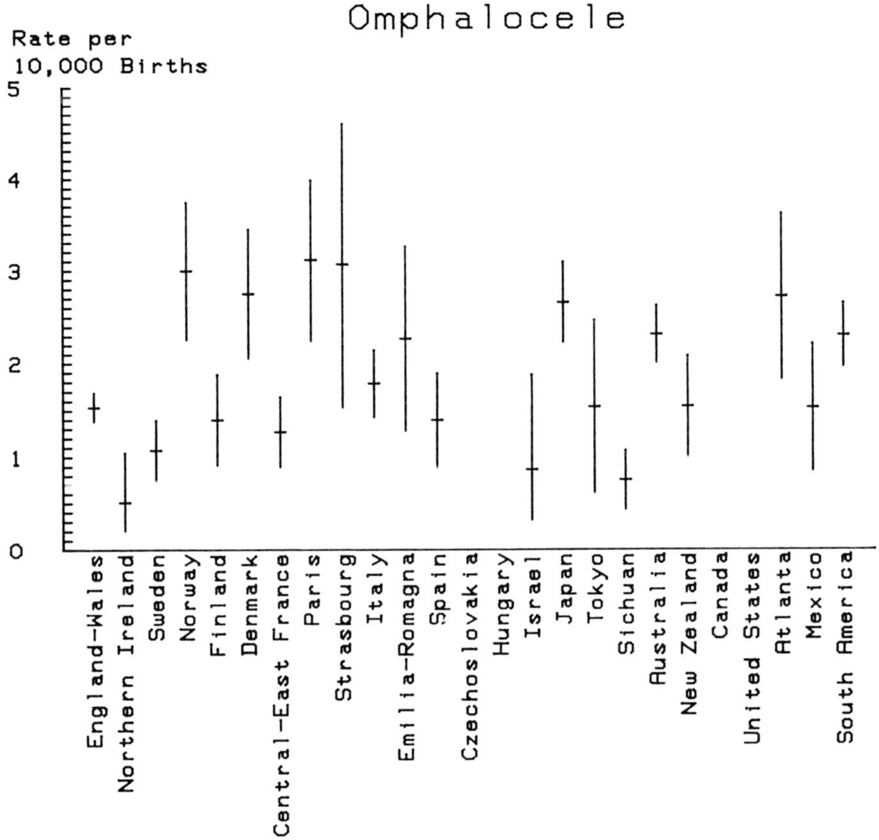

Diagram showing average rates of omphalocele in different programs for the years 1985-1988. Vertical lines indicate 95% confidence intervals of the recorded rates.

Comments

Not all programs have been able to report separately infants with omphalocele or gastroschisis. For those that did, omphalocele tends to follow the pattern of total abdominal wall defects, as omphaloceles make up the majority of the cases. However, in England-Wales the rate of omphalocele, while not unusually low, is only one-fourth of the rate of total abdominal wall defects.

Atlanta shows a marked decrease in omphalocele rates, especially notable during the last two years, without a corresponding decrease in the rates of total abdominal defects. In Tokyo the rate of total abdominal wall defects and of omphalocele both decrease during the observation period. The peak in abdominal wall defect in Norway, described above, is mirrored in the omphalocele rates. Increasing rates of omphaloceles are seen in some programs, including Paris, Strasbourg, Japan, and South America.

Gastroschisis

Definition: A congenital malformation (para-umbilical hernia) characterized by visceral herniation through an abdominal wall defect lateral to an intact umbilical cord.

A. Number of infants born with gastroschisis																
Monitoring program	1974	1975	1976	1977	1978	1979	1980	1981	1982	1983	1984	1985	1986	1987	1988	Total
Atlanta	2	1	3	5	6	7	4	4	7	8	3	5	7	2	16	80
Australia								12	23	17	23	20	22	35	35	187
Central-East France			7	4	1	4	4	7	5	7	8	8	4	7	12	78
Denmark										5	6	6	2	7	8	34
Emilia-Romagna					0	0	0	3	1	2	3	1	3	3	0	16
England-Wales						188	184	166	162	168	122	126	125	134	147	1522
Finland											6	4	3	1	3	17
Israel					0	0	0	1	0	1	2	3	1	1	0	9
Italy					1	2	4	4	5	5	9	7	5	7	4	53
Japan					16	11	15	9	13	9	10	14	21	14	15	147
Mexico							5	6	5	8	1	2	4	4	9	44
New Zealand								0	0	0	1	6	2	2	6	17
Northern Ireland											1	2				3
Norway	6	8	9	5	5	5	7	3	7	4	10	3	2	8	14	96
Paris									4	2	7	9	4	8	2	36
Sichuan												10	16	10	15	51
South America	1	0	0	0	1	2	0	7	8	4	11	13	20	20	11	98
Spain			0	0	0	2	3	7	5	3	4	2	2	6	3	37
Strasbourg									0	1	1	5	1	4	2	14
Sweden	11	10	11	9	8	6	8	7	5	6	7	7	6	2	4	107
Tokyo							1	0	0	0	2	1	4	2	1	11

B. Rate per 10,000 infants.

Monitoring program	1974	1975	1976	1977	1978	1979	1980	1981	1982	1983	1984	1985	1986	1987	1988	Average
Atlanta	0.8	0.4	1.3	2.1	2.5	2.7	1.5	1.5	2.5	2.9	1.0	1.6	2.1	0.6	4.4	1.9
Australia								1.1	1.0	0.7	1.0	0.8	0.9	1.4	1.4	1.0
Central-East France			1.1	0.6	0.1	0.6	0.5	0.9	0.7	0.8	0.9	0.9	0.4	0.8	1.3	0.8
Denmark										1.0	1.2	1.1	0.4	1.2	1.4	1.0
Emilia-Romagna					0	0	0	2.1	0.5	0.9	1.3	0.4	1.3	1.3	0	0.8
England-Wales						2.9	2.8	2.6	2.6	2.7	1.9	1.9	1.9	2.0	2.1	2.3
Finland											0.9	0.6	0.5	0.2	0.5	0.6
Israel					0	0	0	0.5	0	0.5	1.1	1.7	0.6	0.6	0	0.5
Italy					0.2	0.3	0.5	0.4	0.4	0.4	0.7	0.5	0.4	0.5	0.3	0.4
Japan						0.7	1.0	0.6	1.1	0.7	0.8	1.1	1.3	1.0	1.1	1.1
Mexico							1.2	1.7	1.4	2.1	0.3	0.8	1.6	1.0	2.2	1.4
New Zealand								0	0	0	0.2	1.2	0.4	0.4	1.1	0.6
Northern Ireland											0.4	0.7				0.5
Norway	1.0	1.4	1.7	1.0	1.0	1.0	1.4	0.6	1.4	0.8	2.0	0.6	0.4	1.5	2.4	1.2
Paris								0	1.0	0.5	1.8	2.2	1.0	2.0	0.5	1.1
Sichuan												1.6	2.0	1.2	2.3	1.7
South America	0.1	0	0	0	0.1	0.3	0	1.3	0.6	0.3	0.6	0.7	0.9	1.0	0.6	0.5
Spain			0	0	0	0.3	0.5	1.2	0.8	0.4	0.6	0.3	0.3	1.2	0.6	0.5
Strasbourg									0	0.8	0.8	3.9	0.8	3.1	1.5	1.5
Sweden	1.0	1.0	1.1	0.9	0.9	0.6	0.8	0.7	0.5	0.7	0.7	0.7	0.6	0.2	0.4	0.7
Tokyo							0.5	0	0	0	1.0	0.5	2.2	1.1	0.6	0.7

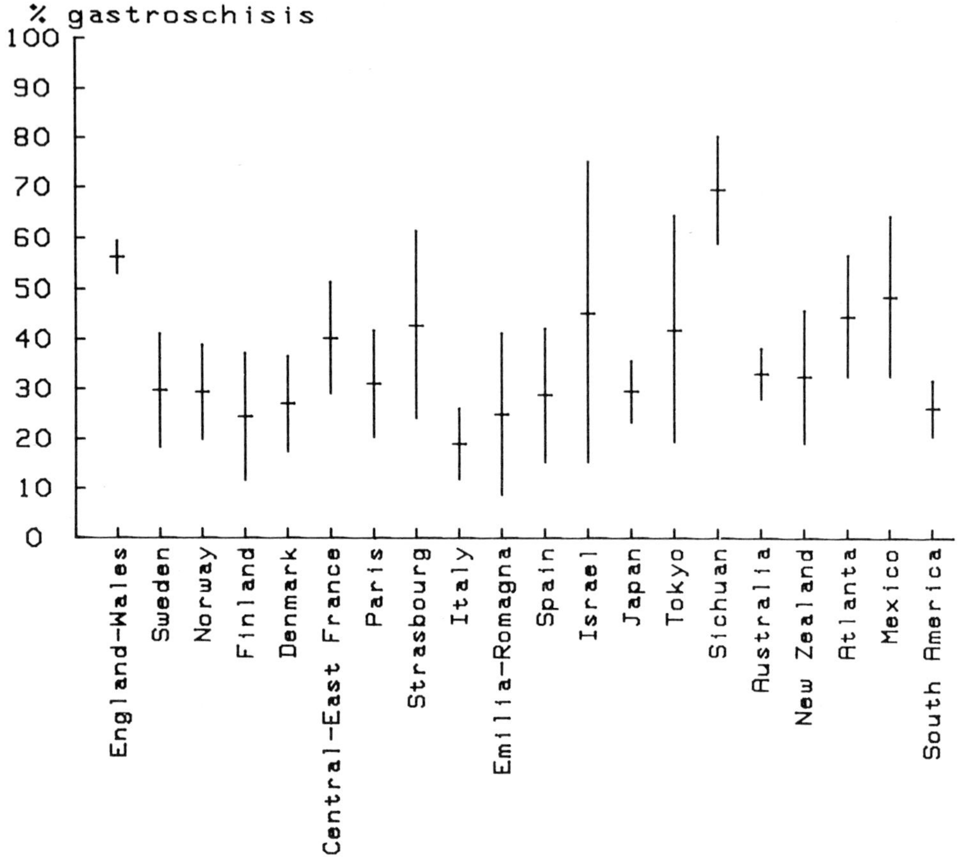

Diagram showing the percentage of gastroschisis among the sum of omphaloceles and gastroschisis in programs that have reported both types. Based on data for 1985-1988. Proportions are given with 95% confidence intervals marked as vertical bars.

Comments

Most programs report about 30% of these malformations as gastroschisis. Two programs (England-Wales and Sichuan) have markedly higher proportions. Some of the variations can be explained by different maternal age distributions, as gastroschisis is associated with a low maternal age and omphalocele with a high maternal age; however, this can explain only part of the difference.

Gastroschisis

Three-year Moving Averages, 1974-1988

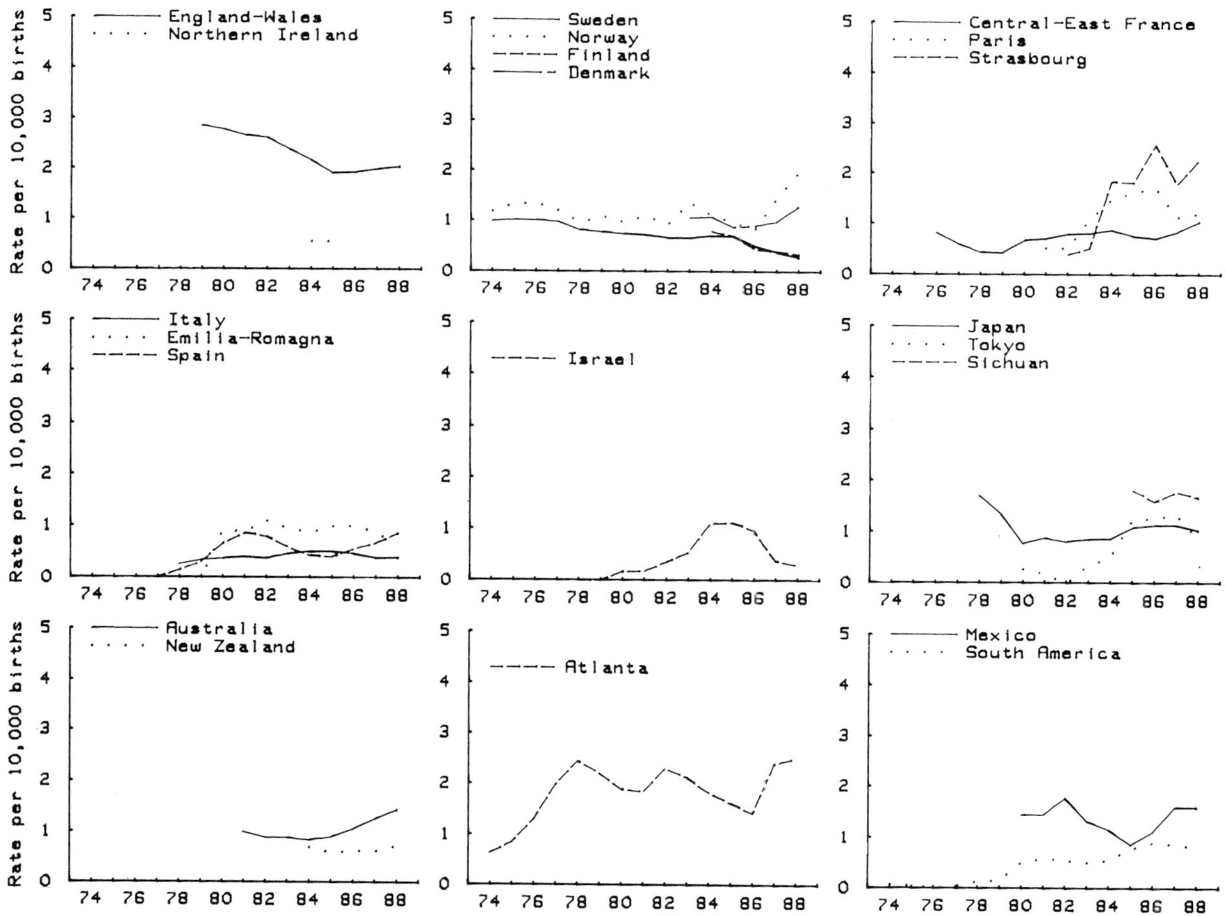

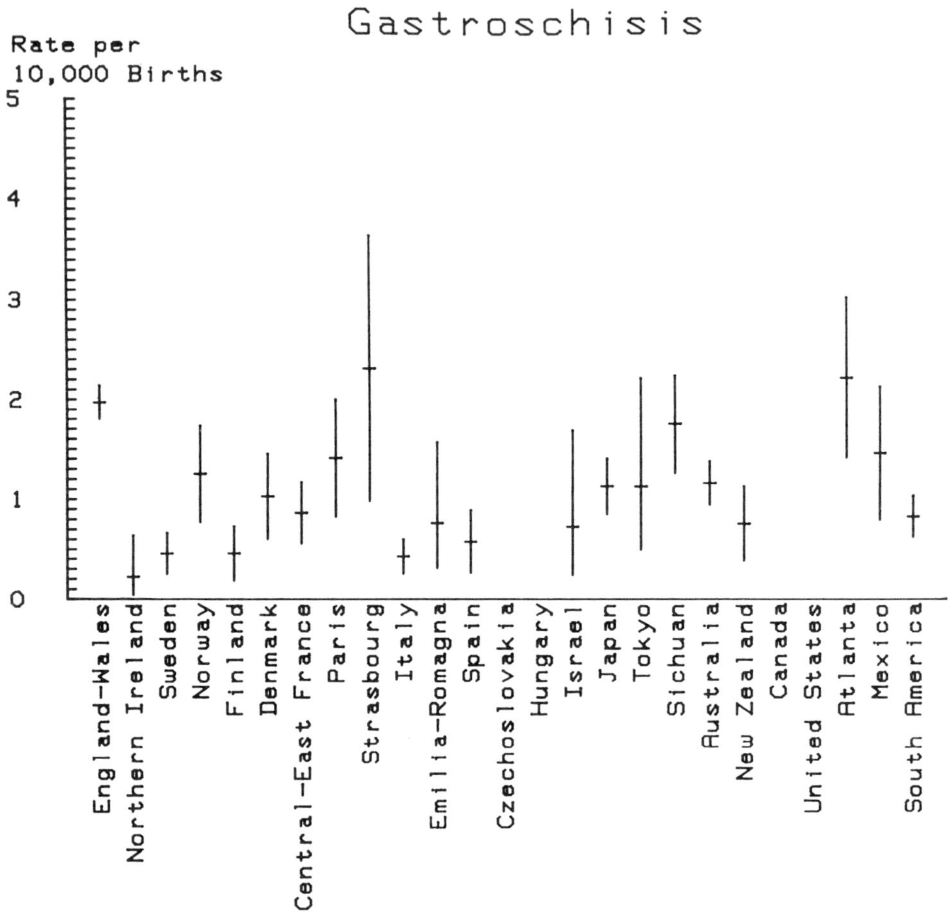

Diagram showing average rates of gastroschisis in different programs for the years 1985-1988. Vertical lines indicate 95% confidence intervals of the recorded rates.

Comments

England-Wales, Strasbourg, and Atlanta show average rates of gastroschisis somewhat higher than the other programs. Increasing rates are also seen elsewhere, e.g., the French programs, Emilia-Romagna, Spain, Israel, Tokyo, Australia, and South America. Such increasing trends of gastroschisis have been described in other populations around the world and are probably not artifacts.

Conjoined twins

This phenomenon arises during the process of monozygotic twinning. The two bodies formed from the same inner embryonic cell mass of the blastula do not separate completely, or a partial doubling of the head process from the primitive streak causes a partial doubling of the body. Many different forms are present. In one group one of the twins is rudimentary and is attached to its co-twin as a parasitic twin. In other forms a relatively normal body has two heads (dicephalus). The most common type consists of twins joined in the thoracic area (thoracopagus). In association with the abnormal area of fusion, malformations are regularly seen, e.g., heart malformations in thoracopagus twins, or anencephalus in dicephalus. Malformations are also common in areas other than the site of fusion. There is an excess of females.

If the twins survive delivery, surgical separation can be contemplated; its success depends on the degree of fusion and the presence of life-threatening malformations.

No heredity exists for conjoined twinning and no exogenous cause has been identified.

Prenatal diagnosis with ultrasound can be made and elective abortion can be carried out.

Conjoined twins

Definition: A congenital malformation characterized by the non-separation of a pair of monozygotic twins. Parasitic twins are not counted.

A. Number of infants conjoined twins

Monitoring program	1974	1975	1976	1977	1978	1979	1980	1981	1982	1983	1984	1985	1986	1987	1988	Total
Atlanta	0	0	2	0	0	0	0	0	0	1	0	0	1	2	0	6
Australia								0	1	6	2	3	3	4	2	21
Canada	9	4	8	6	5	4	3	1	3	3	3	5	7	1	3	65
Central-East France			0	0	1	0	0	1	1	0	0	1	1	0	2	7
Czechoslovakia	2	2	1	2	2	5	5	1	0	4	2	3	1	3	2	35
Denmark										2	1	0	0	1	0	4
Emilia-Romagna					0	0	1	0	0	0	1	0	0	0	1	3
England-Wales	9	6	4	5	6	5	5	5	6	3	4	2	1	1	0	62
Hungary	1	1	3	3	4	3	1	4	4	2	1	0	3	0	0	30
Italy					1	0	0	0	5	1	3	1	3	0	3	17
Japan					1	0	3	1	6	12	5	2	3	7	6	46
Mexico							0	0	0	1	1	2	0	1	1	6
New Zealand									1	2	0	1	0	0	0	4
Norway	0	1	0	1	0	0	0	1	0	2	1	0	0	0	2	8
Paris								0	0	1	0	1	2	0	0	4
Sichuan															1	1
South America	2	0	1	0	3	1	0	0	2	5	4	2	2	0	4	26
Spain			0	0	1	0	0	1	2	1	2	0	0	1	4	12
Strasbourg									0	0	0	0	0	0	0	0
Sweden	0	1	1	0	0	0	1	0	1	1	0	0	1	2	0	8
Tokyo							0	0	0	0	0	0	0	0	1	1
United States	20	18	31	25	17	28	12	15	12	5	13	13	5	8	1	223

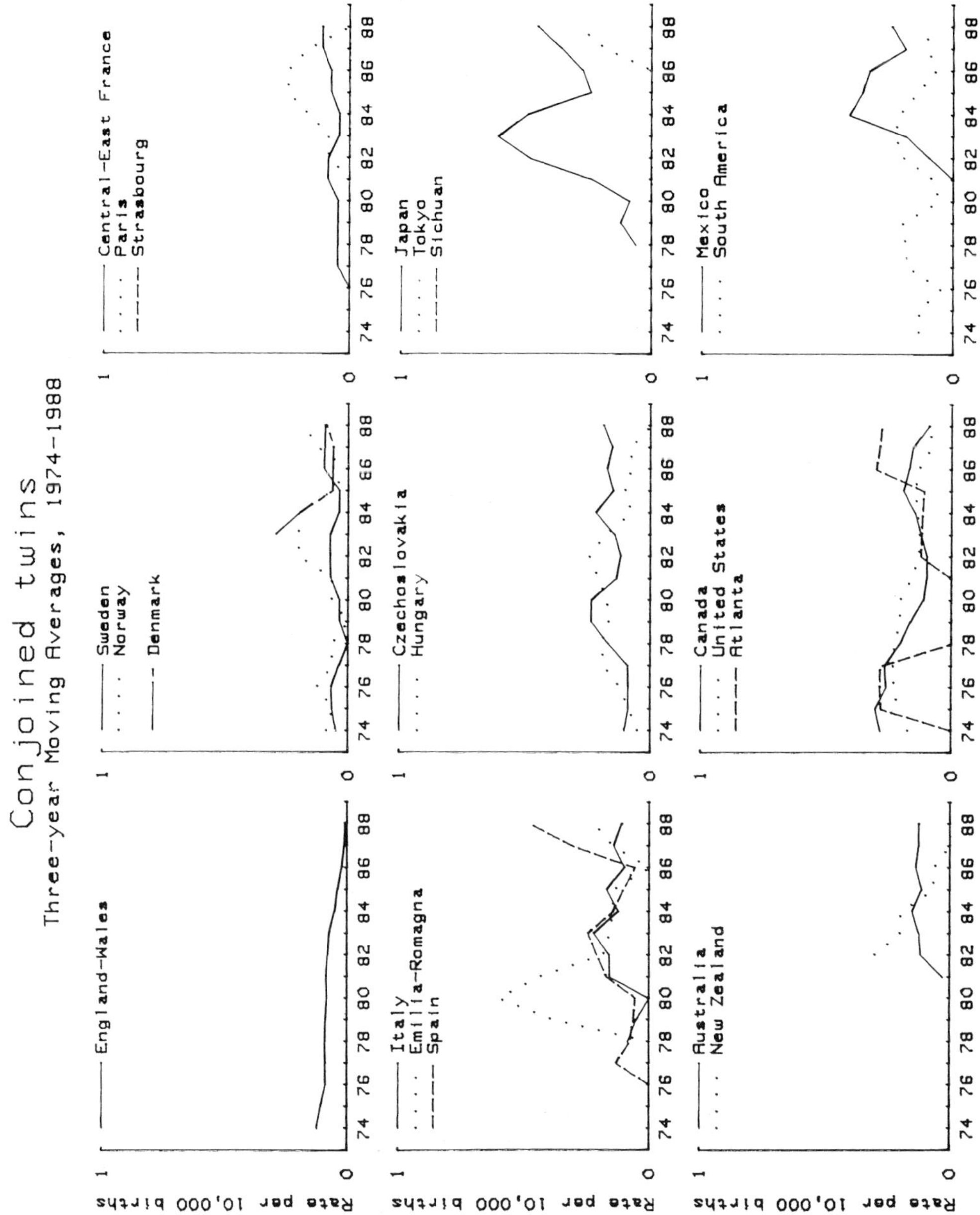
Conjoined twins
Three-year Moving Averages, 1974-1988
Rate per 10,000 births
England-Wales
Sweden
Norway
Denmark
Central-East France
Paris
Strasbourg
Italy
Emilia-Romagna
Spain
Czechoslovakia
Hungary
Japan
Tokyo
Sichuan
Australia
New Zealand
Canada
United States
Atlanta
Mexico
South America
74 76 78 80 82 84 86 88
0
1

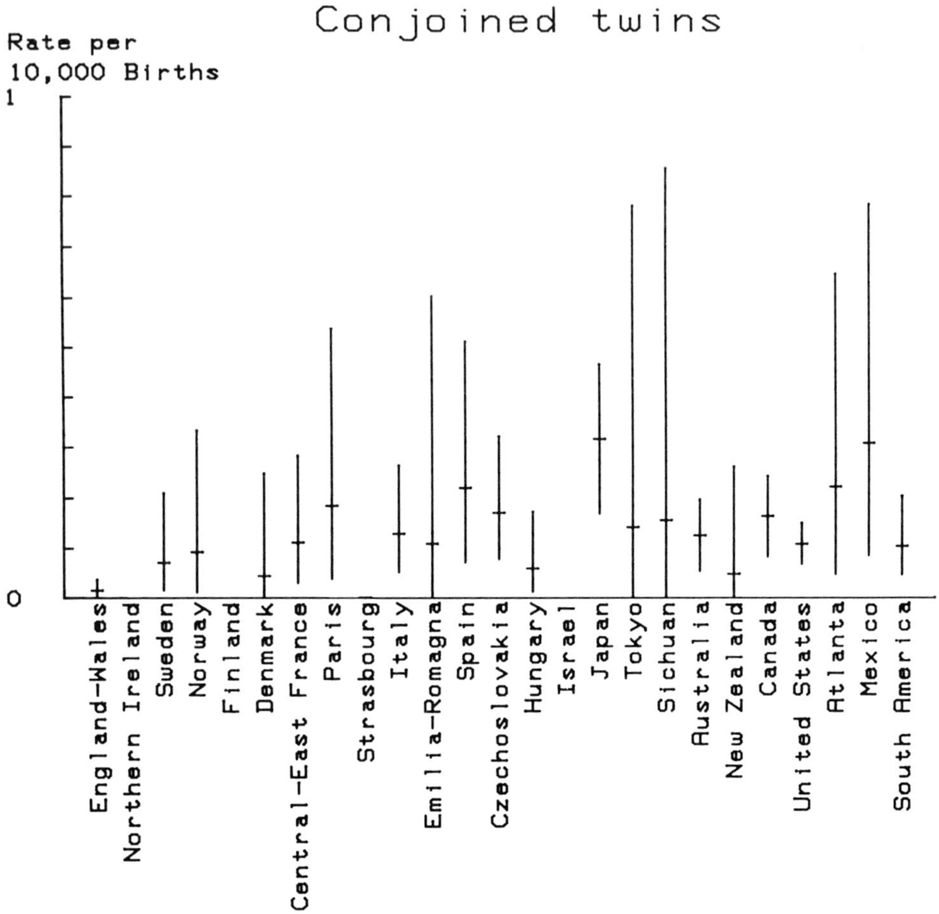

Diagram showing average rates of conjoined twins in different programs for the years 1985-1988. Vertical lines indicate 95% confidence intervals of the recorded rates.

Comments

This is an extremely rare malformation with a rate of 0.1-0.2 per 10,000 births. The only exception is Japan with a somewhat higher rate.

Down syndrome

Down syndrome is caused by an excess of chromosome 21 material, usually as a trisomy 21. The extra chromosome material causes disturbances of development that result in a physical appearance that usually makes the diagnosis simple immediately after birth, an increased risk for various types of malformations, mental retardation, increased sensitivity to infections, increased rate of leukemia, premature aging and death. Among typical dysmorphic features can be mentioned small round head, flat face, large tongue, abundant neck skin, oblique palpebral fissures, epicanthic folds, simian lines, white iris spots. Cardiac malformations (notably endocardial cushion defects) are very common. Other common congenital malformations are duodenal atresia and megacolon.

The typical risk factor for Down syndrome is high maternal age, and the importance of paternal age has also been discussed - some of the trisomies are of paternal origin. A small percentage are caused by chromosomal translocation, about half of which are inherited, and a few have chromosomal mosaicism. The recurrence risk at parental translocation may be considerable; at ordinary trisomy a slight recurrence risk exists independent of the maternal age-specific risk. Nothing is known about possible exogenous causes of the non-disjunction process underlying Down syndrome.

Major malformations can be treated with surgery. Mental development can be increased by adequate care, but normality is never reached.

Prenatal diagnosis can be made but is usually restricted to women of higher age (e.g., above 35 or 37). Ultrasound findings and alphafetoprotein screening may help to identify Down fetuses.

Down syndrome

Definition: A generalized malformation syndrome characterized by a well-known pattern of minor and major anomalies and associated with an excess of chromosome 21 material.

A. Number of infants born with Down syndrome

Monitoring program	1974	1975	1976	1977	1978	1979	1980	1981	1982	1983	1984	1985	1986	1987	1988	Total
Atlanta	27	22	18	16	17	27	32	36	27	32	26	30	31	30	36	407
Australia								111	265	269	240	292	327	288	304	2096
Canada	207	176	177	187	263	274	264	237	269	331	324	347	352	325	296	4029
Central-East France			91	99	96	62	98	76	93	87	102	101	97	113	95	1210
Czechoslovakia	137	145	150	130	130	140	146	113	121	106	126	91	107	124	102	1868
Denmark												41	44	43	46	174
Emilia-Romagna					15	14	17	22	26	20	35	34	26	24	37	270
England-Wales	408	452	394	418	438	458	481	475	527	497	505	442	445	459	428	6827
Finland	27	39	37	47	42	38	60	56	55	65	55	57	69	53	48	748
Hungary	175	167	174	174	154	131	147	128	124	97	78	109	95	102	92	1947
Israel	8	11	11	10	18	19	12	19	14	21	22	24	27	21	18	255
Italy					78	92	127	145	164	470	141	162	187	177	173	1616
Japan					26	59	89	59	71	64	47	62	102	75	79	733
Mexico							61	47	46	36	46	21	39	54	56	406
New Zealand							37	47	32	44	56	54	47	44	54	415
Northern Ireland							0	41	39	40	42	43				205
Norway	68	57	41	47	47	61	50	57	51	48	43	70	69	52	63	824
Paris								45	58	55	54	45	50	42	56	405
South America	104	105	102	114	105	111	81	86	213	223	253	288	274	310	298	2667
Spain			22	45	62	103	78	87	93	95	102	110	91	76	87	1051
Strasbourg									14	10	14	17	14	19	25	113
Sweden	150	133	126	113	101	126	137	129	116	130	115	132	135	141	126	1910
Tokyo							18	14	28	13	18	21	19	19	18	168
United States	874	921	778	819	791	805	568	656	652	667	575	701	682	542	495	10526

B. Rate per 10,000 infants.

Monitoring program	1974	1975	1976	1977	1978	1979	1980	1981	1982	1983	1984	1985	1986	1987	1988	Average
Atlanta	10.9	9.6	7.9	6.8	7.0	10.6	11.7	13.4	9.7	11.5	8.9	9.7	9.5	8.5	9.8	9.7
Australia								9.8	11.1	11.2	10.1	12.1	13.5	11.9	12.4	11.7
Canada	9.2	7.6	7.8	8.1	10.6	10.9	11.0	9.8	10.6	13.6	12.9	13.2	13.4	13.1	13.8	11.1
Central-East France			13.7	14.4	14.0	8.8	13.1	9.9	12.4	10.1	11.8	11.2	10.6	12.6	10.4	11.7
Czechoslovakia	7.1	7.6	8.0	7.2	7.3	8.1	9.5	7.8	8.5	7.7	9.2	6.7	8.0	9.5	7.7	7.9
Denmark												7.6	7.9	7.6	7.8	7.7
Emilia-Romagna					21.3	22.0	13.6	15.4	14.2	9.2	15.1	14.2	11.4	10.6	16.2	13.8
England-Wales	6.3	7.4	6.7	7.3	7.3	7.1	7.3	7.4	8.4	7.9	7.9	6.7	6.7	6.7	6.1	7.1
Finland	4.3	6.0	5.6	7.2	6.6	6.0	9.5	8.8	8.3	9.7	8.5	9.1	11.4	8.9	8.0	7.8
Hungary	9.3	8.5	9.3	9.7	9.1	8.1	9.8	8.9	9.2	7.6	6.2	8.3	7.4	8.0	7.4	8.6
Israel	11.4	14.8	13.0	12.3	9.8	10.1	6.5	10.4	7.8	11.5	12.1	13.5	15.4	12.6	10.3	11.1
Italy					17.7	12.8	15.4	13.5	13.0	12.2	10.3	12.4	13.2	12.9	12.5	12.9
Japan						3.7	5.7	4.2	5.8	5.1	3.7	4.8	6.5	5.2	5.7	5.2
Mexico							14.6	13.6	13.3	9.4	13.7	8.7	15.8	13.3	13.7	13.0
New Zealand							8.0	9.4	6.6	8.7	11.2	10.5	9.0	8.1	9.8	9.1
Northern Ireland							0	14.9	14.3	14.6	15.1	15.5				12.3
Norway	11.3	10.0	7.6	9.1	9.0	11.7	9.7	11.2	9.9	9.5	8.5	13.6	13.1	9.6	10.9	10.3
Paris								11.5	14.9	13.8	13.5	11.0	12.3	10.4	13.5	12.6
South America	12.2	16.1	13.1	16.9	14.4	16.0	14.6	15.4	14.8	14.5	14.9	15.8	13.0	15.9	15.8	14.9
Spain			18.0	16.4	17.4	15.0	13.7	15.5	15.2	13.2	14.7	16.5	15.6	14.9	16.5	15.3
Strasbourg									10.3	8.0	11.0	13.1	10.9	14.7	18.7	12.5
Sweden	13.6	12.8	12.7	11.7	10.8	13.0	14.1	13.7	12.5	14.1	12.2	13.4	13.2	13.4	11.2	12.8
Tokyo							9.5	7.7	14.6	6.9	9.2	11.0	10.4	10.8	11.0	10.1
United States	8.1	8.6	7.4	7.6	8.1	7.8	7.4	7.6	7.9	8.2	7.7	9.7	10.0	9.0	9.7	8.2

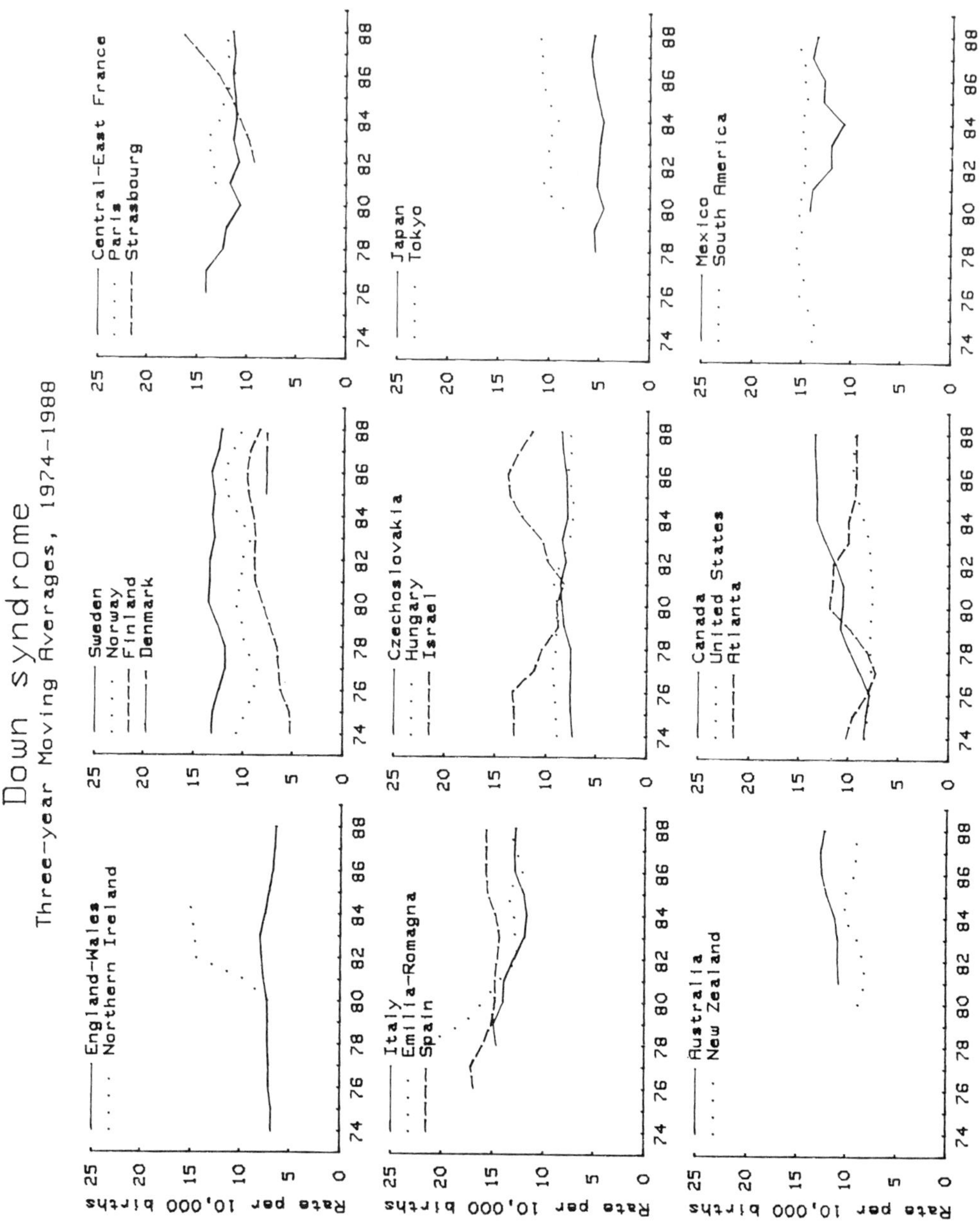
Down syndrome
Three-year Moving Averages, 1974-1988
Rate per 10,000 births
England-Wales
Northern Ireland
Sweden
Norway
Finland
Denmark
Central-East France
Paris
Strasbourg
Italy
Emilia-Romagna
Spain
Czechoslovakia
Hungary
Israel
Japan
Tokyo
Australia
New Zealand
Canada
United States
Atlanta
Mexico
South America
74 76 78 80 82 84 86 88
0 5 10 15 20 25

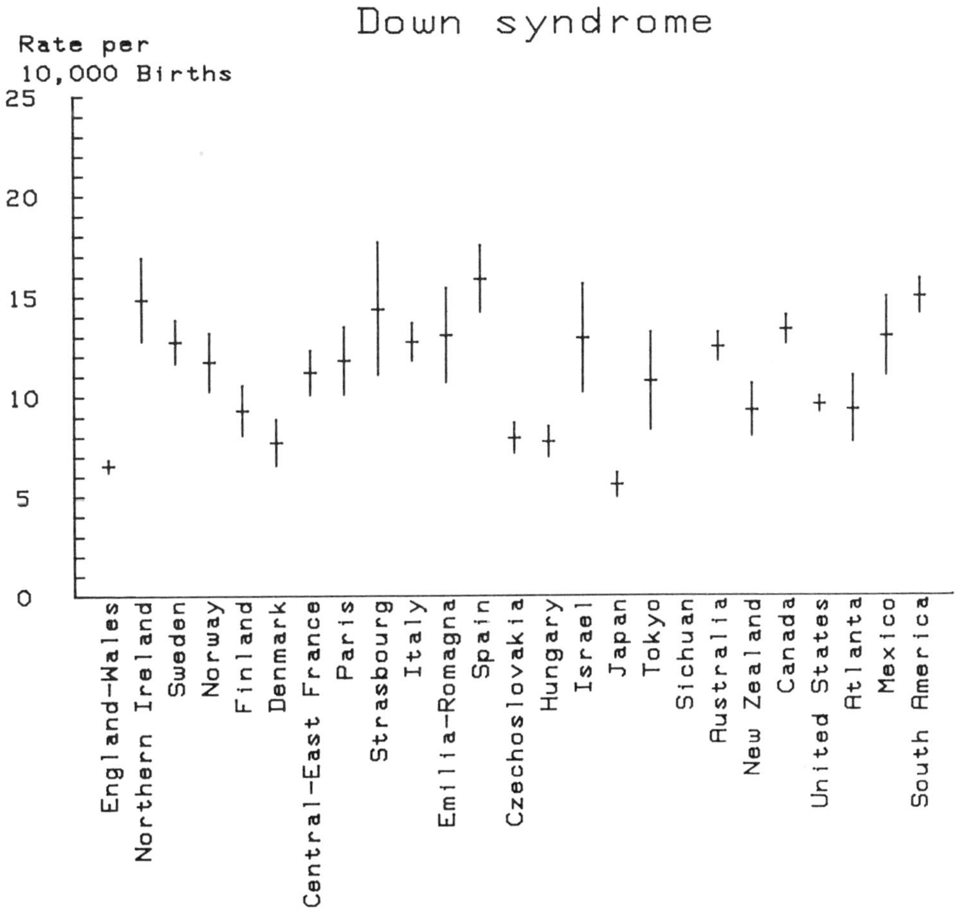

Diagram showing average rates of Down syndrome in different programs for the years 1985-1988. Vertical lines indicate 95% confidence intervals of the recorded rates.

Comments

The rate of Down syndrome in a population is affected by the maternal age distribution and by prenatal diagnosis followed by elective abortion. The recorded rate is also influenced by ascertainment.

The crude rates during 1985-1988 in the various programs center around 13 per 10,000, but the variation is relatively large.

Increasing crude rates are seen in Finland, Strasbourg, and Canada, and decreasing rates in Central-East France and the two Italian programs.

Maternal age-specific rates of Down syndrome, 1981–1988
(logarithmic scale)

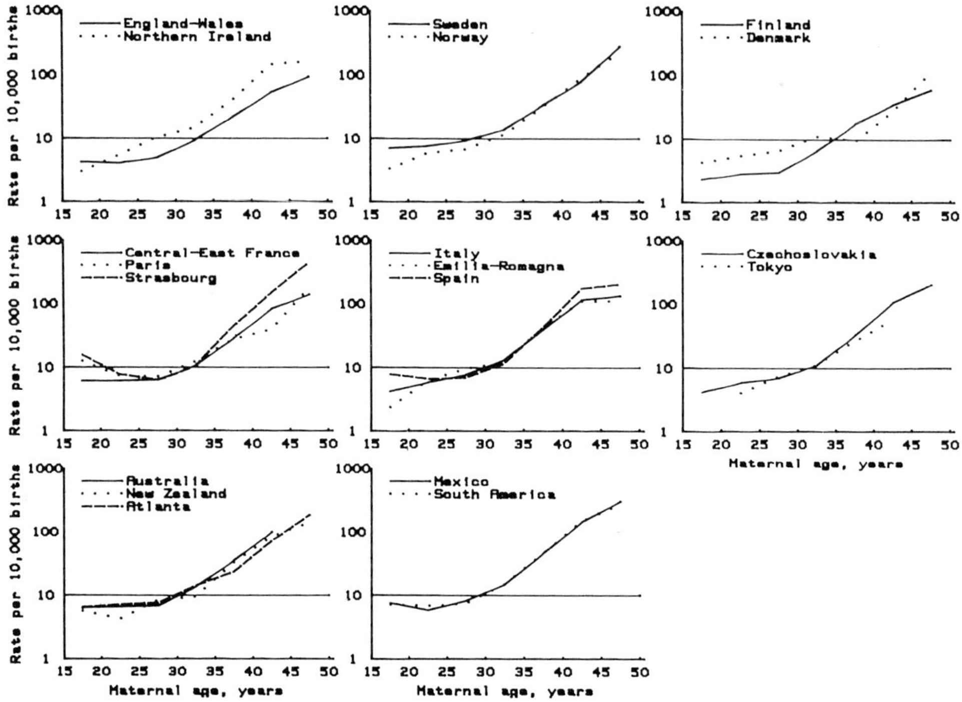

The maternal age-specific rates in the different programs are by and large similar. The low age-specific rate in Finland for young women suggests incomplete ascertainment.

One interesting feature is the slightly increased rate in teenagers seen in Paris and Strasbourg and suggested in Spain, Mexico, and New Zealand. Such a phenomenon has repeatedly been described in the literature. In the majority of programs, no indication is seen of an increased risk for teenage mothers to have a Down infant.

One would expect that intense prenatal diagnosis followed by selective abortion should lower the rate at high maternal age. Some weak indication of this can be seen in the deflection of many graphs at the highest age class.

Chapter V

Two approaches to malformation monitoring: The statistical and the teratological

Since before the first meeting of the *Clearinghouse* in Helsinki in 1974, two opposing philosophies of malformation monitoring have been extant. One stresses the detection of outbreaks or clusters through statistical-epidemiological methods. The foremost proponents for this view are usually found in governmental programs run by health statisticians. The other stresses the importance of clinical details in the search for unusual events - either rare malformations or combinations of malformations - that may indicate the introduction of a new teratogen. Proponents for the latter view are often found in programs run by people with a clinical or research background. The two groups have often had difficulties in communication; the concepts and terms used by one group are often not understood by the other. Perhaps they speak different languages. While one group talks about the best ways to detect spatial or temporal changes in coded data and debates about the advantages and disadvantages of various statistical methods for such a detection, the other group talks about the recognition and classification of specific defects, such as different types of limb reductions or different types of chondrodystrophies.

Let us examine these two approaches to monitoring and see if a reconciliation is possible.

The statistical approach

To monitor malformations the number of observed infants with a specific type of birth defect born during a specified time period is compared with the number of infants expected to be born during that period had no changes in the rate occurred. A difference between the observed and the expected numbers can have many explanations. One is that a real change in rate has occurred, perhaps, but not necessarily, caused by the introduction of a teratogenic agent in the community. Another is that the expected number has been wrongly estimated. A change in the ascertainment can, for instance, result in a difference between the observed and the expected numbers which does not reveal a true change in rate, only a change in the efficiency of detecting and registering the malformed infants. A third explanation of a difference is that the number of infants born with a specific malformation randomly fluctuates over time and just by chance an unusually high (or low) number may have occurred during the period under study. In this approach to malformation monitoring statistical methods are applied to try to detect changes in rates and to sort out those that can be explained by random variations from those that cannot.

Estimating the expected numbers of specific malformations is a crucial point in the monitoring process. The estimates are usually made from "baselines", or data accumulated in the registry, under the assumption that the rates that occurred in the past are the usual rates of occurrence. The baseline rate is then applied to the number of births occurring during the current period of observation. If a baseline rate is derived from relatively few occurrences, its own statistical error will not be negligible, so the baseline may have to be accumulated over a long time. This, however, presents the risk that the estimate is no longer applicable, either because of actual long-term changes in the rate or, more likely, because of changed ascertainment in the system. Changes in ascertainment often do occur – as a result of changing diagnostic routines in the reporting hospitals, changes in the efficiency of the reporting process, or changes in the central handling of the reports. This uncertainty often overrides the importance of taking various confounding factors – like maternal age distribution or seasonality – into consideration when estimating the expected numbers of a malformation.

Often the observed number of malformed infants born in a defined period of time is evaluated by using a very simple statistic: the ratio of the observed to the expected number. This technique assumes that the observed number follows a Poisson distribution and the expected number is fixed without its own error. This is a simple and adequate model to give a momentary picture of the situation, but it does not take into consideration the possibility that previous time periods may have shown similar trends without reaching "statistical significance".

Other and more complicated statistical methods have been applied in order to take into account previous time periods. One method applies techniques originally worked out for industrial quality control. In this model the birth of a malformed infant is regarded as equivalent to a mistake in an industrial production line where a certain number of mistakes are allowed, but if the rate of mistakes increases over a certain level an alarm is given. This approach is exemplified by the so-called CUSUM method and its modifications. This is a sequential method because it takes into consideration both the current and the previous observations. An alternative method is the so-called set technique, which argues that by observing the number of consecutive non-malformed infants born between the birth of two malformed infants (a "set"), a change in the rate of the malformation can be detected. A series of short "sets" indicates that the rate has increased.

Whatever technique is used, the calculations of probability assume the occurrence of only one type of aberration, as in the industrial surveillance process which distinguishes an acceptable product from a faulty one and where any fault in the production has the same significance. To apply this method to malformed infants requires the assumption that all types of malformations are equivalent. This, however, is not a realistic assumption. It is more realistic to assume that if an increase occurs it will occur in one specific type of malformation only. The surveillance procedure must therefore be applied individually to a number of different conditions (malformations) and the probability that one of them will randomly show a deviation at the decided level of significance therefore increases. One can easily compensate by correcting for the number of conditions monitored, but this supposes that a fixed and limited number of conditions - a set of "standard" malformations - is monitored, and the methods can only detect changes in those particular conditions.

The teratological approach

It can be argued that according to present experience most detected human teratogens have caused unusual malformations or combinations of malformations ("syndromes") and that if a new human teratogen appears it may well be expected to behave in a similar way. From this point of view it is important to observe and monitor all types of malformations and combinations of malformations (putative "syndromes") and not to restrict the monitoring process to a fixed number of common conditions that offer themselves to the methods briefly discussed above.

Another argument for this view is that only a small part of the pregnant population is likely to be exposed to a newly introduced teratogen. If the new teratogen causes one of the common malformations (cleft lip, for example) its teratogenic potential must be very high for its effect to be noticed among all the usually occurring malformations of that type. If, on the other hand, the result of the teratogenic exposure is a previously rare condition, the probability of detecting it is much larger. This situation, however, requires that the malformed infants be reported with a degree of detail sufficient to permit identification of an unusual malformation. On the other hand, no formal baseline will be necessary, as the experienced teratologist is on the lookout for phenomena which he more or less intuitively knows should not appear in more than a very few infants. Using an example from the era of thalidomide, the appearance of a cluster of infants with amelia or phocomelia should attract attention, even without knowledge of the exact incidence of these conditions and even if the computer has not been programmed to track them.

Mere codes or even brief diagnoses usually do not provide enough information about the physical appearance of the malformed infants. Detailed descriptions are needed, which requires a dialogue between the monitoring center and the reporting hospitals; if information is incomplete or unspecific, further data must be obtained. A dialogue between the hospital clinicians and the monitoring center may also facilitate the reporting of observed associations between exposures and malformations, which is another way that new teratogens might be detected.

From the teratologist's standpoint, the most important component of monitoring is not the statistical analysis of coded data, but rather the ongoing scrutiny of the population of newborn infants in the search for unusual events. This is best done by consistent handling of the reported data by a teratologically trained person who is able to distinguish between cases that are trivial and can easily be taken care of and the more important ones that may be signals that something is going wrong. The judgment involved in making such distinctions is critical, and the task should not be handed over to a clerical or secretarial staff even if it means that someone with a medical degree has to engage in some tedious routine work.

On the other hand, the teratologist must have sufficient interest in and understanding of statistical methodology to avoid the all too common mistakes of putting too much credence on observations based on too few "interesting" cases and failing to recognize the possibility that "exciting" findings can often be the effects of random fluctuations of small numbers.

Reconciling the differences

The two views expressed above might be thought of not as antagonistic forces but as two phases of a single entity in which the teratologist's version of monitoring detailed and immediate, though perhaps incomplete, information is supplemented by statistical analyses of more complete data in the attempt to describe long-term trends of common malformations and to detect possible "endemic" teratogens, i.e., factors that have been present in society for a long time and therefore do not result in changes in malformation rates. Most individual monitoring programs are restricted in one way or another from fulfilling both functions. It may be the role of the *Clearinghouse* to integrate these two aspects of monitoring.

Since the inception of malformation monitoring during the 1960s in different parts of the world, apparently only a very few teratogenic agents have been introduced into society that should have been detected by the monitoring systems. One such agent is the retinoic acid drugs, but they were already suspected to be teratogenic at their introduction, and pregnancy warnings were given.

If – or when – a new thalidomide-like agent appears in society, the moment of truth will come: Will a monitoring system detect it, and which one will do so first? Will it be a system based exclusively on computerized algorithms aiming at the detection of changes in rates in a number of preselected conditions, or will it be a teratologically inclined system where each reported infant's malformations are scrutinized in the search for unusual characteristics? Regardless of which one does it, it will be the task of the *Clearinghouse* to alert all of the other systems as quickly as possible in order to seek confirmation of the observation and to stop a threatening epidemic of birth defects.

Chapter VI

Multicenter studies: The problem of variability and the beauty of diversity

Multicenter studies are quite common in the fields of cancer and circulatory diseases, but they have been relatively infrequent in the field of birth defects. In recent years, however, the large data sets that have been accumulated by the programs in the *Clearinghouse* have provided source material for joint studies of the epidemiology and etiology of congenital malformations.

Identical protocols are usually employed by all the participants in a multicenter study in order to reduce variability and maximize uniformity of data collection. This basic principle has been followed in the multicenter studies of birth defects conducted in the EUROCAT[1] organization. The *Clearinghouse* works in a different way; it makes use of the already existing large sets of data that have been collected by its members, who are located throughout the world. When such data are to be used for common research, the problems associated with variability, briefly described in previous chapters, come into play. At the same time, the mere fact that data are collected in different ways sometimes gives an extra dimension to the research; a specific artifact may be less likely to be present in all the programs when there is diversity of data collection.

Variability between programs

The Introduction to Chapter IV pointed out some sources of variability in the data collected by different programs, notably as a warning against making hasty comparisons between the recorded rates of various malformations or conclusions about observed time trends.

In planning joint research projects, obviously one must take into consideration the variable nature of the participating programs. A majority of programs in the *Clearinghouse* concentrate on major malformations and give less importance to the recording of mild conditions, partly because of the great variability in their ascertainment when many reporting units are involved in the system. On the other hand, experience has taught that the effects of some human teratogens are

1. European Study of Congenital Anomalies and Twins

often best observed as an increased frequency of mild or clinically insignificant conditions. Examples are the fetal alcohol syndrome and the anticonvulsant syndrome. Studies based on such phenotypical anomalies must then be restricted to those programs that have an interest in recording mild conditions and the facilities for doing so. These are often relatively small programs and programs run by staff interested in dysmorphology.

Congenital heart defects provide another example of the usefulness of having data for research supplied by different monitoring programs. As a group, congenital heart defects are relatively common - about 0.7% of all infants are born with a more or less severe cardiac defect. However, only some of these infants receive a cardiac diagnosis during the newborn period, and still fewer get a specific diagnosis. Studies on the epidemiology and etiology of cardiac defects can therefore best be made in programs where neonatal data are supplemented with data obtained by following the children at least to the age of one. The same applies to other conditions that may not be observable at birth; one major such condition, now included in only a few programs, is mental retardation, the study of which needs a still longer follow-up period.

A few programs - most notably those in the Scandinavian countries - that are easily able to follow up newborn infants can also supply data on long-term survival by means of birth and death record linkage.

It is clear, then, that data for joint research on specific problems may not be available in all of the programs in the *Clearinghouse*. As briefly mentioned in a previous chapter, some programs routinely collect some exposure data for both malformed infants and controls, other programs collect it only for malformed infants, and still other do not routinely collect any exposure data. Even when routinely collected, the data may be biased by the severity and nature of the malformation or if no malformation at all exists (controls). Routine collection of exposure information is usually restricted to a number of specific questions, such as drug use, occupation, socioeconomic level, use of oral contraceptives, chronic diseases. Sufficient detail is often lacking; e.g., for occupation perhaps the term "factory worker" is used, which tells little about actual exposure. Nevertheless, data banks can often supply quick and general information on a suspected relationship, such as between a specific drug and a specific malformation. Information stored in the data banks of several monitoring programs proved useful when the Central-East France program alerted the *Clearinghouse* to its suspicion that an association existed between maternal use of valproic acid and infant spina bifida.

When more detailed exposure information is needed, some programs can go back to medical records or can contact the women who gave birth; programs without this capability have to rely on what has been routinely recorded. In some instances joint research projects have been specially designed to record exposure information for all infants born with a specific malformation and reported to the monitoring systems.

Programs that make use of general medical birth registries containing data on all births in the area monitored may be able to identify cohorts of women with certain characteristics or exposures and study birth defects present in their children. It is thus possible to make combined studies: one program tries to get information on a putative association between exposure and outcome by a case-control method, while another tries to make the study from an exposed cohort.

General medical birth registries are also useful for supplying background information, making it easy to perform epidemiological studies, such as age-parity-specific rates of a certain malformation. Programs with rather scanty background information are hampered in their efforts. Some programs that rely on comparisons between data on the cases and routinely collected controls may not have background information available to them. Therefore, not all program can participate in even relatively simple epidemiological studies.

All these sources of variation - and others - have to be taken into consideration when cooperative studies are to be planned within the *Clearinghouse*.

The beauty of diversity

After having listed so many sources of variation and problems related to data collection, one might ask whether it is worthwhile even to attempt joint studies on birth defect epidemiology with data drawn from such divergent sources. This can be debated, but experience has taught that sometimes the diversity itself has value.

Most etiological studies of birth defects are based on the demonstration of a statistical association between a specific exposure and one or more types of birth defects. In interpreting such associations, the question of causality is often placed in doubt by the presence of confounders. Drugs are nearly always administered because of a disease or a complaint, which, if causally related to a birth defect, can result in a spurious association between the drug and the birth defect. In studies of occupational exposures a strong confounding effect is sometimes seen with socio-economic factors that are related to occupation. When such associations are very strong, it may be difficult to separate direct from indirect effects of drug or occupational exposures. Studies using diverse populations may then help. If a specific disease is treated with different drugs in different parts of the world, there may be an opportunity to dissociate the effects of drug and disease. Similarly, actual exposures within the same occupation may differ widely between populations.

Another interesting aspect of diversity can be found in the different reproductive patterns of different populations. Some birth defects have been associated with parental subfertility, and the impact of this factor will vary with reproductive pattern. In populations with a low reproductive rate because of voluntary restriction of childbearing, the fraction of subfertile couples will be proportionally larger than in other populations. Access to fetal diagnosis and legislation concerning induced abortions also differ between populations and are factors that may help in the analysis of possible effects of contraceptive measures on fetal development.

Little use has so far been made of the diversity among the populations in the causal analysis of environmental factors and birth defects. This area may be a comparatively untapped source of valuable information.

Chapter VII
Joint scientific studies performed in the Clearinghouse

This Chapter will briefly describe some of the joint scientific studies performed by members of the *Clearinghouse*. For details of each study the reader is referred to the original publications.

Follow-up studies of "alarms"

When a member program notices an unusual occurrence while monitoring malformations, or when a possible association between a specific exposure and a birth defect is suggested, the *Clearinghouse* should have the ability to quickly supply information that can shed light on the question raised. This has occurred repeatedly during the history of the *Clearinghouse.* Below are given four examples of the many situations in which the *Clearinghouse* network proved to be efficient for clarifying questions related to the cause of malformations.

The femoral hypoplasia cluster in France

The Central-East France program observed a relatively sudden increase in the number of infants born with femoral hypoplasia, sometimes as part of the femur-fibula-ulna (FFU) syndrome. This "alarm" was reported to the *Clearinghouse*, which responded very quickly by providing the French program with important information: the background rate of this rare malformation in a number of programs around the world. This piece of information made it possible for the Central-East France program to compare both their rate before the observed cluster and the rate during the cluster with the background rates of other programs. These comparisons supported the suspicion that a true increase had occurred.

Reference: Robert, J.M., Guibaud, P., Robert, E. A local outbreak of femoral hypoplasia or aplasia and femoral fibula-ulnar-complex. J. Génét. hum. 29: 379, 1981.

Valproic acid and spina bifida

In a study using data from Central-East France, a possible association was found between maternal use of valproic acid and the occurrence of spina bifida in the child. The finding was reported at a *Clearinghouse* annual meeting before it was published in a scientific journal. On learning of this possible association, the *Clearinghouse* rapidly supplied important information to help evaluate the finding. By compiling data from a number of monitoring systems, it could be shown that although a statistical association probably exists between spina bifida, maternal epilepsy, and use of anticonvulsant drugs of types other than valproic acid, it is much weaker than the association with valproic acid. This information supported the idea that this drug can play a specific role in the etiology of spina bifida. Furthermore, additional case histories, first identified in the Italian program, and subsequently in other programs as well, further supported the finding. Thirdly, by direct contacts made between the *Clearinghouse* members and governmental regulatory agencies, the importance of the finding was probably more rapidly generally recognized and resulted in warnings about the use of valproic acid during pregnancy. In this event the *Clearinghouse* demonstrated its capability to respond to a concern raised by one of its members and by its actions may have prevented the occurrence of further cases of spina bifida caused by maternal use of valproic acid.

Reference: Bjerkedal, T., Czeizel, A., Goujard, J., Kallen, B., Mastroiacovo, P., Nevin, N., Oakley, G. Jr., Robert, E. Valproic acid and spina bifida. Lancet ii: 1096, 1982.

Isotretinoin and a pattern of malformations

Observation of infants born to women who had used isotretinoin during pregnancy revealed a pattern of relatively typical malformations consisting of ear dysplasia, brain malformations, and conotruncal heart defects. By searching their files, a number of *Clearinghouse* members were able to estimate the prevalence of this constellation before the introduction of isotretinoin and found it to be very low.

Gastroschisis

In the early part of the 1970s, the Swedish monitoring program observed an increase of gastroschisis. It was first regarded as an artifact due to a better ascertainment of this relatively rare malformation, but a detailed follow-up study showed that that was not the case and that a true increase had occurred. The observation was reported to the other members of the *Clearinghouse* and some, but not all, programs discovered similar increases in their data. This led to a number of case-control studies which, however, failed to reveal a possible cause of the increases. Although the increased rate has by now been observed in many additional populations, no cause has been identified.

Studies of rare malformations

The aggregate files of the *Clearinghouse* members contain an enormous number of births, providing a unique opportunity to study rare malformations. It should be remembered, however, that not all programs are suitable for studies of such events. Programs based on hospital discharge diagnoses, as opposed to those obtaining complete descriptions of the infants, are seldom able to identify very rare conditions.

Exstrophy of the bladder and epispadias

The prevalence at birth of exstrophy of the bladder has been estimated as between two and five per 100,000 births, but such estimates have been based on relatively small series and therefore have had considerable uncertainty. The *Clearinghouse* collected information on 208 infants with bladder exstrophy from ten programs comprising 6.3 million births and found an average prevalence at birth of 3.3 per 100,000 with no significant variation between programs. Some epidemiological characteristics could be studied. There was a lower male excess (1.5 males for one female) than usually reported in the literature and there was an increased risk at low maternal age and possibly at high parity. The low maternal age dependence resembles the well-known one for gastroschisis, which, interestingly, is a malformation that has pathogenetic mechanisms in common with bladder exstrophy. Thirty percent of the infants had other malformations, mainly those belonging to the cloacal exstrophy sequence (anal atresia, omphalocele, and low spina bifida).

In the same study data on epispadias were also collected. This malformation was present in 148 infants, giving an average rate of 2.4 per 100,000 births. The Atlanta program showed a significantly higher rate than the others, but as can be seen in Chapter V, the rate presently recorded in that program is more consistent with that found elsewhere, suggesting that the high rate was due to misclassification. An increased risk for epispadias was seen at low maternal age, but no parity effect was seen. All but four infants were male, most likely because epispadias in the newborn period is more easily identified in a male infant than in a female infant. This means that the rate estimate is probably too low.

Reference: Epidemiology of bladder exstrophy and epispadias: a communication from the International Clearinghouse for Birth Defects Monitoring Systems. Teratology 36: 221, 1987.

Conjoined twins

Another extremely rare condition is conjoined twinning. The interest in this malformation was increased when a report from the U.S. Food and Drug Administration linked the birth of two cases of conjoined twinning with maternal use of griseofulvin. A survey of conjoined twinning in the data sets of the *Clearinghouse* members identified a total of 232 cases, none of which had been exposed to griseofulvin. With this material at hand, a joint epidemiological study of the condition was conducted. The best estimate of the prevalence at birth was 1.3 per 100,000 births. Sixty percent were females, and the stillbirth rate was close to 50%. A detailed description of type of twinning and associated malformations was produced. This paper is awaiting publication.

Cyclopia and sirenomelia

Eight programs in the *Clearinghouse* collaborated on an epidemiological study of these two rare defects. Material was collected on 102 infants with cyclopia and 99 with sirenomelia (one had both conditions). For each of these conditions the prevalence at birth was about 1 per 100,000. The types of associated malformations as well as various epidemiological characteristics supported the view, previously expressed and based on embryological considerations, that the two conditions are pathogenetically related.

Reference: Källén, B., Castilla, E.E., Lancaster, P.A.L., Mutchinick, O., Knudsen L.B., Martínez-Frías, M.L., Mastroiacovo, P., Robert, E. The cyclops and the mermaid - an epidemiological study of two types of rare malformations. J. med. Genet., in press.

Multimalformed infants

Beginning in 1980, the *Clearinghouse* has collected data on infants with multiple malformations. The data are coded and stored centrally and used for ongoing surveillance, as multimalformed infants are thought to be sensitive indicators of possible new teratogens. During the years a large amount of data on such infants have been collected and analyzed. Various main constellations of malformation associations have been identified, and the material has been especially useful in characterizing the so-called VATER-like associations, composed of vertebral, anal, esophageal and renal malformations. Other constellations have also been described and identified.

Comparative epidemiology of birth defects

Simple comparisons, such as variations in rates between programs, can be made with routinely tabulated data. For more complex epidemiological comparisons further data, including background information, are needed. For the collaborative studies summarized below several programs in the *Clearinghouse* were able to collect such additional information.

Hypospadias

Hypospadias is a rather common condition with enormous variability in recorded rates in different programs (cf. Chapter V). In some programs increases in the prevalence at birth have been observed. In order to further analyze these phenomena, eight of the *Clearinghouse* programs collected detailed information on 8,122 male infants with hypospadias and on the background populations. Efforts were made to see if differences in ascertainment could explain the variable recorded rates. Although ascertainment did vary among the programs, it alone could not explain the large differences in prevalence rates. Interprogram differences were also found in the effect of low maternal age on the occurrence of hypospadias. A detailed analysis of the effects of maternal age and parity, of birthweight and length of gestation, and of associated malformations (present in 9% of the cases) was made.

This descriptive study was followed by a joint case-control study based on interviews with mothers of infants with isolated hypospadias and with the mothers of controls. The study, which was performed in eight different programs, tried to record numerous possible risk factors. The main subject of the study was the possible effects of maternal treatment with hormones and of oral contraceptives, but studies on subfertility were also done. No effect of oral contraceptives on the risk of hypospadias was seen. While hormone treatment during the formative period of hypospadias did carry an approximately doubled risk for the malformation (seen in most published studies), causality in the association was brought into question. There was no correspondence between the time of exposure and the position of the urethral orifice or between hormone exposure and severity of the hypospadias. Furthermore, the main indication for treatment (early pregnancy bleeding) appeared as a stronger confounder in programs where hormones were not used than in programs with a high usage of hormones. This also speaks against causality.

As an adjunct to this study, much was learned about dealing with the problems inherent in multicenter studies, about the marked variability in the rates of various exposures in different populations, and how differences between populations can be used in the interpretation of data. This knowledge may prove useful in future studies.

References: Källén, B., Bertollini, R., Castilla, E., Czeizel, A., Knudsen, L.B., Martínez-Frías, M.L., Mastroiacovo, P., and Mutchinick, O. A joint epidemiological study on the epidemiology of hypospadias. Acta paed. Scand. Suppl. 324, 1986.

Källén, B., Martínez-Frías, M.L., Castilla, E.E., Robert, E., Lancaster, P.A.L., Kringelbach, M., Mutchinick, O., Mastroiacovo, P. Hormone therapy during pregnancy and isolated hypospadias. An international case-control study. Under publication.

Källén, B., Mastroiacovo, P., Lancaster, P.A.L., Mutchinick, O., Kringelbach, M., Martínez-Frías, M.L., Robert, E., Castilla, E.E. Oral contraceptives in the aetiology of isolated hypospadias. Under publication.

Down syndrome

Inter-program variations in the rate of Down syndrome can be readily seen in Chapter V. Four main factors explain these variations: different maternal age distributions, different maternal age-specific risks, different ascertainment, and different use of prenatal diagnosis followed by selective abortion. Data from 19 programs were used in a study that tried to deal with some of these factors. By assuming that the maternal age-specific risks are identical in all populations and that prenatal diagnosis plays a negligible role in the occurrence of Down syndrome in women below the age of 35, the ascertainment in the different populations could be estimated and was found to vary from a little more than 60% upwards. Supposing that ascertainment is the same irrespective of maternal age, the effect of prenatal diagnosis on the Down syndrome rate could be estimated and was found to vary from a 25% reduction to none, with an average of 6%.

Reference: Källén, B., Knudsen, L.B. Effect of maternal age distribution and prenatal diagnosis on the population rates of Down syndrome - a comparative study of nineteen populations. Hereditas 110: 55, 1989.

There are many other aspects of birth defect epidemiology where the data collected by the *Clearinghouse* members could be useful. The routinely collected data would in most instances have to be supplemented with additional information on the cases and the background populations.

Maternal use of anticonvulsants and birth defects

Numerous studies on the teratogenicity of maternal epilepsy and maternal use of anticonvulsant drugs have been published, but most have been too small to analyze possible differences in the effects of specific drugs. Furthermore, in a given population it may be difficult to sort out the effects of a drug from the effects of the disease when certain specific drugs are used for specific types of epilepsy; the different types of epilepsy may have their own effects on embryonic development. A way to reduce this confounding is to study different populations with different therapeutic traditions.

Cohorts of women using anticonvulsants in monotherapy

Three programs in the *Clearinghouse* joined in a study to collect information on pregnancy outcome of epileptic women who received anticonvulsants in monotherapy. Further data were added from a previously published French study. A total of 577 infants born to women on anticonvulsants in monotherapy could be studied. The distribution of drugs used in the different populations varied markedly. No statistically significant difference in the rate of malformations could be seen between the different drugs, but the drugs did show differences in their effects on infant dimensions, with a more marked decrease of birth weight, gestational duration, body length, and head circumference after carbamazepine than after phenobarbital, phenytoin, or valproic acid.

Reference: Bertollini, R., Källén, B., Mastroiacovo, P., Robert, E. Anticonvulsant drugs in monotherapy. Effect on the fetus. Europ. J. Epidemiol. 3: 164, 1987.

Anticonvulsant use and malformations: Is there a drug specificity?

The power of the study described above to detect differences in teratogenic activity of specific anticonvulsant drugs is low because of small numbers. A new study was initiated to compare the type of anticonvulsant drug exposure of 318 malformed infants whose mothers had epilepsy. Data were collected from six of the *Clearinghouse* programs. A significant association was found between the use of valproic acid and spina bifida and a weaker, not statistically significant, association between spina bifida and carbamazepine. Facial clefts were associated with phenobarbital and phenytoin use, as well as with polytherapy.

Reference: Källén, B., Robert, E., Mastroiacovo, P. Martínez-Frías, M.L., Castilla, E.E., Cocchi, G. Anticonvulsant drugs and malformations. Is there a drug specificity? Europ. J. Epidemiol. 5: 31, 1989.

Maternal use of lithium and tricuspid valve malformations

Use of lithium during pregnancy (because of manic-depressive disease) is a rare event. It has been associated with an increased risk for cardiac defects, notably the Ebstein anomaly of the tricuspid valve, a rare malformation. A case-control study was carried out jointly by four *Clearinghouse* programs that together collected data on 69 infants with tricuspid malformations, 25 of which were of the Ebstein type. Drug histories were obtained for the cases and for their controls. No instance of lithium exposure was detected and no significant association was found between any other drug and the tricuspid malformations, which indicates that drugs are not major contributors to these malformations.

Reference: Källén, B. Comments on Teratogen Update: Lithium. Teratology 38: 597, 1988.

Chapter VIII
Thoughts on the future of the Clearinghouse

The final note of Chapter I states that one major achievement of the *Clearinghouse* is to have survived for 17 years. It has survived in spite of uncertain funding and a relatively informal structure - or, perhaps, because of an informal structure.

In this Chapter we will present some thoughts on the future. First of all: Do we need a clearinghouse? If so, what should be its form and functions? And how can we ensure its survival?

Do we need a Clearinghouse?

The primary goal of the *Clearinghouse* is to help identify and to prevent the spread of an epidemic of birth defects by serving as an early warning system. This requires the active cooperation of malformation monitoring programs throughout the world. The effectiveness of the *Clearinghouse* has not been fully tested in a real life situation, as no epidemic similar to that caused by thalidomide has occurred during its 17 years of existence. Likewise, the efficiency of most of the malformation monitoring systems that comprise the *Clearinghouse* has also gone untested. But as long as there is the danger that pregnant women will be exposed to new chemical or physical factors that could cause serious birth defects, vigilant malformation monitoring and international collaboration must be encouraged and maintained. The *Clearinghouse* has successfully provided the means for collaboration at a relatively low cost and with a minimum of bureaucratic impediments. We feel that its continuity should be guaranteed as long as it is working efficiently.

Future form and functions

The commitment of the people who represent the member programs is critical to the survival of the *Clearinghouse*. The representatives, who are usually and ideally the persons actually in charge of their respective programs, are responsible for alerting the *Clearinghouse* of unusual events, for submitting data as required, and for participating in joint activities that are aimed at improving monitoring methods and discovering the nature and causes of birth defects.

The interest, competence, and commitment of such individuals will always be the engine that drives the *Clearinghouse*; they cannot be replaced by a centralized organization with an employed staff. Nevertheless, there still must exist an active central office that not only coordinates the exchange of information, but also initiates and organizes joint studies.

Joint studies have both a stated and an unstated purpose. The stated purpose of a scientific investigation is obvious. The unstated purpose of these activities in the *Clearinghouse* is to maintain a high level of interest among the participants. Just as it is difficult to run an effective malformation monitoring system without active ongoing scientific use of the collected data, it is also almost impossible for the *Clearinghouse* to maintain the active participation and interest of the member programs without conducting collaborative epidemiological studies.

One of the tasks of the *Clearinghouse* laid down in the bylaws is to advance the skills in monitoring birth defects. This is often thought of in terms of courses and seminars or pamphlets and articles on the subject, all of which have been done. More effective, perhaps, have been the participation in joint studies and

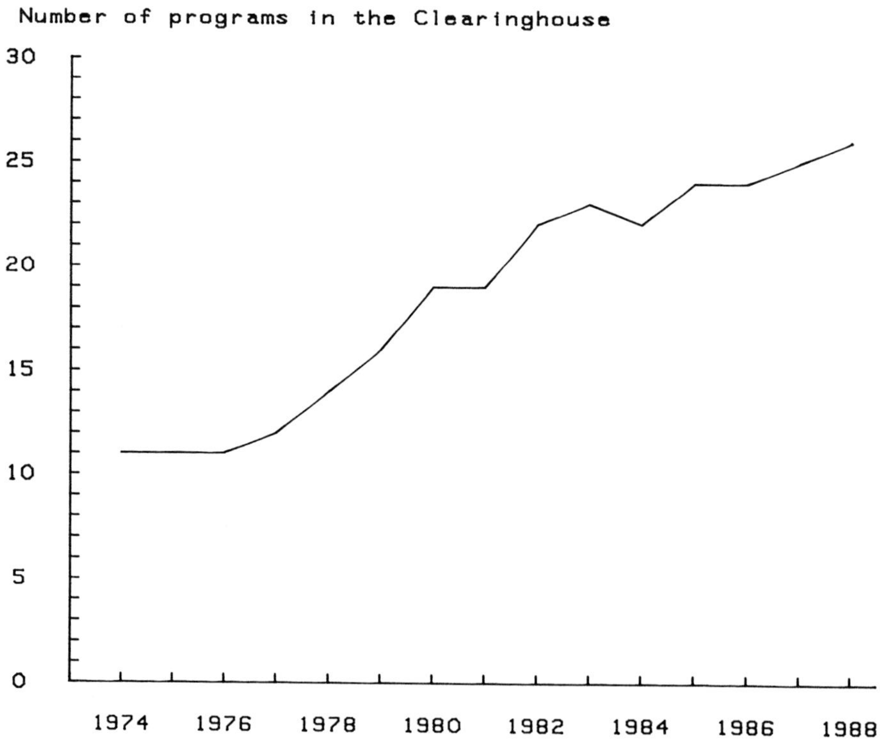

other direct contacts between various programs that often represent different philosophies with regard to the monitoring process. As long as a monitoring system works in an isolated and somewhat protected environment, its faults or inefficiencies may be unnoticed or ignored. When the program participates in joint studies where demands are made on the data and standards of quality are required, defects may be detected and repaired. This important part of the educational process could be expanded by participation of more programs in the joint studies.

The *Clearinghouse* has grown from 11 programs in its first year to 26 programs 17 years later (see figure). To what extent should it continue to expand? There is a natural wish to be as inclusive as possible, and there are still large areas of the world where there is little or no information on the epidemiology of birth defects and where the installation of new programs would be valuable. For example, more information is needed on the occurrence of birth defects in Africa, Southwest Asia, and in heavily polluted parts of Eastern Europe.

Expansion of the *Clearinghouse* network must not, however, be at the expense of the quality requirements placed on the member programs. Perhaps more important than the fulfillment of the formal requirements listed in Chapter II is the need for actively interested, even devoted, program representatives who not only see birth defect monitoring as the quarterly or yearly production and review of statistical tables, but wish to see the biological realities behind the figures and are willing to spend the time needed to make full use of the opportunities for collaboration offered by the *Clearinghouse*.

There is also a risk that if the organization gets too large and impersonal, its effectiveness will diminish. As stressed repeatedly, the most important aspect of the Clearinghouse's activities is not the mere tabulation of routine data, however interesting, but rather it is the reporting of unusual events that might herald an epidemic of birth defects. This reporting, often based on scanty evidence, is encouraged by the existence of a network of people who personally know and trust each other.

Ensuring survival

The member programs have always underwritten part of the work done in the *Clearinghouse* by donating staff time to the various activities, both routine data submission and special projects. In spite of this help, financing the *Clearinghouse* has always been a problem. During the first few years the March of Dimes played a decisive role by supporting most of the organization's functions. Later, annual fees, supplemented by *ad hoc* applications for funds provided enough income to support the basic activities. More recently, a three-year grant from the Norwegian government has at least temporarily relaxed the financial stress of the organization.

This grant, which will run until December 1991, enabled the creation in 1989 of an International Centre for Birth Defects in Bergen, Norway. From its inception this center has been closely connected with the *Clearinghouse* and has served as its office for the past two years. This has fulfilled the long-standing wish of the *Clearinghouse* that its central office would be supplied with a secretarial staff and other facilities. However, the amount of central facilities needed by the organization is limited, and a number of possible future associations between the *Clearinghouse* and various other organizations are presently being discussed. It is important that associations with other entities not overshadow the most important need for survival and development of the *Clearinghouse*: intense collaboration among the participating programs.

Funding is therefore needed both for a central office function and for making collaborative work possible. Not only is such collaboration facilitated by the ability of the participants to meet for planning and discussions, but experience has shown that such meetings are absolutely necessary - though expensive because participants often have to travel long distances.

Thus, to secure continuity of operations and to ensure that important projects are not hampered or delayed by lack of funds, long-term financing of the *Clearinghouse* is essential. Moreover, funding should be multinational. It must be realized that the agents causing birth defects often do not recognize political borders and that results of investigations made in one part of the world may protect infants elsewhere from possible malformations. A contribution to the funding of international cooperation in birth defect monitoring should be regarded as a sound investment for the prevention of birth defects in one's own country.

Chapter IX
Bibliography

Introduction

During the past 15 years a large number of scientific papers on congenital malformations have been published by the member programs of the *Clearinghouse*. This bibliography aims to give a readily available source of references to such articles.

This bibliography contains publications in periodicals and books up to the end of 1990. Letters to journals are also included if they report data from epidemiological studies. Abstracts of papers presented at scientific meetings have not been included.

The references are listed alphabetically according to first author.

References were selected with the scope of this monograph in mind. This naturally implies that there has been a great number and variety of publications in each program than is presented here. The selection criteria for this bibliography are: registration; monitoring, and its methodology; human teratogens, including occupational exposure; structural birth defects. Most articles are in English. In cases where the title is in English and the article is in another language, that language is indicated in brackets.

This bibliography is based on an earlier one with a restricted circulation. The original bibliography was compiled by Jennifer Burn and Paul Lancaster (Sydney). The present bibliography has been completed by ICBD.

The complete bibliography can be obtained on a floppy disk upon request. Send your application to the International Centre for Birth Defects.

ABRATE M BARACCHINI P FULCHERI E LAPERTOSA G PANTAROTTO MF MASTROIACOVO P
STUDIO EPIDEMIOLOGICO DELL'ANENCEFALIA IN ITALIA E RILIEVI ANATOMOPATOLOGICI SUI CASI DI NOSTRA OSSERVAZIONE
PATHOLOGICA 1990 82:133-54

ADAMS C JOHNSTON WP NEVIN NC
FAMILY STUDY OF CONGENITAL HYDROCEPHALUS
DEV MED CHILD NEUROL 1982 24:493-498

ADAMS MJ JR
NEURAL TUBE DEFECTS. A REVIEW FOR THE CLINICIAN
BULL EMORY UN SCH MED 1983 5:30-39

ADAMS MJ JR
HONEYBEE SYNDROME, GLYCOLYSIS AND BIRTH DEFECTS (LETTER)
NEW ENGL J MED 1984 311:860

ADAMS MJ JR WINDHAM GC JAMES LM GREENBERG F CLAYTON-HOPKINS JA REIMER CB OAKLEY GP JR
CLINICAL INTERPRETATION OF MATERNAL SERUM ALPHA-FETOPROTEIN CONCENTRATIONS
AM J OBSTET GYNECOL 1984 148:241-254

ADAMS MM
INCIDENCE OF DOWN SYNDROME
AM J HUM GENET 1987 40:287

ADAMS MM ERICKSON JD LAYDE PM OAKLEY GP JR
DOWN'S SYNDROME RECENT TRENDS IN THE UNITED STATES
JAMA 1981 246:758-760

ADAMS MM FINLEY S HANSEN H JAHIEL RI OAKLEY GP JR SANGER W WELLS G WERTELECKI W
UTILIZATION OF PRENATAL GENETIC DIAGNOSIS IN WOMEN 35 YEARS OF AGE AND OLDER IN THE UNITED STATES 1977-78
AM J OBSTET GYNECOL 1981 139:673-677

ADAMS MM GREENBERG F KHOURY MJ MARKS JS OAKLEY GP JR
TRENDS IN CLINICAL CHARACTERISTICS OF INFANTS WITH SPINA BIFIDA - ATLANTA 1972-1979
AM J DIS CHILD 1985 139:514-517

ADAMS MM GREENBERG F KHOURY MJ MARKS JS OAKLEY GP JR
SURVIVAL OF INFANTS WITH SPINA BIFIDA - ATLANTA 1972-1979
AM J DIS CHILD 1985 139:518-523

ADAMS MM MULINARE J DOOLEY K
RISK FACTORS FOR CONOTRUNCAL CARDIAC DEFECTS IN ATLANTA
JACC 1989 14:432-42

ADAMS MM OAKLEY GP JR MARKS JS
MATERNAL AGE AND BIRTHS IN THE 1980S
JAMA 1982 247:493-494

ADAMS MM WEIS P OAKLEY GP JR FALEK A
USE OF PRENATAL DIAGNOSIS AMONG PARENTS OF INFANTS WITH SPINA BIFIDA IN ATLANTA GEORGIA 1976-79
AM J OBSTET GYNECOL 1984 148:749-751

AHLBORG G JR BJERKEDAL T EGENAES J
DELIVERY OUTCOME AMONG WOMEN EMPLOYED IN THE PLASTICS INDUSTRY IN SWEDEN AND NORWAY
AM J IND MED 1987 12:507-517

ALDERMAN BW LAMMER EG JOSHUA SC CORDERO JF OUIMETTE DR WILSON MJ FERGUSON SW
AN EPIDEMIOLOGIC STUDY OF CRANIOSYNOSTOSIS: RISK INDICATORS FOR CRANIOSYNOSTOSIS OCCURENCE IN COLORADO
AM J EPIDEMIOL 1988 128:431-438

ANDERSON CE EDMONDS LD ERICKSON JD
PATENT DUCTUS ARTERIOSUS AND VENTRICULAR SEPTAL DEFECT: TRENDS IN REPORTED FREQUENCY
AM J EPIDEMIOL 1978 107:281-289

ANONYMOUS
REGISTRATION OF CONGENITAL ABNORMALITIES (DAN)
UGESKR LAEGER 1979 141:3325-3329

ARO T
MATERNAL DISEASES, ALCOHOL CONSUMPTION AND SMOKING DURING PREGNANCY ASSOCIATED WITH REDUCTION LIMB DEFECTS
EARLY HUM DEV 1983 9:49-57

ARO T HAAPAKOSKI J HEINONEN OP
A MULTIVARIATE ANALYSIS OF THE RISK INDICATORS OF REDUCTION LIMB DEFECTS
INT J EPIDEMIOL 1984 13:459-464

ARO T HAAPAKOSKI J HEINONEN OP SAXEN L
LACK OF ASSOCIATION BETWEEN VITAMIN INTAKE DURING EARLY PREGNANCY AND REDUCTION LIMB DEFECTS
AM J OBSTET GYNECOL 1984 150:433

ARO T HEINONEN OP SAXEN L
INCIDENCE AND SECULAR TRENDS OF CONGENITAL LIMB DEFECTS IN FINLAND
INT J EPIDEMIOL 1982 11:239-244

ARO T HEINONEN OP SAXEN L
RISK INDICATORS OF REDUCTION LIMB DEFECTS
J EPIDEMIOL COMMUNITY HEALTH 1983 37:50-56

ASHIZAWA M
BIRTH DEFECTS MONITORING SYSTEM. STEPS TAKEN TOWARDS ORGANIZING BIRTH DEFECTS MONITORING SYSTEM. IN: FUKUYAMA Y ARIMA M MAEKAWA K YAMAGUCHI K (EDS) INTERNATIONAL CONGRESS SERIES NO 579 CHILD NEUROLOGY PROC
AMSTERDAM: ELSEVIER 1981 334-338

ASHIZAWA M BJERKEDAL T CASTILLA E ET AL
CONGENITAL ANOMALIES (FRE) (LETTER)
MED HYG (GENEVE) 1983 41:4136

ASHIZAWA M KURACHI T
MONITORING OF BIRTH DEFECTS AND EPIDEMIOLOGY
CONG ANOM 1986 26:49-54

AVELLAN L
THE INCIDENCE OF HYPOSPADIAS IN SWEDEN
SCAND J PL REC SURG 1975 9:129-139

BAHNA SL BJERKEDAL T
THE COURSE AND OUTCOME OF PREGNANCY IN WOMEN WITH NEUROSES
ACTA OBSTET GYNEC SCAND 1974 53:129-133

BAHNA SL BJERKEDAL T
THE COURSE AND OUTCOME OF PREGNANCY IN WOMEN WITH BRONCHIAL ASTHMA
ACTA ALLERGOLOGICA 1972 27:397-406

BAKKETEIG LS
MEDICAL REGISTRATION OF BIRTH, IMPLICATIONS FOR HEALTH SERVICES ACTIVITIES
JOURNAL OF MIDWIFERY 1974 147-54

BAKKETEIG LS
DETECTION OF TERATOGENS BY MONITORING HUMAN BIRTHS. IN: KLINGBERG M AND WEATHERALL JAC (EDS) CONTRIBUTIONS TO EPIDEMIOLOGY AND BIOSTATISTICS VOL 1: EPIDEMIOLOGIC METHODS FOR DETECTION OF TERATOGENS
BASEL: KARGER, 1978 53-56

BAKKETEIG LS EIK-NES SH JACOBSEN G ULSTEIN MK BRODTKORB CJ BALSTAD P ERIKSEN BC JORGENSEN NP
DIAGNOSTIC ULTRASOUND IN PREGNANCY
LANCET 1984 2:744

BALARAJAN R SONI RALEIGH V BOTTING B
MORTALITY FROM CONGENITAL MALFORMATIONS IN ENGLAND AND WALES: VARIATIONS BY MOTHER'S COUNTRY OF BIRTH
ARCH DIS CHILD 1989 64:1457-62

BALTZAR B ERICSON A KALLEN B
DELIVERY OUTCOME IN WOMEN EMPLOYED IN MEDICAL OCCUPATIONS IN SWEDEN
J OCCUP MED 1979 21:543-548

BALTZAR B ERICSON A KALLEN B
PREGNANCY OUTCOME AMONG WOMEN WORKING IN SWEDISH HOSPITALS (LETTER)
NEW ENGL J MED 1979 300:627-628

BANISTER P
CONGENITAL MALFORMATIONS: PRELIMINARY REPORT OF AN INVESTIGATION OF REDUCTION DEFORMITIES OF THE LIMBS TRIGGERED BY A PILOT SURVEILLANCE SYSTEM
CAN MED ASSOC J 1970 103:466-472

BANISTER P
EVALUATION OF VITAL RECORD USAGE FOR CONGENITAL ANOMALY SURVEILLANCE. IN: HOOK EB JANERICH DT PORTER IH (EDS) MONITORING BIRTH DEFECTS AND ENVIRONMENT: THE PROBLEM OF SURVEILLANCE
NEW YORK: ACADEMIC PRESS INC 1971 119-136

BANISTER P
VALIDITY OF DATA FOR ANENCEPHALUS (LETTER)
TERATOLOGY 1979 19:269

BAO GZ LI XP XIAO KZ
CONGENTIAL HYDROCEPHALY OF PERINATES IN SICHUAN PROVINCE
HEREDITY DIS 1989 6:132

BAO GZ WAN CH XIAO KZ
NEURAL TUBE DEFECTS OF 92.301 PERINATES IN CHENGDU AREA
J PRAC OBSTET GYNECOL 1989 5:25-6

BECERRA JE KHOURY MJ CORDERO JF ERICKSON JD
DIABETES MELLITUS DURING PREGNANCY AND THE RISKS FOR SPECIFIC BIRTH DEFECTS: A POPULATION-BASED CASE-CONTROL STUDY
PEDIATRICS 1990 85:1-9

BELLYEI A CZEIZEL A
A HIGHER INCIDENCE OF CONGENITAL STRUCTURAL TALIPES EQUINOVARUS IN GIPSIES
HUM HERED 1983 33:58-59

BEN-ARI Y SHUPER A MIMOUNI M ROSEN D GRUNEBAUM M MERLOB P
AGENESIS OF CORPUS CALLOSUM ASSOCIATED WITH DOUBLE URINARY COLLECTING SYSTEM TRIGONOCEPHALY AND OTHER MINOR ANOMALIES: A NEW ASSOCIATION (LETTER)
EUR J PEDIATR 1989 148:787-8

BERRY RJ BUEHLER JW STRAUSS LT
BIRTH WEIGHT-SPECIFIC INFANT MORTALITY DUE TO CONGENITAL ANOMALIES 1960-80
PUBLIC HEALTH REP 1987 102:171-81

BERTOLLINI R DI LALLO D MASTROIACOVO P PERUCCI CA
REDUCTION OF BIRTHS IN ITALY AFTER THE CHERNOBYL ACCIDENT
SCAND J WORK ENVIRON HEALTH 1990 16:96-100

BERTOLLINI R KALLEN B MASTROIACOVO P ROBERT E
ANTICONVULSANT DRUGS IN MONOTHERAPY: EFFECT ON THE FETUS
EUR J EPIDEMIOL 1987 3:164-71

BERTOLLINI R MASTROIACOVO P SEGNI G
MATERNAL EPILEPSY AND BIRTH DEFECTS: A CASE-CONTROL STUDY IN THE ITALIAN MULTICENTRIC REGISTRY OF BIRTH DEFECTS (IPIMC)
EUR J EPIDEMIOL 1985 1:67-72

BJERKEDAL T
CONGENITAL MALFORMATIONS REGISTERED AT BIRTH IN NORWAY 1967-1976 MEDICAL BIRTH REGISTRY BERGEN (NOR)
TIDSSKR NOR LAEGEFOREN 1980 100:202-205

BJERKEDAL T
OUTCOME OF PREGNANCY IN WOMEN WITH EPILEPSY, NORWAY 1967 TO 1978.
IN: JANSZ D EPILEPSY PREGNANCY AND THE CHILD
NEW YORK: RAVEN PRESS 1982 75-80

BJERKEDAL T
OCCUPATION AND OUTCOME OF PREGNANCY: A POPULATION-BASED STUDY IN NORWAY
PROG CLIN BIOL RES 1985 163B:265-268

BJERKEDAL T BAKKETEIG LS
MEDICAL REGISTRATION OF BIRTHS IN NORWAY DURING THE 5 YEAR PERIOD: 1967-71
UNIVERSITY OF BERGEN, BERGEN 1975

BJERKEDAL T BAKKETEIG LS
PRELIMINARY REPORT ON A CASE-CONTROL STUDY BASED ON AN INCREASED FREQUENCY OF HYPOSPADIAS (NOR)
TIDSSKR NOR LAEGEFOREN 1975 95:1436-37

BJERKEDAL T BAHNA SL LEHMANN EH
THE COURSE AND OUTCOME OF PREGNANCY IN WOMEN WITH PULMONARY TUBERCULOSIS
SCAND J RESP DIS 1975 56, 245-250

BJERKEDAL T EGENAES J
IL RISCHIO TERATOGENA LEGATO ALL'ATTIVITÁ LAVORATIVA. UN TENTATIVA DE STIMARE IL RISCHIO RELATIVO E ATTRIBUTIBLE.
PROSPECTTIVE PEDIATRIA 1982 45: 39-43

BJERKEDAL T BAHNA SL
THE COURSE AND OUTCOME OF PREGNANCY IN WOMEN WITH EPILEPSY
ACTA OBST GYNE SCAND 1973 52:245-248

BJERKEDAL T BAKKETEIG LS
SURVEILLANCE OF CONGENITAL MALFORMATIONS AND OTHER CONDITIONS IN THE NEWBORN
INT J EPIDEMIOL 1975 4:31-36

BJERKEDAL T CZEIZEL A GOUJARD J KALLEN B MASTROIACOVO P NEVIN N OAKLEY GP JR ROBERT E
INTERNATIONAL CLEARINGHOUSE FOR BIRTH DEFECTS MONITORING SYSTEMS: VALPROIC ACID AND SPINA BIFIDA (LETTER)
LANCET 1982 1096

BLOMQUIST U ERICSON A KALLEN B WESTERHOLM P
DELIVERY OUTCOME FOR WOMEN WORKING IN THE PULP AND PAPER INDUSTRY
SCAND J WORK ENVIRON HEALTH 1981 7:114-118

BOD M CZEIZEL A
CONGENITAL MALFORMATION SURVEILLANCE
TERATOLOGY 1981 24:277-283

BOD M CZEIZEL A LENZ W
INCIDENCE AT BIRTH OF DIFFERENT TYPES OF LIMB REDUCTION ABNORMALITIES IN HUNGARY 1975-1977
HUM GENET 1983 65:27-33

BOD M CZEIZEL A LENZ W
CHARACTERISTICS OF CERTAIN TYPES OF LIMB REDUCTION ABNORMALITIES (HUN)
ORV HETIL 1985 126:1917-1920

BORMAN B CHAPMAN C HOWARD K BUCKFIELD P FINDLAY J
USING A NATIONAL REGISTER FOR THE EPIDEMIOLOGICAL STUDY OF CONGENITAL HEART DEFECTS
NZ MED J 1987 100:404-6

BORMAN B CRYER C
THE FALLACIES OF INTERNATIONAL AND NATIONAL COMPARISONS OF DISEASE OCCURRENCE IN THE EPIDEMIOLOGY OF NEURAL TUBE DEFECTS
TERATOLOGY 1990 42:405-12

BORMAN B HOWARD JK CHAPMAN CJ
THE EPIDEMIOLOGICAL STUDY OF BIRTH DEFECTS
NZ MED J 1984 97:602

BORMAN B HOWARD JK CHAPMAN CJ
SECULAR TRENDS IN THE PREVALENCE OF ANENCEPHALUS IN NEW ZEALAND
NZ MED J 1986 99:183-5

BORMAN B SMITH AH HOWARD JK
RISK FACTORS IN THE PREVALENCE OF ANENCEPHALUS AND SPINA BIFIDA IN NEW ZEALAND
TERATOLOGY 1986 33:221-30

BORMAN B VEALE AMO FINDLAY J
MAJOR BIRTH DEFECTS IN NEW ZEALAND: PREVALENCE AND PATTERNS
PATIENT MAN 1987 16:113-22

BRADSHAW T WEALE J WEATHERALL J
CONGENITAL MALFORMATIONS OF THE CENTRAL NERVOUS SYSTEM
POPULATION TRENDS 1980 12:HMSO LONDON

BUGGE M HAUGE M
GASTROSCHISIS AND OMPHALOCELE IN DENMARK AN EPIDEMIOLOGICAL INVESTIGATION (DAN)
UGESKR LAEGER 1983 145:1323-1327

CALZOLARI E CAVAZZUTI GB COCCHI G CONTRINO C MAGNANI C MORETTI M RONCARATO E SALVIOLI GP VOLPATO S
CONGENITAL MALFORMATIONS IN 100,000 CONSECUTIVE BIRTHS IN EMILIA ROMAGNA REGION NORTHERN ITALY: COMPARISON WITH THE EUROCAT DATA
EUR J EPIDEMIOL 1987 3:423-30

CALZOLARI E CONTIERO MR RONCARATI E MATTIUZ L VOLPATO S
AETIOLOGICAL FACTORS IN HYPOSPADIAS
J MED GENET 1986 23:333-339

CALZOLARI E MILAN M CAVAZZUTI GP COCCHI G GANDINI E MAGNANI C MORETTI M GARANI GP SALVIOLI GP VOLPATO S
EPIDEMIOLOGICAL AND GENETIC STUDY OF 200 CASES OF ORAL CLEFT IN THE EMILIA ROMAGNA REGION OF NORTHERN ITALY
TERATOLOGY 1988 38:559-64

CAMERA G CLERICI BAGOZZI D SALMOIRAGHI MG LEZZI GB RUSSO A D'ARMIENTO P MASTROIACOVO P
CRANIO A TRIFOGLIO DESCRIZIONE DI QUATTRO CASI
PATHOLOGICA 1988 80/1086:459-68

CAMERA G GIORDANO F MASTROIACOVO P
PYKNOACHONDROGENESIS: AN ASSOCIATION OF SKELETAL DEFECTS RESEMBLING ACHONDROGENESIS WITH GENERALIZED BONE SCLEROSIS. A NEW CONDITION?
CLIN GENET 1986 30:335-7

CAMERA G MASTROIACOVO P
BIRTH PREVALENCE OF SKELETAL DYSPLASIAS IN THE ITALIAN MUTLICENTRIC MONITORING SYSTEM FOR BIRTH DEFECTS
PROG CLIN BIOL RES 1982 104:441-9

CAMERA G MASTROIACOVO P
BIRTH PREVALENCE AND MUTATION RATE OF ACHONDROPLASIA IN THE ITALIAN MULTICENTRIC MONITORING SYSTEM FOR BIRTH DEFECTS. IN: HUMAN ACHONDROPLASIA: A MULTIDISCIPLINARY APPROACH. NICOLETTI (ED)
PLENUM PRESS 1988 :10-4

CAMPBELL H NEWCOMBE RG WEATHERALL JA
EPIDEMIOLOGY OF SIMPLE HYPOSPADIAS (LETTER)
BR MED J 1973 3:52-53

CARLGREN LE ERICSON A KALLEN B
MONITORING OF CONGENITAL CARDIAC DEFECTS
PEDIATR CARDIOL 1987 8:247-256

CASTILLA E
VALPROIC ACID AND SPINA BIFIDA (LETTER)
LANCET 1983 2:683

CASTILLA E CZEIZEL A KALLEN B MASTROIACOVO P OAKLEY GP JR TAKESHITA K DEWALS P KULIEV A
METHODOLOGY FOR BIRTH DEFECTS MONITORING
BIRTH DEFECTS ORIGINAL ARTICLE SERIES 1986 22:1-43

CASTILLA E MUTCHINICK O PAZ J MUNOZ E GELMAN Z
LATIN AMERICAN STUDY OF CONGENITAL MALFORMATIONS (SPA)
BOL OF SANIT PANAM 1974 76:494-502

CASTILLA E ORIOLI-PARREIRAS IM MEDEIROS-SIMOES MA
STUDIES ON RISK FACTORS IN THE DOWN SYNDROME (SPA)
PEDIATRIA (SANTIAGO) 1980 23:89-105

CASTILLA E PAZ J MUTCHINICK O MUNOZ E GIORGIUTTI E GELMAN Z
POLYDACTYLY: A GENETIC STUDY IN SOUTH AMERICA
AM J HUM GENET 1973 25:405-412

CASTILLA E PAZ J ORIOLI-PARREIRAS IM
PREGNANCY BLEEDING AND EARLIER ABORTIONS AS RISK FACTORS FOR MALFORMATIONS (SPA)
PEDIATRIA (SANTIAGO) 1980 23:117-123

CASTILLA EE DUTRA M ORIOLI-PARREIRAS IM
EPIDEMIOLOGY OF CONGENITAL PIGMENTED NAEVI: 1 INCIDENCE RATES AND RELATIVE FREQUENCIES
BR J DERMATOL 1981 104:307-315

CASTILLA EE DUTRA M ORIOLI-PARREIRAS IM
EPIDEMIOLOGY OF CONGENITAL PIGMENTED NAEVI: 2 RISK FACTORS
BR J DERMATOL 1981 104:421-427

CASTILLA EE LOPEZ-CAMELO JS
THE SURVEILLANCE OF BIRTH DEFECTS IN SOUTH AMERICA: I THE SEARCH FOR TIME CLUSTERS: EPIDEMICS
ADV MUTAG RES 1990 VOL II 1990 191-210

CASTILLA EE LOPEZ-CAMELO JS ORIOLI IM SANCHEZ O PAZ JE
THE EPIDEMIOLOGY OF CONJOINED TWINS IN LATIN-AMERICA
ACTA GENET MED GEMELL 1988 37:111-118

CASTILLA EE MARTINEZ-FRIAS ML PAZ JE
PATTERNS OF COMBINED LIMB MALFORMATIONS
TERATOLOGY 1977 16:203-210

CASTILLA EE MUTCHINICK O
MALFORMACIONES CONGENITAS EN: PEDIATRIA CLINICA Y SOCIAL
MENEGHELLO J ET AL. (EDS) INTERMEDICA, BUENOS AIRES 1973

CASTILLA EE MUTCHINICK O
GENETICA-NOCIONES GENERALES EN: ENFERMEDADES DE LA BOCA GRISPAN D ET AL.(EDS)
BUENOS AIRES: MUNDI 1970

CASTILLA EE ORIOLI IM
COLABORACION INTERNACIONAL EN LA MONITORIZACION DE DEFECTOS CONGENITOS (SPA)
CIENC CULT SAO PAULO 1983 35:569-576

CASTILLA EE ORIOLI IM
EL ESTUDIO COLABORATIVO LATINOAMERICANO DE MALFORMACIONES CONGENITAS:ECLAMC/MONITOR (SPA)
INTERCIENCIA 1983 8:271-278

CASTILLA EE ORIOLI IM
SECULAR TRENDS FOR CONGENITAL LIMB DEFECTS IN SOUTH-AMERICA
PREVENTION OF PHYSICAL AND MENTAL CONGENITAL DEFECTS, PART C
NEW YORK: ALAN R LISS INC 1985 91-94

CASTILLA EE ORIOLI IM
EPIDEMIOLOGY OF NEURAL TUBE DEFECTS IN SOUTH AMERICA
AM J MED GENET 1985 22:695-702

CASTILLA EE ORIOLI IM
PREVALENCE RATES OF MICROTIA IN SOUTH-AMERICA
INT J EPIDEMIOL 1986 15:364-368

CASTILLA EE ORIOLI IM LOPEZ-CAMELO JS
ON MONITORING THE MULTIPLY MALFORMED INFANT 1: CASE-FINDING, CASE-RECORDING AND DATA HANDLING IN A LATIN AMERICAN PROGRAM
AM J MED GENET 1985 22:717-725

CASTILLA EE ORIOLI IM LUGARINHO R DUTRA G
EPIDEMIOLOGY OF AMBIGUOUS GENITALIA IN SOUTH AMERICA
AM J MED GENET 1987 27:337-343

CASTILLA EE ORIOLI IM LUGARINHO R DUTRA GP LOPEZ-CAMELO JS CAMPANA HE SPAGNOLO A MASTROIACOVO P
MONTHLY AND SEASONAL VARIATIONS IN THE FREQUENCY OF CONGENITAL ANOMALIES
INT J EPIDEMIOL 1990 19:399-404

CASTILLA EE ORIOLI-PARREIRAS IM
MALFORMATIONS AND INBREEDING
BOL GENET INST FITOTEC CASTELAR 1982 11:19-24

CASTILLA EE ORIOLI-PARREIRAS IM DUTRA MG FUENTES ML
EPIDEMIOLOGY OF CONGENITAL PIGMENTED NAEVI: III HEREDITABILITY
ARCH ARGENT DERMATOL 1982 32:413-418

CASTILLA EE PAZ JE MARTINEZ-FRIAS ML
INCIDENCE OF CONGENITAL MALFORMATIONS IN LATIN AMERICA RESULTS OF A COOPERATIVE STUDY (SPA)
REV MED CHIL 1975 103:331-334

CASTILLA EE PAZ JE ORIOLI IM
PECTORALIS MAJOR MUSCLE DEFECT AND POLAND COMPLEX
AM J MED GENET 1979 4:263-269

CASTILLA EE PAZ JE ORIOLI-PARREIRAS IM
SYNDACTYLY: FREQUENCY OF SPECIFIC TYPES
AM J MED GENET 1980 5:357-364

CASTILLA EE SOD R
THE SURVEILLANCE OF BIRTH DEFECTS IN SOUTH-AMERICA:II THE SEARCH FOR GEOGRAPHIC CLUSTERS: ENDEMICS
ADV MUTAG RES VOL II 1990 211-230

CASTILLA EE SOD R ANZORENA O TEXIDO J
NEONATAL TESTICULAR TORSION IN TWO BROTHERS
J MED GENET 1975 12:112-113

CEREIJO AI SALVADOR J ALONSO MD PRIETO L MARTINEZ-FRIAS ML
MATERNAL INFLUENZA AND DEFECTS IN NEURAL TUBE CLOSURE IN THE NEWBORN (SPA)
PROG OBSTET GINECOL 1985 28:279-284

CHAVEZ GF CORDERO JF BECERRA JE
LEADING MAJOR CONGENITAL MALFORMATIONS AMONG MINORITY GROUPS IN THE UNITED STATES 1981-86
JAMA 1989 261:205-209

CHAVEZ GF CORDERO JF BECERRA JE
PATENT DUCTUS ARTERIOSUS, PREMATURITY AND RESPIRATORY DISTRESS SYNDROME
JAMA 1989 261:3410

CHAVEZ GF MULINARE J CORDERO JF
MATERNAL COCAINE USE DURING EARLY PREGNANCY AS A RISK FACTOR FOR CONGENITAL UROGENITAL ANOMALIES
JAMA 1989 262:795-798

CHEMKE J CHEN R KLINGBERG MA LEVIN S
SOME INDICATIONS FOR GENETIC FACTORS IN CONGENITAL MALFORMATIONS
ISR J MED SCI 1973 9:1400-1403

CHEN R
A SURVEILLANCE SYSTEM FOR CONGENITAL MALFORMATIONS
JASA 1978 73:323-327

CHEN R
STATISTICAL TECHNIQUES IN BIRTH DEFECTS SURVEILLANCE IN:KLINGBERG MA WEATHERALL JAC (EDS) CONTRIBUTIONS TO EPIDEMIOLOGY AND BIOSTATISTICS VOL 1 EPIDEMIOLOGIC METHODS FOR THE DETECTION OF TERATOGENS
BASEL:KARGER, 1979 :184-189

CHEN R WEISSMAN SL SALAMA R KLINGBERG MA
CONGENITAL DISLOCATION OF THE HIP (CDH) AND SEASONALITY: THE GESTATIONAL AGE OF VULNERABILITY TO SOME SEASONAL FACTORS
AM J EPIDEMIOL 1970 92:287-293

CNATTINGIUS S ERICSON A GUNNARSKOG J KALLEN B
A QUALITY STUDY OF A MEDICAL BIRTH REGISTRY
SCAND J SOC MED 1990 143-8

CNATTINGIUS S ERICSON A KALLEN B
THE MEDICAL BIRTH RECORD - EVALUATION OF CONTENTS AND PROPOSAL FOR IMPROVEMENT (SWE)
JORDEMODERN 1989 102:18-23

COCCHI G CALZOLARI E CONTRINO C MAGNANI C RONCARATI E
THE EMILIA-ROMAGNA CONGENITAL MALFORMATIONS STUDY GROUP: COVERAGE AND GEOGRAPHIC DISTRIBUTION OF CONGENITAL MALFORMATIONS IN EMILIA-ROMAGNA (ITA)
PEDIATR MED CHIR 1982 4:501-4

COCCHI G MORINI MS
CENTRAL NERVOUS SYSTEM MALFORMATIONS NEONATAL MEDICAL PROBLEMS
FETAL THER 1986 1:83-86

COCCHI G MORINI MS CALZOLARI E MAGNANI C RONCARATI E CONTRINO C
SENSITIVITY OF ULTRASOUND IN DETECTION OF CENTRAL NERVOUS SYSTEM CONGENITAL MALFORMATIONS
EUR J EPIDEMIOL 1986 2:329

COCCHI G BERRA E MORINI MS RICCI R SALVIOLI GP
STILLBIRTH AND CONGENITAL MALFORMATIONS: A 6 YEAR SURVEY IN THE IMER CENTER OF BOLOGNA (ITA)
ACTA PAEDIATRICA LATINA 1988 41:895-98

COCCHI G MORINI MS RICCI R LANARI M CACCIARI A RIZZO N BOVICELLI L SALVIOLI GP
URINARY TRACT ABNORMALITIES: THE IMPACT OF PRENATAL DIAGNOSIS. DATA OF IMER CENTER OF BOLOGNA (ITA)
ACTA PAEDIATRICA LATINA 1988 41:82-88

COCCHI G MORINI MS SANDRI F
BIRTH DEFECTS OF CENTRAL NERVOUS SYSTEM: EPIDEMIOLOGICAL AND CLINICAL REMARKS (ITA)
DOCTOR PED 1987 10:57-64

COCCHI G RICCI R MORINI MS SANDRI F FOSCHI F SALVIOLI GP
AGENESIS OF THE CORPUS CALLOSUM. EPIDEMIOLOGICAL AND CLINICAL DATA IN 13 NEWBORN INFANTS (ITA)
ACTA PAEDIATRICA LATINA 1990 43:104-10

COCCHI G RICCI R MORINI MS SALVIOLO GP
THE KLIPPEL-TRENAUNAY-WEBER SYNDROME. REPORT OF 3 CASES (ITA)
ACTA PAEDIATRICA LATINA 1986 39:465-71

COCHI SL EDMONDS LD DYER K GREAVES WL MARKS JS ROVIRA EZ PREBLUD SR ORENSTEIN WA
CONGENITAL RUBELLA SYNDROME IN THE UNITED STATES 1970-85: ON THE VERGE OF ELIMINATION
AM J EPIDEMIOL 1989 129:349-261

COMELLINI L PICCHIO FM PRANDSTRALLER D COCCHI G LAMBERTI A LUCCHI A SALVIOLI GP MAGNANI B
CONGENITAL HEARTH DISEASES IN THE NEWBORN. CRITICAL REVIEW OF OUR EXPERIENCE IN 208 CASES II ANALYSIS OF CASE RECORDS AND CLINICO-DIAGNOSTIC AND THERAPEUTIC CONSIDERATIONS (ITA)
MINERVA PEDIATR 1984 36:621-34

COMELLINI L PICCHIO FM PRANDSTRALLER D COCCHI G LAMBERTI A LUCCHI A SALVIOLI GP MAGNANI B
CONGENITAL HEART DISEASES IN THE NEWBORN INFANT. CRITICAL REVIEW OF OUR EXPERIENCES IN 208 CASES I PREVENTION OF CASE REPORTS (ITA)
MINERVA PEDIATR 1984 36:863-71

CONNOLLY JH NEVIN NC SIMPSON DM O'NEILL HJ
OUTCOME OF PREGNANCY IN A RUBELLA OUTBREAK IN NORTHERN IRELAND 1978-79
ULSTER MED J 1984 53:65-73

CORDERO JF
ISSUES CONCERNING AIDS EMBRYOPATHY? (LETTER)
AM J DIS CHILD 1988 142:9

CORDERO JF
DRUGS AS TERATOGENS: CLINICAL FINDINGS (SPA)
IDEPSA 1988 28-35

CORDERO JF
EFFECT OF ENVIRONMENTAL AGENTS ON PREGNANCY OUTCOMES: DISTURBANCES OF PRENATAL GROWTH AND DEVELOPMENT
MED CLIN NORTH AM 1990 74:279-90

CORDERO JF LAYDE PM
VAGINAL SPERMICIDES. CHROMOSOMAL ABNORMALITIES AND LIMB REDUCTION DEFECTS
FAMILY PLANNING PERSP 1983 15:16-18

CORDERO JF OAKLEY GP JR
DRUG EXPOSURE DURING PREGNANCY: SOME EPIDEMIOLOGIC CONSIDERATIONS
CLIN OBSTET GYNECOL 1983 26:418-428

CORDERO JF OAKLEY GP JR GREENBERG F JAMES LM
IS BENDECTIN A TERATOGEN?
JAMA 1981 245:2307-2310

CORDIER S GOUJARD J
METHODOLOGICAL ISSUES FOR THE STUDY OF THE RISK ASSOCIATED WITH OCCUPATIONAL EXPOSURE TO POTENTIAL TERATOGENS IN: DE WALS PH LECHAT M (EDS) EUROCAT REPORT 2 SURVEILLANCE OF CONGENITAL ANOMALIES YEARS
BRUXELLES, 1987 228-234

CORDIER S GOUJARD DE WALS PH
COLLABORATIVE STUDY ON ENVIRONNMENT AND PREGNANCY
EUROCAT GUIDE 4, UNIVERISTY CATHOLIC OF LOUVAIN BRUSSELS 1989

CZEIZEL A
COXSACKIEVIRUS AND CONGENITAL MALFORMATION
J AMER MED ASS 1967 201:142

CZEIZEL A
EFFECTS OF INFLUENZA ON PREGNANCY
LANCET 1967 II:517

CZEIZEL A
MAJOR MALFORMATIONS OF THE CENTRAL NERVOUS SYSTEM IN HUNGARY
BR J PREV SOC MED 1970 24:205

CZEIZEL A
AN EPIDEMIOLOGIC STUDY OF CLEFT LIP WITH OR WITHOUT CLEFT PALATE AND POSTERIOR CLEFT PALATE IN HUNGARY
HUM HERED 1971 21:17

CZEIZEL A
INCIDENCE OF CONGENITAL HEART DEFECTS IN BUDAPEST
ACTA PAED ACAD SCI HUNG 1972 13:191

CZEIZEL A
INCIDENCE AND RECURRENCE RISK OF COMMON CONGENITAL MALFORMATIONS IN BUDAPEST IN THE SIXTIES
ACTA UNIV CAROL (MED MONOGR , PRAHA) 1973 56:49-51

CZEIZEL A
THE HUNGARIAN CONGENITAL MALFORMATION REGISTER
ACTA UNIV CAROL (MED MONOGR , PRAHA) 1973 56:53-57

CZEIZEL A
SURVEILLANCE OF CONGENITAL ANOMALIES IN HUNGARY
ACTA PAED ACAD SCI HUNG 1976 17:123-134

CZEIZEL A
DIAZEPAM PHENYTOIN AND AETIOLOGY OF CLEFT LIP AND/OR CLEFT PALATE (LETTER)
LANCET 1976 1:810

CZEIZEL A
INCREASE OF UPPER LIMB REDUCTION DEFORMITIES IN HUNGARY
LANCET 1976 I:701

CZEIZEL A
MULTIFACTORIAL AETIOLOGY OF COMMON CONGENITAL MALFORMATIONS
BUDAPEST: MEDICAL GENETICS, EDS, SZABÒ G, PAPP Z, AKADÈMIAI KIADÒ 1977 411

CZEIZEL A
THE BASELINE DATA OF THE HUNGARIAN CONGENITAL MALFORMATION REGISTER 1970-1976
ACTA PAED ACAD SCI HUNG 1978 19:149-156

CZEIZEL A
THE HUNGARIAN CONGENITAL MALFORMATION MONITORING SYSTEM
ACTA PAED ACAD SCI HUNG 1978 19:225-238

CZEIZEL A
RECURRENCE RISK OF OMPHALOCELE (LETTER)
LANCET 1979 2:470

CZEIZEL A
ARE CONTRACEPTIVE PILLS TERATOGENIC?
ACTA MORPH ACAD SCI HUNG 1980 28:177-188

CZEIZEL A
STUDIES OF CLEFT LIP AND CLEFT PALATE IN EAST EUROPEAN POPULATIONS
PROG CLIN BIOL RES 1980 46:249-296

CZEIZEL A
TERATOGENESIS
PERINATAL MED 1980 :193-225

CZEIZEL A
SCHISIS-ASSOCIATION
AM J MED GENET 1981 10:25-35

CZEIZEL A
DEFINITION OF MULTIPLE CONGENITAL ABNORMALITIES
ACTA MORPH ACAD SCI HUNG 1981 29:251-258

CZEIZEL A
BIRTH PREVALENCES OF MORE FREQUENT CONGENITAL ABNORMALITIES IN HUNGARY
HUMANBIOL 1982 11:123-5

CZEIZEL A
SPINA BIFIDA AND ANENCEPHALY (LETTER)
BR MED J 1983 287:429

CZEIZEL A
NEW LETHAL OMPHALOCELE-CLEFT PALATE SYNDROME?
HUM GENET 1983 64:99

CZEIZEL A
FURTHER INVESTIGATIONS WHEN ABDOMINAL WALL DEFECTS ARE DIAGNOSED IN UTERO
LANCET 1983 II:1084

CZEIZEL A
SPINA BIFIDA AND ANENCEPHALY
LANCET 1983 II:429

CZEIZEL A
RE: INCIDENCE AND PREVALENCE AS MEASURES OF THE FREQUENCY OF BIRTH DEFECTS (LETTER)
AM J EPIDEMIOL 1984 119:141-142

CZEIZEL A
TERATOEPIDEMIOLOGY
PROG CLIN BIOL RES 1985 163 B:7-10

CZEIZEL A
INCREASING TRENDS IN CONGENITAL MALFORMATIONS OF MALE EXTERNAL GENITALIA (LETTER)
LANCET 1985 I:462-463

CZEIZEL A
CASE-CONTROL SURVEILLANCE SYSTEM OF CONGENITAL ANOMALIES IN RELATION TO OCCUPATIONAL EXPOSURES
NEW YORK: ALAN R LISS INC 1986:195-199

CZEIZEL A
POLYCYSTIC KIDNEY AND CARDIOVASCULAR MALFORMATION ASSOCIATION
AM J MED GENET 1986 SUPPL 2:17-21

CZEIZEL A
GENITAL ANOMALIES OF MALES (GAM-COMPLEX)
EUR J PEDIATR 1987 146:181-183

CZEIZEL A
PRENATAL DIAGNOSIS POLICY IN NEURAL TUBE DEFECTS (LETTER)
AM J MED GENET 1987 27:991-2

CZEIZEL A
FAMILIAL SITUS INVERSUS AND CONGENITAL HEART DEFECTS
AM J MED GENET 1987 28:227-228

CZEIZEL A
BILIARY DYSGENESIS AND CONGENITAL CARDIOVASCULAR MALFORMATION ASSOCIATION
ACTA PAED ACAD SCI HUNG 1987 28:63-80

CZEIZEL A
LACK OF EVIDENCE OF TERATOGENICITY OF BENZODIAZEPINE DRUGS IN HUNGARY
REPROD TOXICOL 1988 1:183-8

CZEIZEL A
NEURAL TUBE DEFECTS (LETTER)
JAMA 1988 259:3562

CZEIZEL A
RESERPINE IS NOT A HUMAN TERATOGEN
J MED GENET 1988 25:787

CZEIZEL A
ADDITIVE CONGENITAL ANOMALY PATTERNS
AM J MED GENET 1988 29:727-738

CZEIZEL A
SOME EPIDEMIOLOGICAL CHARACTERISTICS OF DOWN'S SYNDROME IN HUNGARY
ACTA MORPH ACAD SCI HUNG 1988 36:63-77

CZEIZEL A
THE ACTIVITIES OF THE HUNGARIAN CENTRE FOR CONGENITAL ANOMALY CONTROL
WHO STAT REP QUART 1988 41:219-27

CZEIZEL A
MATERNAL MORTALITY, FETAL DEATH, CONGENITAL ANOMALIES AND INFANT MORTALITY AT AN ADVANCED MATERNAL AGE
MATURITAS 1988 SUPPL 1:73-81

CZEIZEL A
POPULATION SURVEILLANCE OF SENTINEL ANOMALIES
MUTAT RES 1989 212:3-9

CZEIZEL A
TERATOGENICITY OF ERGOTAMINE
J MED GENET 1989 26:69-70

CZEIZEL A
A FAMILY STUDY OF CASES WITH UNIDENTIFIED MULTIPLE CONGENITAL ABNORMALITY
ACTA PAED ACAD SCI HUNG 1989 29:317-29

CZEIZEL A
DRUG USE DURING PREGNANCY IN HUNGARY
ACTA MED HUNG 1989 46:53-62

CZEIZEL A
HUNGARIAN SURVEILLANCE OF GERMINAL MUTATIONS. LACK OF DETECTABLE INCREASE IN INDICATOR CONDITIONS CAUSED BY GERMINAL MUTATIONS FOLLOWING THE CHERNOBYL ACCIDENT
HUM GENET 1989 82:359-66

CZEIZEL A
OVULATION INDUCTION AND NEURAL TUBE DEFECTS (LETTER)
LANCET 1989 II:167

CZEIZEL A BELLYEI A KRANICZ J MOCSAI L TUSNADY G
CONFIRMATION OF THE MULTIFACTORIAL THRESHOLD MODEL FOR CONGENITAL STRUCTURAL TALIPES EQUINOVARUS
J MED GENET 1981 18:99-100

CZEIZEL A BOD M LENZ W
FAMILY STUDY OF CONGENITAL LIMB REDUCTION ABNORMALITIES IN HUNGARY 1975-77
HUM GENET 1983 65:34-45

CZEIZEL A BROOSER G
POSTAXIAL POLYDACTYLY AND PROGRESSIVE MYOPIA SYNDROME OF AUTOSOMAL DOMINANT INHERITANCE
CLIN GENET 1986 30:406-8

CZEIZEL A ERODI E TOTH J
AN EPIDEMIOLOGICAL STUDY ON UNDESCENDED TESTIS
J UROL 1981 126:524-27

CZEIZEL A FRITZ G
ETHICS OF A RANDOMIZED TRIAL OF PERICONCEPTUAL VITAMINS (LETTER)
JAMA 1989 262:1634

CZEIZEL A GOBLYOS P
FAMILIAL COMBINATION OF BRACHYDACTYLY TYPE E AND ATRIAL DEFECT TYPE II
EUR J PEDIATR 1989 149:117-9

CZEIZEL A HUISKES N
A CASE-CONTROL STUDY TO EVALUATE THE RISK OF CONGENITAL ANOMALIES AS A RESULT OF ALLYLESTRENOL THERAPY DURING PREGNANCY
CLIN THERAPEUTICS 1988 LO:725-39

CZEIZEL A KAMARAS J BALOGH O SZENTPETERI J
INCIDENCE OF CONGENITAL HEART DEFECTS IN BUDAPEST
ACTA PAED ACAD SCI HUNG 1972 13:191-202

CZEIZEL A KARIG G
ANALYSIS OF THE CHANGING BIRTH PREVALENCE OF NEURAL TUBE DEFECTS IN HUNGARY
ACTA MORPH ACAD SCI HUNG 1985 33:89-99

CZEIZEL A KELLER I BOD M
AN AETIOLOGICAL EVALUATION OF INCREASED OCCURRENCE OF CONGENITAL LIMB REDUCTION ABNORMALITIES IN HUNGARY 1975-78
J EPIDEMIOL 1983 12:445-9

CZEIZEL A KEREKES L MERETEY K OSZTOVICS M SOBEL M STUBER A TARRO S
NATIONAL PROGRAMME FOR PREVENTION OF THE RECURRENCE OF NEURAL TUBE DEFECTS
ACTA PAED ACAD SCI HUNG 1979 20:315-319

CZEIZEL A KISS P OSZTOVICS M PAZONYI I
NATIONWIDE INVESTIGATION OF MULTIPLE MALFORMATIONS
ACTA PAED ACAD SCI HUNG 1978 19:275-280

CZEIZEL A KISS R RACZ K MOHORI K GLAZ EDIT
CASE-CONTROL CYTOGENETIC STUDY IN OFFSPRING OF MOTHERS TREATED WITH BROMOCRIPTINE DURING EARLY PREGNANCY
MUTAT RES 1989 210:23-7

CZEIZEL A KOVACS M
A FAMILY STUDY OF CONGENITAL DIAPHRAGMATIC DEFECTS
AM J MED GENET 1985 21:105-117

CZEIZEL A KOVACS M KISS P MEHES K SZABO L OLAH E KOSZTOLANYI G SCEMERE G KOVACS H FEKETE G
A NATIONWIDE EVALUATION OF MULTIPLE CONGENITAL ABNORMALITIES IN HUNGARY
GENET EPIDEMIOL 1988 5:183-202

CZEIZEL A LENDVAY A
IN UTERO EXPOSURE TO BENZODIAZEPINES
LANCET 1987 I:627

CZEIZEL A LENDVAY A
ATTEMPTED SUICIDE AND PREGNANCY
AM J OBSTET GYNECOL 1989 161:497

CZEIZEL A LOSONCI A
SPLIT HAND, OBSTRUCTIVE URINARY ANOMALIES AND SPINA BIFIDA OR DIAPHRAGMATIC DEFECT SYNDROME WITH AUTOSOMAL DOMINANT INHERITANCE
HUM GENET 1987 77:203-4

CZEIZEL A LUDANYI I
VACTERL-ASSOCIATION
ACTA MORPH ACAD SCI HUNG 1984 32:75-96

CZEIZEL A LUDANYI I
AN AETIOLOGICAL STUDY OF THE VACTERL-ASSOCIATION
EUR J PEDIATR 1985 144:331-337

CZEIZEL A MESZAROS M
TWO FAMILY STUDIES OF CHILDREN WITH VENTRICULAR SEPTAL DEFECT
EUR J PEDIATR 1981 136:81-85

CZEIZEL A METNEKI J
EMPIRICAL RECURRENCE RISK AFTER UNIDENTIFIED MULTIPLE CONGENITAL ABNORMALITIES
J MED GENET 1983 20:367-371

CZEIZEL A METNEKI J
RECURRENCE RISK AFTER NEURAL TUBE DEFECTS IN A GENETIC COUNSELLING CLINIC
J MED GENET 1984 21:413-416

CZEIZEL A METNEKI J
EVALUATION OF COUNSELLING FOR PREGNANT WOMEN EXPOSED TO POTENTIALLY HAZARDOUS ENVIRONMENTAL FACTORS
ACTA PAED ACAD SCI HUNG 1985 26:175-185

CZEIZEL A NAGY E
A RECENT AETIOLOGICAL STUDY ON FACIAL CLEFTING IN HUNGARY
ACTA PAED ACAD SCI HUNG 1986 27:145-66

CZEIZEL A PAZONYI I
INCREASE OF UPPER-LIMB REDUCTION DEFORMITIES IN HUNGARY (LETTER)
LANCET 1976 1:701

CZEIZEL A PAZSY A PUSZTAI J NAGY M
AETIOLOGICAL MONITOR OF CONGENITAL ABNORMALITIES: A CASE-CONTROL SURVEILLANCE SYSTEM
ACTA PAED ACAD SCI HUNG 1983 24:91-9

CZEIZEL A PAZSY A TELEGDI L TUSNADY G
CLASSIFICATION AND REGISTRATION OF MULTIPLE CONGENITAL ABNORMALITIES
ACTA MORPH ACAD SCI HUNG 1981 29:377-390

CZEIZEL A PORNOI A PETERFFY E TARCAL E
STUDY OF CHILDREN OF PARENTS OPERATED ON FOR CONGENITAL CARDIOVASCULAR MALFORMATIONS
BR HEART J 1982 47:290-293

CZEIZEL A REVESZ C
MAJOR MALFORMATIONS OF THE CENTRAL NERVOUS SYSTEM IN HUNGARY
BR J PREV SOC MED 1970 24:205-222

CZEIZEL A RODE K
TRIAL TO PREVENT FIRST OCCURRENCE OF NEURAL TUBE DEFECTS BY PERICONCEPTIONAL MULTIVITAMIN SUPPLEMENTATION (LETTER)
LANCET 1984 2:40

CZEIZEL A SANKARANARAYANAN K
THE LOAD OF GENETIC AND PARTIALLY GENETIC DISORDERS IN MAN. I CONGENITAL ANOMALIES: ESTIMATES OF DETRIMENT IN TERMS OF YEARS OF LIFE LOST ANY YEARS OF IMPAIRED LIFE
MUTAT RES 1984 128:73-103

CZEIZEL A SZABUKA M BOD M PAZONYI I VACZO GY TUSNADY G
ETIOLOGICAL EVALUATION OF BABIES WITH CONGENITAL LIMB REDUCTION MALFORMATIONS BORN IN 1975 (HUN)
ORV HETIL 1978 119:1025-1029

CZEIZEL A SZENTESI I MOLNAR G
LACK OF EFFECT OF SELF-POISONING ON SUBSEQUENT REPRODUCTIVE OUTCOME
MUTAT RES 1984 127:175-82

CZEIZEL A SZENTESI I SZEKERES I GLAUBER A BUCSKI P MOLNÀR GY
PREGNANCY OUTCOME AND HEALTH CONDITIONS OF OFFSPRING OF SELF-POISONING PREGNANT WOMEN
ACTA PAED ACAD SCI HUNG 1984 25:209-36

CZEIZEL A TELEGDI L TUSNADY G
A MULTIDIMENSIONAL THRESHOLD MODEL FOR MULTIPLE CONGENITAL ABNORMALITIES
ACTA PAED ACAD SCI HUNG 1986 27:189-204

CZEIZEL A TELEGDI L TUSNADY G (EDS)
MULTIPLE CONGENITAL ABNORMALITIES
BUDAPEST: AKADEMIAI KIADO 1988 1-463

CZEIZEL A TOTH J CZVENITS E
INCREASED BIRTH PREVALENCE OF ISOLATED HYPOSPADIAS IN HUNGARY
ACTA PAED ACAD SCI HUNG 1986 27:329-37

CZEIZEL A TOTH J ERODI E
AETIOLOGICAL STUDIES OF HYPOSPADIAS IN HUNGARY
HUM HERED 1979 29:166-171

CZEIZEL A TUSNADI G
AN EPIDEMIOLOGIC STUDY OF CLEFT LIP WITH OR WITHOUT CLEFT PALATE AND POSTERIOR CLEFT PALATE IN HUNGARY
HUM HERED 1971 21:17-38

CZEIZEL A TUSNADY G
A FAMILY STUDY ON CLEFT LIP WITH OR WITHOUT CLEFT PALATE AND POSTERIOR CLEFT PALATE IN HUNGARY
HUM HERED 1972 22:405-416

CZEIZEL A TUSNADY G
AETIOLOGICAL STUDIES OF ISOLATED COMMON CONGENITAL ABNORMALITIES IN HUNGARY
BUDAPEST:AKADEMIAI KIADO, 1984

CZEIZEL A VITEZ M
BIRTH PREVALENCE OF FIVE CONGENITAL ABNORMALITIES OF MEDIUM FREQUENCY IN BUDAPEST
ACTA PAED ACAD SCI HUNG 1981 22:299-308

CZEIZEL A VITEZ M
ETIOLOGICAL STUDY OF OMPHALOCELE
HUM GENET 1981 58:390-395

DANZON A ROBERT E COLLET JP ROBERT JM
ATRESIA OF THE ESOPHAGUS STUDY OF A CLUSTER OBSERVED IN 1984 IN THE RHONE-ALPES REGION (FRE)
ARCH FR PEDIATR 1988 45:231-5

DE LA MATA I DE WALS P DOLK H LECHAT MF BECKERS R BORLEE I LYS F ZORI R GOUJARD J STOLL C ET AL
INCIDENCE OF CONGENITAL RUBELLA SYNDROME IN 19 REGIONS OF EUROPE IN 1980-86
EUR J EPIDEMIOL 1989 5:106-9

DENES J ZISZI K BOGNAR M SCHLAFFER E TOTH J
CONGENITAL SHORT COLON ASSOCIATED WITH IMPERFORATE ANUS (ZACHARY-MORGAN SYNDROME)
ACTA PAED ACAD SCI HUNG 1984 25:377-383

DESSEMOND M BOSCHETTI R MAMELLE N
SYSTEMATIC REGISTRATION OF MALFORMATIONS (FRE)
J GENET HUM 1975 SUPPL 23:50-57

DOLK H DE WALS P LECHAT MF GOUJARD J STOLL C ET AL
PRELIMINARY EVALUATION OF THE IMPACT OF THE CHERNOBYL RADIOLOGICAL CONTAMINATION ON THE FREQUENCY OF CENTRAL NERVOUS SYSTEM MALFORMATIONS IN 18 REGIONS OF EUROPE
PAEDIATR PERINATAL EPIDEMIOL 1988 2:253-64

DOMANY Z SEREGELY G CZEIZEL A
CHROMOSOME EXAMINATIONS FOLLOWING TREATMENT WITH CONTRACEPTIVE PILLS PRODUCED IN HUNGARY (HUNG)
HUNG MED J 1975 23:50

DUDORKINOVA D KUCERA J
SYNDROME OF CAUDAL REGRESSION WITH ARTHROGRYPOSIS MULTIPLEX CONGENITA AND SIGNS OF OTHER SYNDROMES IN A BABY OF DIABETIC MOTHER (CZE)
PRAKT LEK 1983 64:758-760

EDMONDS L WINDHAM G
TRENDS IN THE INCIDENCE OF NEURAL TUBE DEFECTS IN THE US. PROCEEDINGS BIRTH DEFECTS INSTITUTE SYMPOSIUM XIV 1983. IN: MIZEJEWSKI GJ PORTER IH (EDS) ALPHA-FETOPROTEIN AND CONGENITAL DISORDERS
FLORIDA, ACADEMIC PRESS INC 1985 295-308

EDMONDS LD ANDERSON CE FLYNT JW JR JAMES LM
CONGENITAL CENTRAL NERVOUS SYSTEM MALFORMATIONS AND VINYL CHLORIDE MONOMER EXPOSURE: A COMMUNITY STUDY
TERATOLOGY 1978 17:137-142

EDMONDS LD FALK H NISSIM JE
CONGENITAL MALFORMATIONS AND VINYL CHLORIDE (LETTER)
LANCET 1975 1098

EDMONDS LD JAMES LM
TEMPORAL TRENDS IN THE INCIDENCE OF MALFORMATIONS IN THE UNITED STATES SELECTED YEARS 1970-71 1982-83
MMWR SURVEILL SUMM 1985 34:1

EDMONDS LD LAYDE PM
CONJOINED TWINS IN THE UNITED STATES 1970-1977
TERATOLOGY 1982 25:301-308

EDMONDS LD LAYDE PM ERICKSON JD
AIRPORT NOISE AND TERATOGENESIS
ARCH ENVIRON HEALTH 1979 34:243-247

EDMONDS LD LAYDE PM ERICKSON JD FLYNT JW JR ERICKSON JD OAKLEY GB JR
CONGENITAL MALFORMATIONS SURVEILLANCE: TWO AMERICAN SYSTEMS
INT J EPIDEMIOL 1981 10:247-252

EDSTROM R KALLEN B
DATA DISPLAY SCREEN OPERATORS DURING PREGNANCY-NO CONCLUSIVE EVIDENCE FOR DAMAGE TO FETUS (SWE)
LAKARTIDNINGEN 1985 82:687-8

EGENAES J BJERKEDAL T
OCCURRENCE OF GASTROSCHISIS AND OMPHALOCELE IN NORWAY 1967-1979 (NOR)
TIDSSKR NOR LAEGEFOREN 1982 102:172-176

ELWOOD JH NEVIN NC
FACTORS ASSOCIATED WITH ANENCEPHALUS AND SPINA BIFIDA IN BELFAST
BR J PREV SOC MED 1973 27:73-80

ELWOOD JH NEVIN NC
ANENCEPHALUS AND SPINA BIFIDA IN BELFAST
ULSTER MED J 1973 42:213-222

ENSLEIN K LANDER TR STRANGE JR
TERATOGENESIS: A STATISTICAL STRUCTURE-ACTIVITY MODEL
TERATO CARCINOG MUTAG 1983 3:289-309

ERICKSON JD
RACIAL VARIATIONS IN THE INCIDENCE OF CONGENITAL MALFORMATIONS
ANN HUM GENET 1976 39:315-20

ERICKSON JD
DOWN SYNDROME PATERNAL AGE, MATERNAL AGE AND BIRTH ORDER
ANN HUM GENET 1978 41:289-98

ERICKSON JD
PATERNAL AGE AND DOWN SYNDROME
AM J HUM GENET 1979 31:489-497

ERICKSON JD
DOWN SYNDROME, WATER FLUORIDATION AND MATERNAL AGE
TERATOLOGY 1980 21:177-180

ERICKSON JD
EPIDEMIOLOGY AND DEVELOPMENTAL TOXICOLOGY. IN: KIMMEL CA BUELKE-SAM J (EDS) MONOGRAPH ON DEVELOPMENTAL TOXICOLOGY
NEW YORK: RAVEN PRESS, 1981 289-301

ERICKSON JD
PARENTAL OCCUPATION AND BIRTH DEFECTS
R SOC MED 1983

ERICKSON JD
ASSESSING OCCUPATIONAL HAZARDS AND REPRODUCTION: USES OF EXISTING DATA SETS. IN: LOCKEY JE LEMASTERS GK KEYE WR (EDS) REPRODUCTION: THE NEW FRONTIER IN OCCUPATIONAL AND ENVIRONMENTAL HEALTH AND RESEARCH
NEW YORK: ALAN R LISS INC 1984

ERICKSON JD
BIRTH DEFECTS AND PARENTAL OCCUPATION. IN: CHAMBERLAIN G (ED) PREGNANT WOMEN AT WORK
LONDON: THE MACMILLAN PRESS 1984 61-72

ERICKSON JD BJERKEDAL T
DOWN SYNDROME ASSOCIATED WITH FATHER'S AGE IN NORWAY
J MED GENET 1981 18:22-28

ERICKSON JD COCHRAN WM ANDERSON CE
BIRTH DEFECTS AND PRINTING (LETTER)
LANCET 1978 1:385

ERICKSON JD COCHRAN WM ANDERSON CE
PARENTAL OCCUPATION AND BIRTH DEFECTS. A PRELIMINARY REPORT
CONTR EPIDEMIOL BIOSTAT 1979 1:107-17

ERICKSON JD MULINARE J
VIETNAM VETERANS' RISK FOR FATHERING CHILDREN WITH BIRTH DEFECTS (LETTER)
JAMA 1985 254:609-610

ERICKSON JD MULINARE J
AGENT ORANGE AND RISKS TO REPRODUCTION: THE LIMITS OF EPIDEMIOLOGY (LETTER)
TERATO CARCINOG MUTAG 1987 7:197-200

ERICKSON JD MULINARE J JAMES LM FITCH TG
DESIGN AND EXECUTION OF A VERY LARGE BIRTH-DEFECTS CASE-CONTROL STUDY
PROG CLIN BIOL RES 1985 163B:273-7

ERICKSON JD MULINARE J MCCLAIN PW FITCH TG JAMES LM MCCLEARN AB ADAMS MJ JR
VIETNAM VETERANS' RISKS FOR FATHERING BABIES WITH BIRTH DEFECTS
JAMA 1984 252:903-12

ERICKSON JD OAKLEY GP JR FLYNT JW JR HAY S
WATER FLUORIDATION AND CONGENITAL MALFORMATIONS: NO ASSOCIATION
J AM DENT ASSOC 1976 84:244-246

ERICSON A ERIKSSON M KALLEN B WESTERHOLM P ZETTERSTROM R
DELIVERY OUTCOME OF WOMEN WORKING IN LABORATORIES DURING PREGNANCY
ARCH ENVIRON HEALTH 1984 39:5-10

ERICSON A ERIKSSON M KALLEN B ZETTERSTROM R
MATERNAL OCCUPATION AND DELIVERY OUTCOME: A STUDY USING CENTRAL REGISTRY DATA
ACTA PAEDIATR SCAND 1987 76:512-518

ERICSON A ERIKSSON M KALLEN B ZETTERSTROM R
SOCIO-ECONOMIC VARIABLES AND PREGNANCY OUTCOME BIRTHWEIGHT IN SINGELTONS
ACTA PAEDIATR SCAND (SUPPL) 1989 360:48-55

ERICSON A ERIKSSON M WESTERHOLM P ZETTERSTROM R
PREGNANCY OUTCOME AND SOCIAL INDICATORS IN SWEDEN
ACTA PAEDIATR SCAND 1984 73:69-74

ERICSON A ERIKSSON M ZETTERSTROM R
THE INCIDENCE OF CONGENITAL MALFORMATIONS IN VARIOUS SOCIOECONOMIC GROUPS IN SWEDEN
ACTA PAEDIATR SCAND 1984 73:664-666

ERICSON A KALLEN B
GEOGRAPHICAL DISTRIBUTION OF ABNORMALITIES AND PERINATAL MORTALITY IN SWEDEN (SWE)
LAKARTIDNINGEN 1977 74:2189-2190

ERICSON A KALLEN B
SURVEY OF INFANTS BORN IN 1973 OR 1975 TO SWEDISH WOMEN WORKING IN OPERATING ROOMS DURING THEIR PREGNANCIES
ANESTH ANALG 1979 58:302-305

ERICSON A KALLEN B
HOSPITALIZATION FOR MISCARRIAGE AND DELIVERY OUTCOME AMONG SWEDISH NURSES WORKING IN OPERATING ROOMS 1973-1978
ANESTH ANALG (CLEVE) 1985 64:981-988

ERICSON A KALLEN B
AN EPIDEMIOLOGICAL STUDY OF WORK WITH VIDEO SCREENS AND PREGNANCY OUTCOME I A REGISTRY STUDY
AM J IND MED 1986 9:447

ERICSON A KALLEN B
AN EPIDEMIOLOGICAL STUDY OF WORK WITH VIDEO SCREENS AND PREGNANCY OUTCOME II A CASE-CONTROL STUDY
AM J IND MED 1986 9:459

ERICSON A KALLEN B
PREGNANCY OUTCOME IN WOMEN WORKING AS DENTISTS, DENTAL ASSISTANTS OR DENTAL TECHNICIANS
INT ARCH OCCUP ENVIRON HEALTH 1989 61:329

ERICSON A KALLEN B LINDSTEN J
LACK OF CORRELATION BETWEEN CONTRACEPTIVE PILLS AND DOWN'S SYDROME
ACTA OBST GYNE SCAND 1983 62:511-514

ERICSON A KALLEN B LOFKVIST E
ENVIRONMENTAL FACTORS IN THE ETIOLOGY OF NEURAL TUBE DEFECTS: A NEGATIVE STUDY
ENVIRON RES 1988 45:38-47

ERICSON A KALLEN B MEIRIK O WESTERHOLM P
GASTROINTESTINAL ATRESIA AND MATERNAL OCCUPATION DURING PREGNANCY
J OCCUP MED 1982 24:515-518

ERICSON A KALLEN B MEYER-LIE AK
DELIVERY OF MALFORMED CHILDREN AND PERINATAL MORTALITY IN VARMLAND - STUDY WITH THE USE OF CENTRAL REGISTRIES (SWE)
LAKARTIDNINGEN 1977 74:634-636

ERICSON A KALLEN B WESTERHOLM P
CIGARETTE SMOKING AS AN ETIOLOGIC FACTOR IN CLEFT LIP AND PALATE
AM J OBSTET GYNECOL 1979 135:348-351

ERICSON A KALLEN B WESTERHOLM P
CLUSTERS OF MALFORMATIONS IN SWEDEN: A STUDY WITH CENTRAL REGISTERS
ENVIRON RES 1983 30:466-79

ERICSON A KALLEN B WESTERHOLM P
THE HEALTH INSURANCE STUDY: NO INCREASED RISK FOR FETAL ABNORMALITIES IN WOMEN WORKING WITH VIDEO DISPLAY TERMINALS (SWE)
LAKARTIDNINGEN 1985 82:2180-4

ERICSON A KALLEN B WINBERG J
SURVEILLANCE OF MALFORMATIONS AT BIRTH: A COMPARISON OF TWO RECORD SYSTEMS RUN IN PARALLEL
INT J EPIDEMIOL 1977 6:35-41

ERICSON A WESTERHOLM B WESTERHOLM P
COMMITTEE OF THE NATIONAL BOARD OF HEALTH AND SOCIAL WELFARE ON DEFORMITY PROBLEMS - A RETROSPECTIVE STUDY (SWE)
LAKARTIDNINGEN 1980 77:324-6

ETESON DJ ADOMIAN GE ORNOY A KOIDE T SUGIURA Y CALABRO A LUNGAROTTI S MASTROIACOVO P LACHMAN RS RIMOIN DL
FIBROCHONDROGENESIS: RADIOLOGIC AND HISTOLOGIC STUDIES
AM J MED GENET 1984 19:277-90

EUROCAT WORKING GROUP
PRELIMINARY EVALUATION OF THE CHERNOBYL RADIOLOGICAL CONTAMINATION OM THE FREQUANCY OF CENTRAL NERVOUS SYETM MALFORMATIONS IN 18 REGIONS OF EUROPE
PERINATAL EPIDEMIOLOGY 1988 2:252-264

EUROCAT WORKING GROUP
THE PREVALENCE AT BIRTH OF DOWN SYNDROME IN 19 REGIONS OF EUROPE 1980-1986. IN: KEY ISSUES IN MENTAL RETADATION RESEARCH
LONDON: FRASER 1990 3-11

FABRIS C PRANDI GM GARZENA E LICATA D MASTROIACOVO P
INIENCEFALIA
RIV ITAL PEDIATR 1988 14:133-4

FAVIER M FAVIER A ROBERT E GUIGNIER M MALINAS Y
CAN ZINC DEFICIENCY IN THE MOTHER BE RESPONSIBLE FOR THE OCCURRENCE OF SPINA BIFIDA APERTA IN THE FETUS? (FRE)
REV FR GYNECOL OBSTET 1987 82:575-81

FERNHOFF PM BLACKSTON RD OAKLEY GP JR
INTRAUTERINE GROWTH RETARDATION. ABNORMAL FACIAL APPEARANCE SYNDROME IDENTIFICATION VI:10-11
WHITE PLAINS: MARCH OF DIMES BIRTH DEFECTS FOUNDATION 1980

FERNHOFF PM LAMMER EJ
CRANIOFACIAL FEATURES OF ISOTRETINOIN EMBRYOPATHY
J PEDIATR 1984 105:595-7

FERNHOFF PM OAKLEY GP JR
ALPHA-FETOPROTEIN AS PREDICTOR OF FETAL NEURAL-TUBE DEFECTS (LETTER)
LANCET 1975 2:368

FINNE PH HANSEN E STEEN J RUUD E BJERKEDAL T
RETROLENTAL FIBROPLASY IN NORWAY (NOR)
TIDSSKR NOR LAEGEFOREN 1981 101:193-196

FLYNT JW JR
TRENDS IN SURVEILLANCE OF CONGENITAL MALFORMATIONS. CONGENITAL DEFECTS: NEW DIRECTIONS IN RESEARCH
NEW YORK: ACAD PRESS 1974:119-128

FLYNT JW JR
TECHNIQUES FOR ASSESSING TERATOGENIC EFFECTS: EPIDEMIOLOGY
ENVIRON HEALTH PERSPECT 1976 18:117-123

FLYNT JW JR EBBIN AJ OAKLEY GP JR FALEK A HEATH CW JR
METROPOLITAN ATLANTA CONGENITAL DEFECTS PROGRAM. MONITORING BIRTH DEFECTS AND ENVIRONMENT: THE PROBLEM OF SURVEILLANCE
NEW YORK: ACAD PRESS INC 1971 155-158

FLYNT JW JR HAY S
INTERNATIONAL CLEARINGHOUSE FOR BIRTH DEFECTS MONITORING SYSTEMS CONTRIBUTIONS TO EPIDEMIOLOGY AND BIOSTATISTICS VOL 1 EPIDEMIOLOGIC METHODS FOR THE DETECTION OF TERATOGENS
BASEL:KARGER, 1979 :44-52

FOSTER FH
CONGENITAL ANOMALY MONITORING SYSTEM IN NEW ZEALAND
NZ MED J 1979 90:509-510

FOSTER FH
CONGENITAL ANOMALY MONITORING IN NEW ZEALAND 1979-81
NZ MED J 1982 95:780-781

FOSTER FH
THE NEW ZEALAND CONGENITAL ANOMALY REGISTER
NZ MED J 1984 97:150-153

FRANCANNET C LEFRANCOIS P DECHELOTTE P ROBERT E MALPUECH G ROBERT JM
FRASER SYNDROME WITH RENAL AGENESIS IN TWO CONSANGUINEOUS TURKISH FAMILIES
AM J MED GENET 1990 36:477-9

FRASER FC CZEIZEL A HANSON C
INCREASED FREQUENCY OF NEURAL TUBE DEFECTS IN SIBS OF CHILDREN WITH OTHER MALFORMATIONS
LANCET 1982 II:144-5

FRIAS JL MARTINEZ FRIAS ML
BIRTH DEFECTS: CLINICAL AND EPIDEMILOGICAL ASPECTS (SPA)
CUADERNOS DE SALUD ED. SERVICIO VASCO DE SALUD, BILBAO 1989 1:65-87

GADOW EC PAZ JE CASTILLA EE SOD R
DEFINICION DE RECURRENCIA ANORMAL Y RIESGO DE REPETICION DEL ABORTO ESPONTANEO
OBST GINEC LATINOAMERIC 1976 34:46-52

GADOW EC PAZ JE JIMENEZ J CASTILLA EE MENDIZABAL AF
DIAGNOSTICO PRENATAL DE LAS ANOMALIAS GENETICAS
REV ARGENT GINECOL OBSTET 1974 723:377-379

GARCIA-ALONSO F RODRIGUES-PINILLA E MARTINEZ-PRIAS ML MARCOS-HERRERO F SALVADOR J LEVY-MAFHODA M DAL RE SAAVEDRA M
USE OF SEXUAL HORMONES IN PREGNANT WOMEN I SPAIN DURING THE 1976-1984 PERIOD (SPA)
MED CLIN 1988 90:183-185

GARDENT J GOUJARD J FARDEAU M CROST M
ECONOMICS OF THE DIFFUSION OF PRENATAL DIAGNOSIS BY AMNIOCENTESIS PART ONE: EPIDEMIOLOGIC MEDICAL AND SOCIO-ECONOMIC BASES (FRE)
REV EPIDEM SANTE PUBL 1984 32:88-96

GARZA A CORDERO JF MULINARE J
EPIDEMIOLOGY OF EARLY AMNION RUPTURE SPECTRUM OF DEFECTS. ATLANTA 1968-82
AM J DIS CHILD 1988 142:541-544

GJERUM NIELSEN K PILGAARD B MIKKELSEN M
PREVALENCE AND SURVIVAL OF NEWBORNS WITH DOWN SYNDROME IN DENMARK 1980-1985 (DAN)
UGESKR LAEGER 1987 149:2170-2173

GLAUBER A BUCSKI P
A STUDY OF ADVERSE EFFECTS ON THE PROGENY AFTER INTOXICATION DURING PREGNANCY
ARCH TOXICOL 1988 62:1-7

GOLDBERG MF CHEN ATL AHN YW REIDY JA
FIRST TRIMESTER FETAL CHROMOSOMAL DIAGNOSIS USING ENDOCERVICAL LAVAGE: A NEGATIVE EVALUATION
AM J OBSTET GYNECOL 1980 138:436-40

GOLDBERG MF EDMONDS LD OAKLEY GP JR
REDUCING BIRTH DEFECT RISK IN ADVANCED MATERNAL AGE
JAMA 1979 242:2292-94

GOLDBERG MF OAKLEY GP JR
INTERPRETING ELEVATED AMNIOTIC FLUID ALPHA-FETOPROTEIN LEVELS IN CLINICAL PRACTICE: USE OF THE PREDICTIVE VALUE POSITIVE CONCEPT
AM J OBSTET GYNECOL 1979 133:126-32

GOLDBERG MF OAKLEY GP JR
PRENATAL SCREENING FOR ANENCEPHALY-SPINA BIFIDA: SOME EPIDEMIOLOGIC PROJECTIONS FOR A NATIONAL PROGRAM. IN: PORTER IH HOOK EB (EDS) SERVICE AND EDUCATION IN MEDICAL GENETICS
NEW YORK: ACAD PRESS 1979 55-58

GONZALEZ ER
TERATOGEN MAY BE IMPLICATED IN LETHAL CONGENITAL SYNDROME
JAMA 1979 242:1119-1120

GOODMAN RM TRILLING R HERTZ M HOROSZOWSKI H MERLOB P REISNER SH
NEW CLINICAL OBSERVATIONS IN THE TRICHORHINOPHALANGEAL SYNDROME
J CRANIO GEN DEV BIO 1981 1:15-29

GOUJARD J
ESTIMATION OF THE TERATOGENIC RISK ASSOCIATED WITH THE TAKING OF DRUGS AT THE BEGINNING OF PREGNANCY (FRE)
ACQUIS MED RECENT 1981 157-71

GOUJARD J
LES REGISTRES ORIENTES SUR UNE AFFECTION. IN: VOIES NOUVELLES DE L'EVALUATION SCIENTIFIQUE ET REGLEMENTAIRE DU MEDICAMENT
INSERM 1983 112:459-69

GOUJARD J
REGISTRATION OF CONGENITAL ANOMALIES IN PARIS AND YVELINES (FRANCE). IN: REGISTRATING OF CONGENITAL ANOMALIES IN EUROCAT CENTERS 1979-83
DE WALS PH WEATHERALL JAC LECHAT MF (EDS)
BRUSSELS: CABAY 1985 29-39

GOUJARD J
ADVERSE DRUG REACTIONS MONITORING THE CHOICE OF DRUG SURVEILLANCE METHODS IN TERATOLOGY (FRE)
THERAPIE 1985 40:287-292

GOUJARD J
REGISTRES ET PHARMACOVIGILANCE. IN: PHARMACOVIGILANCE ET EPIDEMIOLOGIE
PARIS:INSERM 1985 63-77

GOUJARD J
DOWN'S SYNDROME AND NEURAL TUBE DEFECTS. IN: ELIMINATION OR REDUCTION OF DISEASES? OPPORTUNITIES FOR HEALTH SERVICE ACTIONS IN EUROPE SILMAN AJ ALWRIGHT SPA (EDS)
OXFORD UNIVERSITY PRESS 1988 181-210

GOUJARD J
RESEARCH ON TERATOGENIC RISKS USING A REGISTER OF CONGENITAL MALFORMATIONS (FRE)
REV EPIDEM SANTE PUBL 1988 36:283-91

GOUJARD J
LA MUCOVISCIDOSE: ASPECTS EPIDEMIOLOGIQUES
REV EPIDEM SANTE PUBL 1988 36:71 82

GOUJARD J
LES FACTEURS TERATOGENES DE L'ENVIRONNEMENT: APPROCHES METHODOLOGIQUES. IN: MALFORMAZIONI CONGENITE GALANTI ET FIORETTO I (EDS) REGGION EMILIA 1988 41 SUPPL NO 3
ACTA PAEDIATRICA LATINA 1988 694-706

GOUJARD J
APPROCHE EPIDEMIOLOGIQUE DES MALFORMATIONS CONGENITALES. IN: DIAGNOSTIC ANTENATAL DES MALFORMATIONS FOETALES PAR L'ECHOGRAPHIE GILLET JY BOOG G DUMEZ Y NISAND I VALETTE C (EDS)
PARIS: VIGOT 1990 1-8

GOUJARD J DU MAZAUBRUN C MAILLARD F
LE DIAGNOSTIC ECHOGRAPHIQUE DES ANOMALIES FOETALES. LE POINT DE VUE DE L'EIDEMIOLOGISTE. IN: APPORT DE L'ECHOGRAPHIE EN OBSTETRIQUE TOURNAIRE M (ED)
PARIS: VIGOT 1987 275-88

GOUJARD J GRACCO DE LAY MO CROST M MAILLARD F
MALFORMATION CONGENITALES ET PATHOLOGIE NEONATALE. IN: NAITRE EN FRANCE: 10 ANS D'EVOLUTION RUMEAU-ROQUETTE C DU MAZAUBRUN CH RABARISON Y (EDS) GRANDES ENQUETES EN SANTE PUBLIQUE ET EPIDEMIOLOGIE
INSERM 1984 45-53

GOUJARD J MAILLARD F ANCELIN C DU MAZAUBRUN CH ANDRE F
ENREGISTREMENT DES MALFORMATIONS CONGENITALES A PARIS. BILAN ET PERSPECTIVES DE L'ETUDE PLACEE SOUS L'EGIDE DE LA C E E
J GYN OBST BIOL REPR 1983 12:805-17

GOUJARD J MAILLARD F DU MAZAUBRUN C
EVALUATION DES ACTIONS DE DEPISTAGE DES MALFORMATIONS CONGENITALES: LE POINT DE VUE DE L'EPIDEMIOLOGISTE. IN: CHERCHER POUR AGIR; RECHERCHE D'AUHOURD'HUI, MEDECINE D'AUJOURD'HUI ET DE DEMAIN
INSERM 1988 187:201-10

GOUJARD J MAILLARD F DU MAZAUBRUN C PASSAVY AM
THE IMPACT OF PRENATAL DIAGNOSIS ON THE PREVALENCE RATE OF CONGENITAL ANOMALIES AT BIRTH
EUR J EPIDEMIOL 1986 2:321

GOUJARD J SAFAR A ROLLAND A JOB JC
EPIDEMIOLOGY OF HYPOTHYROIDISM DUE TO CONGENITAL MALFORMATION OF THE GLAND: ATHYREOSIS OR ECTOPIC THYROID (FRE)
ARCH FR PEDIATR 1981 38:875-9

GOUJARD J STOLL CL ET AL.
PREVALENCE OF NEURAL TUBE DEFECTS IN 16 REGIONS OF EUROPE 1980-83
INT J EPIDEMIOL 1987 16 2:246-251

GRANROTH G
DEFECTS OF THE CENTRAL NERVOUS SYSTEM IN FINLAND: IV ASSOCIATIONS WITH DIAGNOSTIC X-RAY EXAMINATIONS
AM J OBSTET GYNECOL 1979 133:191-194

GREENBERG F
PRENATAL DIAGNOSIS OF CONGENITAL ADRENAL HYPERPLASIA (LETTER)
LANCET 1979 I:908

GREENBERG F JAMES LM OAKLEY GP JR
ESTIMATES OF BIRTH PREVALENCE RATES OF SPINA BIFIDA IN THE UNITED STATES FROM COMPUTER GENERATED MAPS
AM J OBSTET GYNECOL 1983 145:570-73

GREENBERG G INMAN WH WEATHERALL JA ADELSTEIN AM
HORMONAL PREGNANCY TESTS AND CONGENITAL MALFORMATIONS (LETTER)
BR MED J 1975 2 191-192

GREENBERG G INMAN WH WEATHERALL JA ADELSTEIN AM HASKEY JC
MATERNAL DRUG HISTORIES AND CONGENITAL ABNORMALITIES
BR MED J 1977 2:853-856

HALVORSEN L BJARTVEIT KRUGER M KRUGER Y BAKKETEIG LS
SMOKING HABITS AMONG PREGNANT WOMEN IN TRONDELAG (NOR)
TIDSSKR NOR LAEGEFOREN 1979 99:575-79

HAMALAINEN T OHRNBERG R SAXEN L
MATERNAL AGE AND CONGENITAL DEFECTS (FIN)
DUODECIM (HELSINKI) 1970 86:719-729

HANSON JW OAKLEY GP
SPRAY ADHESIVES AND BIRTH DEFECTS (LETTER)
JAMA 1976 236:1010

HANSON JW OAKLEY GP JR
HALOPERIDOL AND LIMB DEFORMITY (LETTER)
JAMA 1975 231:26

HANSSON E JANSA S WANDE H KALLEN B OSTLUND E
PREGNANCY OUTCOME FOR WOMEN WORKING IN LABORATORIES IN SOME OF THE PHARMACEUTICAL INDUSTRIES IN SWEDEN
SCAND J WORK ENVIRON HEALTH 1980 6:131-134

HARJULEHTO T ARO T SAXEN L
LONG-TERM CHANGES IN MEDICATION DURING PREGNANCY
TERATOLOGY 1988 37:145-148

HEATH CW JR FLYNT JW JR OAKLEY GP JR FALEK A
THE ROLE OF BIRTH DEFECT SURVEILLANCE IN CONTROL OF FETAL ENVIRONMENTAL HAZARDS
POSTGRAD MED J (SUPP II) 1975 51:69-77

HEMMINKI K KYYRONEN P LINDBOHM ML
SPONTANEOUS ABORTIONS AND MALFORMATIONS IN THE OFFSPRING OF NURSES EXPOSED TO ANAESTHETIC GASES, CYTOSTATIC DRUGS AND OTHER POTENTIAL HAZARDS IN HOSPITALS BASED ON REGISTERED INFORMATION OF OUTCOME
J EPIDEMIOL COMMUNITY HEALTH 1985 39:141-147

HEMMINKI K LINDBOHM ML HEMMINKI T VAINIO H
REPRODUCTIVE HAZARDS AND PLASTICS INDUSTRY
PROG CLIN BIOL RES 1984 141:79-87

HEMMINKI K MUTANEN P LUOMA K SALONIEMI I
CONGENITAL MALFORMATIONS BY THE PARENTAL OCCUPATION IN FINLAND
INT ARCH OCCUP ENVIRON HEALTH 1980 46:93-98

HEMMINKI K MUTANEN P SALONIEMI I
SMOKING AND THE OCCURRENCE OF CONGENITAL MALFORMATIONS AND SPONTANEOUS ABORTIONS: MULTIVARIATE ANALYSIS
AM J OBSTET GYNECOL 1983 145:61-66

HEMMINKI K SALONIEMI I KYYRONEN P KEKOMAKI M
GASTROSCHISIS AND OMPHALOCELE IN FINLAND IN THE 1970S: PREVALENCE AT BIRTH AND ITS CORRELATES
J EPIDEMIOL COMMUNITY HEALTH 1982 36:289-293

HILL GB SPICER CC WEATHERALL JA
THE COMPUTER SURVEILLANCE OF CONGENITAL MALFORMATIONS
BR MED BULL 1968 24:215-218

HILL L MURPHY M MCDOWALL M PAUL AH
MATERNAL DRUG HISTORIES AND CONGENITAL MALFORMATIONS, LIMB REDUCTION DEFECTS AND ORAL CLEFTS
J EPIDEMIOL COMMUNITY HEALTH 1988 42:1-7

HOGUE CJ CATES W TIETZE C
THE EFFECTS OF INDUCED ABORTION ON ON SUBSEQUENT REPRODUCTION
EPIDEMIOL REV 1982 4:66-94

HOLMBERG PC
CENTRAL NERVOUS DEFECTS IN TWO CHILDREN OF MOTHERS EXPOSED TO CHEMICALS IN THE REINFORCED PLASTICS INDUSTRY. CHANCE OR A CAUSAL RELATION?
SCAND J WORK ENVIRON HEALTH 1977 4:212-214

HOLMBERG PC
CENTRAL-NERVOUS-SYSTEM DEFECTS BORN TO MOTHERS EXPOSED TO ORGANIC SOLVENTS DURING PREGNANCY
LANCET 1979 2:177-179

HOLMBERG PC
CONGENITAL DEFECTS AND ENVIRONMENTAL FACTORS DURING PREGNANCY: NATIONWIDE SURVEILLANCE
PROG CLIN BIOL RES 1985 163B:287-289

HOLMBERG PC HERNBERG S
CONGENITAL DEFECTS AND OCCUPATIONAL FACTORS A COMPARISON OF TWO DIFFERENT METHODOLOGICAL APPROACHES
SCAND J WORK ENVIRON HEALTH 1979 5:328-332

HOLMBERG PC HERNBERG S KURPPA K RANTALA K RIALA R
ORAL CLEFTS AND ORGANIC SOLVENT EXPOSURE DURING PREGNANCY
INT ARCH OCCUP ENVIRON HEALTH 1982 50:371-376

HOLMBERG PC KURPPA K
AN EPIDEMIOLOGIC APPROACH TO THE STUDY OF POSSIBLE TERATOGENIC EFFECTS OF CHEMICAL AND PHYSICAL ENVIRONMENTS
SCAND J WORK ENVIRON HEALTH 1982 8 SUPPL 1:89-91

HOLMBERG PC KURPPA K RIALA R RANTALA K KUOSMA E
SOLVENT EXPOSURE AND BIRTH DEFECTS: AN EPIDEMIOLOGIC SURVEY
PROG CLIN BIOL RES 1986 220:179-185

HOLMBERG PC NURMINEN M
CONGENITAL DEFECTS OF THE CENTRAL NERVOUS SYSTEM AND OCCUPATIONAL FACTORS DURING PREGNANCY: A CASE-REFERENT STUDY
AM J IND MED 1980 1:167-176

HOWITZ P KNUDSEN LB
BUILDING UP OF A NEW MALFORMATION REGISTER BY THE HEALTH BOARD (DAN)
UGESKR LAEGER 1982 144:1506-7

HULTIN H
REGISTRATION OF CONGENITAL MALFORMATIONS (FIN)
KATILOLEHTI 1971 76:398-399

INGALLS TH KLINGBERG MA
IMPLICATIONS OF EPIDEMIC EMBRYOPATHY FOR PUBLIC HEALTH
AM J PUBLIC HEALTH 1965 55:200-208

INTERNATIONAL CLEARINGHOUSE FOR BIRTH DEFECTS MONITORING SYSTEMS
A COMMUNICATION FROM THE INTERNATIONAL CLEARINGHOUSE FOR BIRTH DEFECTS MONITORING SYSTEMS
INT J EPIDEMIOL 1981 10:245-246

INTERNATIONAL CLEARINGHOUSE FOR BIRTH DEFECTS MONITORING SYSTEMS
EPIDEMIOLOGY OF BLADDER EXSTROPHY AND EPISPADIAS: A COMMUNICATION FROM THE INTERNATIONAL CLEARINGHOUSE FOR BIRTH DEFECTS MONITORING SYSTEMS
TERATOLOGY 1987 36:221-227

INTERNATIONAL CLEARINGHOUSE FOR BIRTH DEFECTS MONITORING SYSTEMS
TERATOGENICITY OF ISOTRETINOIN (LETTER)
LANCET 1988 II:1254-5

IRGENS LM LIE RT
BIRTH DEFECTS MONITORING SYSTEM
AM J EPID (LETTER) 1988 128:679

IRGENS LM SKJAERVEN R
OCCURRENCE OF BIRTH DEFECTS IN VARIOUS CATEGORIES OF NORWEGIAN MUNICIPALITIES
EUR J EPIDEMIOL 1989 5:255

ITURBE ALESSIO I FONSECA MC MUTCHINICK O SANTOS MA ZAJARIAS A SALAZAR E
RISK OF ANTICOAGULANT THERAPY IN PREGNANT WOMEN WITH ARTIFICIAL HEART VALVES
NEW ENG J MED 1986 315:1390-3

JABER L MERLOB P
THE PREVALENCE OF SUPERNUMERARY NIPPLES IN ARAB INFANTS AND CHILDREN (LETTER)
EUR J PEDIATR 1988 147:443

JELINEK R KUCERA J
EMBRYOTOXICITY AS A PART OF ENVIRONMENTAL RISK (CZE)
CAS LEK CESK 1981 120:1299-1304

JERVELL J BJERKEDAL T MOE N
OUTCOME FOR PREGNANCIES IN DIABETIC MOTHERS IN NORWAY 1967-1976
DIABETOLOGIA 1980 18:131-134

JERVELL J MOE N BJERKEDAL T
DIABETES MELLITUS AND PREGNANCY (NOR)
TIDSSKR NOR LAEGEFOREN 1979 99:784-786

KALLEN B
MATERNAL EPILEPSY, ANTIEPILEPTIC DRUGS AND BIRTH DEFECTS
PATHOLOGICA 1986 78:757-768

KALLEN B
HEXACHLOROPHENE TERATOGENICITY IN HUMANS DISPUTED (LETTER)
JAMA 1978 240:1585-1586

KALLEN B
DELIVERY TURNOUT AMONG EMPLOYEES IN MEDICAL CARE (EDITORIAL)(SWE)
LAKARTIDNINGEN 1978 75:3769-3770

KALLEN B
STRATEGIES IN ANALYSIS OF THE TERATOGENIC EFFECT OF DRUGS (EDITORIAL)(SWE)
LAKARTIDNINGEN 1979 76:2476

KALLEN B
WORKING IN A LABORATORY AND PREGNANCY (SWE)
LAKARTIDNINGEN 1979 76:2535-2536

KALLEN B
MODELLING MATERNAL BIRTH COHORT EFFECTS ON MALFORMATION RATES - A REPLY (LETTER)
INT J EPIDEMIOL 1983 12:378

KALLEN B
COMPUTER OPERATORS AND PREGNANCY (SWE)
LAKARTIDNINGEN 1985 82:1339-1342

KALLEN B
CONGENITAL MALFORMATIONS IN TWINS: A POPULATION STUDY
ACTA GENET MED GEMEL (ROMA) 1986 35:167-178

KALLEN B
A REGISTER STUDY OF MATERNAL EPILEPSY AND DELIVERY OUTCOME WITH SPECIAL REFERENCE TO DRUG USE
ACTA NEUROL SCAND 1986 73:253-259

KALLEN B
CAUDAL APLASIA
HANDBOOK OF CLINICAL NEUROL 1987

KALLEN B
HYPEREMESIS DURING PREGNANCY AND DELIVERY OUTCOME: A REGISTRY STUDY
EUR J OBST GYNE REP 1987 26:291-302

KALLEN B
POPULATION SURVEILLANCE OF MULTIMALFORMED INFANTS - EXPERIENCE WITH THE SWEDISH REGISTRY OF CONGENITAL MALFORMATIONS FIRST PART
J GENET HUM 1987 35:205-215

KALLEN B
POPULATION SURVEILLANCE OF MULTIMALFORMED INFANTS EXPERIENCE WITH THE SWEDISH REGISTRY OF CONGENITAL MALFORMATIONS SECOND PART
J GENET HUM 1987 35:321-338

KALLEN B
SEARCH FOR TERATOGENIC RISKS WITH THE AID OF MALFORMATION REGISTRIES
TERATOLOGY 1987 35:47-52

KALLEN B
EPIDEMIOLOGY OF HUMAN REPRODUCTION
CRC PRESS, BOCA RATON 1988

KALLEN B
MALFORMAZIONI MULTIPLE NON SYNDROMICHE: APPROCCIO PER L IDENTIFICATIONE DI NUOVE SYNDROMI
PROSPECTTIVE PEDIATRIA 1988 18:151

KALLEN B
CASE CONTROL STUDY OF HYPOSPADIAS BASED ON REGISTRY INFORMATION
TERATOLOGY 1988 38:45-50

KALLEN B
COMMENTS ON TERATOGEN UPDATE: LITHIUM
TERATOLOGY 1988 38:597

KALLEN B
DOWN'S SYNDROME AND MATERNAL CANCER. A PRELIMINARY STUDY
APMIS 1988 96:168-70

KALLEN B
MATERNAL USE OF ORAL CONTRACEPTIVES AND DOWN SYNDROME
CONTRACEPTION 1989 39:503-6

KALLEN B
A PROSPECTIVE STUDY OF SOME AETIOLOGICAL FACTORS IN LIMB REDUCTION DEFECTS IN SWEDEN
J EPIDEMIOL COMMUNITY HEALTH 1989 43:86-91

KALLEN B
POPULATION SURVEILLANCE OF CONGENITAL MALFORMATIONS: POSSIBILITIES AND LIMITATIONS
ACTA PAEDIATR SCAND 1989 78:657-63

KALLEN B BERTOLLINI R CASTILLA E CZEIZEL A KNUDSEN L MARTINEZ-FRIAS ML MASTROIACOVO P MUTCHINICK O
A JOINT INTERNATIONAL STUDY ON THE EPIDEMIOLOGY OF HYPOSPADIAS
ACTA PAEDIATR SCAND 1986 324:1-51

KALLEN B HAY S KLINGBERG M
BIRTH DEFECTS MONITORING SYSTEMS: ACCOMPLISHMENTS AND GOALS IN: ISSUES AND REVIEWS IN TERATOLOGY VOL 2
NEW YORK: PLENUM PRESS, 1984 1-22

KALLEN B KNUDSEN LB
EFFECT OF MATERNAL AGE DISTRIBUTION AND PRENATAL DIAGNOSIS ON THE POPULATION RATES OF DOWN SYNDROME-A COMPARATIVE STUDY OF NINETEEN POPULATIONS
HEREDITAS 1989 110:55-60

KALLEN B LINDHAM S
A WOMEN'S BIRTH COHORT EFFECT ON MALFORMATION RATES
INT J EPIDEMIOL 1982 11:398-401

KALLEN B LOFKVIST E
TIME TRENDS OF SPINA BIFIDA IN SWEDEN 1947-81
J EPIDEMIOL COMMUNITY HEALTH 1984 38:103-7

KALLEN B MALMQUIST G MORITZ U
DELIVERY OUTCOME AMONG PHYSIOTHERAPISTS IN SWEDEN: IS NON-IONIZING RADIATION A FETAL HAZARD?
ARCH ENVIRON HEALTH 1982 37:81-5

KALLEN B MASBACK A
DOWN SYNDROME. SEASONALITY AND PARITY EFFECTS
HEREDITAS 1988 109:21-7

KALLEN B RAHMANI TM WINBERG J
INFANTS WITH CONGENITAL LIMB REDUCTION REGISTERED IN THE SWEDISH REGISTER OF CONGENITAL MALFORMATIONS
TERATOLOGY 1984 29:73-85

KALLEN B ROBERT E MASTROIACOVO P MARTINEZ-FRIAS ML CASTILLA EE COCCHI G
ANTICONVULSANT DRUGS AND MALFORMATIONS IS THERE A DRUG SPECIFICITY?
EUR J EPIDEMIOL 1989 5:31-6

KALLEN B RYBO G
CONJOINED TWINNING IN SWEDEN
ACTA OBST GYNE SCAND 1978 57:257-259

KALLEN B TANDBERG A
LITHIUM AND PREGNANCY. A SHORT STUDY ON MANIC-DEPRESSIVE WOMEN
ACTA PSYCHIATR SCAND 1983 68:134-9

KALLEN B THORBERT G
A STUDY OF PREGNANCY OUTCOME IN A SMALL AREA AROUND A CHEMICAL FACTORY AND A CHEMICAL DUMP
ENVIRON RES 1985 37:313-9

KALLEN B WINBERG J
EXPERIENCES WITH CONTINUOUS REGISTRATION OF MALFORMATIONS (SWE)
LAKARTIDNINGEN 1966 63:1941-1951

KALLEN B WINBERG J
A SWEDISH REGISTER OF CONGENITAL MALFORMATIONS EXPERIENCE WITH CONTINUOUS REGISTRATION DURING 2 YEARS WITH SPECIAL REFERENCE TO MULTIPLE MALFORMATIONS
PEDIATRICS 1968 41:765-776

KALLEN B WINBERG J
MULTIPLE MALFORMATIONS STUDIED WITH A NATIONAL REGISTER OF MALFORMATIONS
PEDIATRICS 1969 44:410-417

KALLEN B WINBERG J
CAUDAL MESODERM PATTERN OF ANOMALIES: FROM RENAL AGENESIS TO SIRENOMELIA
TERATOLOGY 1974 9:99-111

KALLEN B WINBERG J
DEALING WITH SUSPICIONS OF MALFORMATION FREQUENCY INCREASE EXPERIENCE WITH THE SWEDISH REGISTER OF CONGENITAL MALFORMATIONS
ACTA PAEDIATR SCAND (SUPPL) 1979 275:66-74

KALLEN B WINBERG J
AN EPIDEMIOLOGICAL STUDY OF HYPOSPADIAS IN SWEDEN
ACTA PAEDIATR SCAND (SUPPL) 1982 293:1-2

KAPLAN KM COCHI SL EDMONDS LD
A PROFILE OF MOTHERS GIVING BIRTH TO INFANTS WITH CONGENITAL RUBELLA SYNDROME: AN ASSESSMENT OF RISK FACTORS
AM J DIS CHILD 1990 144:118-23

KATO K YOKOCHI M YOSHIMURA K FUJIKI K KUROSA T SHIMAMURA M
BIRTH DEFECTS MONITORING IN TOKYO METROPOLITAN HOSPITALS, 10 YEARS REPORT, 1979-1988 (JAP)
TOKYO: METROP INST NEUROSC 1990

KHOURY MJ
THE USE OF BIOMARKERS IN EPIDEMIOLOGIC STUDIES OF BIRTH DEFECTS AND DEVELOPMENTAL DISABILITIES
PROC ENVIRON HEALTH CONF 1989

KHOURY MJ
EPIDEMIOLOGY OF BIRTH DEFECTS: AN UPDATE
EPIDEMIOL REV 1989 11:244-8

KHOURY MJ ADAMS M FLANDERS WD
AN EPIDEMIOLOGIC APPROACH TO ECOGENETICS
AM J HUM GENET 1988 42:89-95

KHOURY MJ ADAMS MM RHODES P ERICKSON JD
MONITORING FOR MULTIPLE MALFORMATIONS IN THE DETECTION OF EPIDEMICS OF BIRTH DEFECTS
TERATOLOGY 1987 36:345-53

KHOURY MJ BEATY TH
RECURRENCE RISKS IN THE PRESENCE OF GENETIC SUSCEPTIBILITY TO ENVIRONMENTAL AGENTS
AM J MED GENET 1987 28:159-69

KHOURY MJ BECERRA JE CORDERO JF ERICKSON JD
CLINICAL-EPIDEMIOLOGIC ASSESSMENT OF PATTERN OF BIRTH DEFECTS ASSOCIATED WITH HUMAN TERATOGENS: APPLICATION TO DIABETIC EMBRYOPATHY
PEDIATRICS 1989 84:658-65

KHOURY MJ BECERRA JE D'ALMADA PJ
MATERNAL THYROID DISEASE AND RISK OF BIRTH DEFECTS IN OFFSPRING: A POPULATION-BASED CASE-CONTROL STUDY
PAEDIATR PERINATAL EPIDEMIOL 1989 3:402-20

KHOURY MJ CORDERO JF GREENBERG F JAMES LM ERICKSON JD
A POPULATION STUDY OF THE VACTERL ASSOCIATION: EVIDENCE FOR ITS ETIOLOGIC HETEROGENEITY
PEDIATRICS 1983 71:815-20

KHOURY MJ CORDERO JF MULINARE J OPTIZ JM
SELECTED MIDLINE DEFECT ASSOCIATIONS: A POPULATION STUDY
PEDIATRICS 1989 84:266-72

KHOURY MJ CORDERO JF RASMUSSEN S
ECTOPIA CORDIS, MIDLINE DEFECTS AND CHROMOSOMAL ABNORMALITIES: AN EPIDEMIOLOGIC PERSPECTIVE
AM J MED GENET 1988 30:811-17

KHOURY MJ EDMONDS LD WATERS G JAMES LM
SPINA BIFIDA AS A RISK FACTOR TO NECROTIZING ENTEROCOLITIS (LETTER)
J PEDIATR 1989 115:337-8

KHOURY MJ ERICKSON JD CORDERO JF MCCARTHY BJ
CONGENITAL MALFORMATIONS AND INTRAUTERINE GROWTH RETARDATION: A POPULATION STUDY
PEDIATRICS 1988 82:83-90

KHOURY MJ ERICKSON JD JAMES LM
ETIOLOGIC HETEROGENEITY OF NEURAL TUBE DEFECTS: CLUES FROM EPIDEMIOLOGY
AM J EPIDEMIOL 1982 115:538-548

KHOURY MJ ERICKSON JD JAMES LM
ETIOLOGIC HETEROGENEITY OF NEURAL TUBE DEFECTS: II CLUES FROM FAMILY STUDIES
AM J HUM GENET 1982 34:980-987

KHOURY MJ ERICKSON JD JAMES LM
MATERNAL FACTORS IN CLEFT LIP WITH OR WITHOUT PALATE: EVIDENCE FROM INTERRACIAL CROSSES IN THE UNITED STATES
TERATOLOGY 1983 27:351-57

KHOURY MJ FLANDERS WD BEATY TH
PENETRANCE IN THE PRESENCE OF GENETIC SUSCEPTIBILITY TO ENVIRONMENTAL FACTORS
AM J MED GENET 1988 29:397-403

KHOURY MJ FLANDERS WD JAMES LM ERICKSON JD
HUMAN TERATOGENS: PRENATAL MORTALITY AND SELECTION BIAS
AM J EPIDEMIOL 1989 130:361-70

KHOURY MJ GOMEZ-FARIAS M MULINARE J
DOES MATERNAL CIGARETTE SMOKING DURING PREGNANCY CAUSE CLEFT LIP AND PALATE IN OFFSPRING?
AM J DIS CHILD 1989 143:33-7

KHOURY MJ HOLTZMAN NA
ON THE ABILITY OF BIRTH DEFECTS MONITORING TO DETECT NEW TERATOGENS
AM J EPIDEMIOL 1987 126:136-43

KHOURY MJ HOLTZMAN NA
ON THE ABILITY OF BIRTH DEFECTS MONITORING TO DETECT NEW TERATOGENS. REPLY TO LETTER BY IRGENS AND LIE
AM J EPIDEMIOL 1988 128:679

KHOURY MJ STEWART W WEINSTEIN A PANNY S
RESIDENTIAL MOBILITY DURING PREGNANCY: IMPLICATIONS FOR ENVIRONMENTAL TERATOGENESIS
J CLIN EPIDEMIOL 1988 41:15-20

KHOURY MJ WEINSTEIN A PANNY S HOLTZMAN NA
CIGARETTE SMOKING AND ORAL CLEFTS: A POPULATION-BASED STUDY
AM J PUBLIC HEALTH 1987 77:623-5

KIMURA M
BIRTH DEFECTS MONITORING SYSTEM AND EPIDEMIOLOGICAL STUDY
CONGEN ANOMS (TOKYO) 1982 22:411-413

KISS P OSZTOVICS M PAZONYI I CZEIZEL A
CLINICAL STUDY OF CONGENITAL MULTIPLE MALFORMATIONS REGISTERED IN HUNGARY 1970-74. IN: SZABO G PAPP Z (EDS) MEDICAL GENETICS
AMSTERDAM: EXCERPTA MEDICA 1977 487-493

KLEMETTI A
REGISTRY FOR CONGENITAL MALFORMATIONS (FIN)
DUODECIM (HELSINKI) 1971 87:1409-1411

KLEMETTI A
CONGENITAL DEFECTS IN A COHORT FOLLOWED FOR SEVEN YEARS
ACTA PAEDIATR SCAND 1978 67:601-605

KLEMETTI A SAXEN L
THE FINNISH REGISTER OF CONGENITAL MALFORMATIONS. HEALTH SERVICES RESEARCH OF THE NATIONAL BOARD OF HEALTH IN FINLAND, HELSINKI
1970

KLINGBERG MA CHEMKE J CHEN R LEVIN S
A SURVEY OF CONGENITAL MALFORMATIONS IN ISRAEL THE EFFECT OF SOME FACTORS ASSOCIATED WITH ETHNIC ORIGIN
ISR J MED SCI 1971 7:1529-1534

KLINGBERG MA CHEN R CHEMKE J LEVIN S
AN EPIDEMIOLOGIC STUDY OF CONGENITAL MALFORMATIONS AMONG DIFFERENT ETHNIC AND SOCIAL GROUPS IN ISRAEL
DEV MED CHILD NEUROL 1971 13:735-745

KLINGBERG MA CHEN R CHEMKE J LEVIN S
RISING RATES OF CONGENITAL DISLOCATION OF THE HIP (LETTER)
LANCET 1976 1:298

KLINGBERG MA CHEN R CHEMKE J LEVIN S
RISING RATES OF CONGENITAL DISLOCATION OF THE HIP? (LETTER)
LANCET 1976 2:583

KLINGBERG MA CHEN R PAPIER CM CHEMKE J AMIZUR G
PATERNAL AGE AND DOWN SYNDROME
CONGEN ANOMS (TOKYO) 1982 22:1-6

KLINGBERG MA FARA GM CHEN R CHEMKE J
EPIDEMIOLOGICAL FINDINGS IN THE STUDY OF CONGENITAL MALFORMATIONS (ITA)
MINERVA MED 1975 66:2189-2199

KLINGBERG MA PAPIER CM
ENVIRONMENTAL TERATOGENS: THEIR SIGNIFICANCE AND EPIDEMIOLOGIC METHODS OF DETECTION CONTRIBUTIONS TO EPIDEMIOLOGY AND BIOSTATISTICS VOL 1 EPIDEMIOLOGIC METHODS FOR THE DETECTION OF TERATOGENS
BASEL:KARGER, 1979 1-22

KLINGBERG MA PAPIER CM HART J
BIRTH DEFECTS MONITORING
AM J IND MED 1983 4:309-328

KNUDSEN LB BORLUM KRISTENSEN F
MONITORING PERINATAL MORTALITY AND PERINATAL CARE WITH A NATIONAL REGISTER: CONTENT AND USAGE OF THE DANISH MEDICAL BIRTH REGISTER
COMMUN MED 1986 8:29-36

KNUDSEN LB KALLEN B
GASTRIC BYPASS, PREGNANCY AND NEURAL TUBE DEFECTS (LETTER)
LANCET 1986 2:227

KNUDSEN LB KALLEN B
INTESTINAL BYPASS OPERATION AND PREGNANCY OUTCOME
ACTA OBST GYNE SCAND 1986 65:831-4

KOFMAN-ALFARO S MUTCHINICK O VALDES E PEREZ-PALACIOS G
SEX DIFFERENTIATION II ABNORMALITIES OF THE SEX CHROMOSOMES AND CHANGES IN GONADAL DIFFERENTIATION (SPA)
REV INVEST CLIN 1984 36:53-70

KONDO K KATO K AKITA T HENMI I KUROSA T
BIRTH DEFECTS MONITORING IN THE TOKYO METROPOLITAN HOSPITALS, 5 YEARS REPORT, 1978-1982 (JAP)
TOKYO: METROP INST NEUROSC 1984

KUCERA J
REGISTRACE VROZENYCH VYVOJOVYCH VAD V CESKOSLOVENSKU
PRAKT LEK 1960 41:487-90

KUCERA J
FREKVENCE VROZENYCH VAD V CESKYCH KRAJICH A VLIVY KTERE NA NI PUSOBI I FREKVENCE TYP Y A VLASTNOSTI
CAS LEK CESK 1961 100:1609-14

KUCERA J
PORUCHY NITRODELOZNIHO VYVOJE CLOVEKA
PRAHA SZDN 1964 pp 1-238

KUCERA J
NOVE CHARAKTERISTIKY DOWNOVA SYNDROMU V CESKOSLOVENSKU A JEJICH VYZNAM TEORETICKY A PRAKTICKY
CAS LEK CESK 1964 103:1354-9

KUCERA J
DIE ERFASSUNG DER ANGEBORENEN MISSBILDUNGEN IN DER CSSR
ANN PAEDIATR (BASEL) 1965 204:141-51

KUCERA J
SHLUKOVANI VROZENYCH VAD JAKO NEPRIMY DUKAZ JEJICH SPOLECNE PRICINY?
CESK PEDIATR 1965 20:873-6

KUCERA J
EPIDEMIOLOGY OF CONGENITAL DEFECTS (CZE)
CAS LEK CESK 1968 107:968-972

KUCERA J
SYNDROM KAUDALNI REGRESE A JEHO VYZNAM PRO STUDIUM ETIOLOGIE A PREVENCE VROZENYCH VAD
CESK PEDIATR 1968 23:17-25

KUCERA J
EXPOSURE TO FAT SOLVENTS: A POSSIBLE CAUSE OF SACRAL AGENESIS IN MAN
J PEDIATR 1968 72:857-8

KUCERA J
DOWN'S SYNDROME AND INFECTIOUS HEPATITIS
LANCET 1970 1:569-70

KUCERA J
LEUKAEMIA AND TWINNING TENDENCY IN FAMILIES OF CHILDREN WITH DOWN'S SYNDROME
J MENT DEFIC RES 1971 15:77-80

KUCERA J
MOVEMENTS OF FREQUENCIES OF CONGENITAL MALFORMATIONS IN TIME AND SPACE
SOC BIOL 1971 18:422-30

KUCERA J
PATTERNS OF CONGENITAL ANOMALIES OF THE OFFSPRING OF WOMEN EXPOSED TO DIFFERENT DRUGS AND/OR CHEMICALS DURING PREGNANCY
TERATOLOGY 1971 4:492

KUCERA J
DOWN'S SYNDROME AND INFECTIVE HEPATITIS IN BOHEMIA
TERATOLOGY 1971 4:492-3

KUCERA J
RATE AND TYPE OF CONGENITAL ANOMALIES AMONG OFFSPRING OF DIABETIC WOMEN
J REPROD MED 1971 7:61-70

KUCERA J
ZPRAVA O DOBROVOLNE REGISTRACI VROZENYCH VAD V CESKYCH KRAJICH
CESK PEDIATR 1972 17:1119-21

KUCERA J
CONCORDANCE OF LEUKAEMIA AND TWINNING IN DOWN'S SYNDROME FAMILIES
LANCET 1972 1:150

KUCERA J
PREPARATION OF INTERNATIONAL SYSTEM FOR FOLLOW-UP OF CONGENITAL DEFECTS (CZE)
CESK PEDIATR 1973 28:270-271

KUCERA J
PROSPECTS AND LIMITATIONS OF EPIDEMIOLOGY IN HUMAN TERATOLOGY
ACTA UNIV CAROL (MED MONOGR , PRAHA) 1973 56:7-20

KUCERA J
VROZENE VADY VYVOLANE LEKY
CESK PEDIATR 1973 28:664-6

KUCERA J
CONGENITAL ANOMALIES IN DOWN'S SYNDROME (CZE)
CESK PEDIATR 1974 29:389-393

KUCERA J
EPIDEMIOLOGIE VROZENYCH NADORU A NADORU V KOJENECKEM VEKU V CSSR ZA LETA 1959-71
CAS LEK CESK 1975 114:681-6

KUCERA J
EPIDEMIE VROZENYCH SRDECNICH VAD NA OKRESE KLADNO V R 1972
CESK PEDIATR 1975 30:481-5

KUCERA J
POPULATION TERATOLOGY - METHOD AND NEW DISCIPLINE (CZE)
REV CZECH MED 1977 23:228-235

KUCERA J
MONITOR OF INBORN DEFECTS IN CZECHOSLOVAKIA RESULTS AND EXPERIENCES DURING THE FIRST YEAR OF ITS EXISTENCE (CZE)
CESK PEDIATR 1977 32:178-180

KUCERA J
RELATION BETWEEN POPULATION GENETICS AND POPULATION TERATOLOGY
MEDICAL GENETICS
AMSTERDAM: EXC MED-AKAD KIADO 1977:449-73

KUCERA J
EPIDEMIOLOGY AND PHENOTYPE OF CONGENITAL ARTERY CORONARIAL ANOMALIES
COR VASA 1978 20:369-78

KUCERA J
DECREASE IN THE RATE OF ANENCEPHALY IN CZECHOSLOVAKIA 1961-1975 (CZE)
CESK PEDIATR 1979 34:495-497

KUCERA J
THE ROLE OF POPULATION TERATOLOGY IN DETECTION OF XENOBIOTICS (CZE)
CAS LEK CESK 1980 119:637-638

KUCERA J
POPULATION TERATOLOGY THROWS SOME LIGHT ON THE ISCHEMIC HEART DISEASE
ACTA MORPHOL 1980 28:213-5

KUCERA J
EPIDEMIOLOGY OF DOWN'S SYNDROME (TRISOMY 21)(CZE)
CESK PEDIATR 1980 35:702-4

KUCERA J
DOWN'S SYNDROME - TWINNING - CANCER: A THREEFOLD EFFECT OF ONE COMMON CAUSE IN WOMEN 35-39 YEARS OLD? (CZE)
CESK GYNECOL 1980 45:755-758

KUCERA J
DOWNUV SYNDROM - MODEL A PROBLEM
PRAHA: AVICENUM 1981 1-141

KUCERA J
POPULATION TERATOLOGY AND ITS PART IN CHEMICAL TERATOGENESIS RISK ASSESSMENT (CZE)
CAS LEK CESK 1981 120:1318-21

KUCERA J
SECONDARY PREVENTION OF CONGENITAL DEFECTS IN THE WORLD AND IN CZECHOSLOVAKIA (CZE)
CAS LEK CESK 1982 121:1478-84

KUCERA J
SECONDARY PREVENTION OF DOWN'S SYNDROME IN CZECHOSLOVAKIA 1975-80 (CZE)
CESK PEDIATR 1982 37:404-8

KUCERA J
THE ASSESSMENT OF EMBRYOTOXICITY RISKS IN MAN-MADE ECOLOGY: A PERMANENT MULTIDISCIPLINARY INQUIRY
PROG CLIN BIOL RES 1985 163B:69-73

KUCERA J
POPULATION EVOLUTION IN THE CSR FROM THE POINT OF VIEW OF A POPULATION TERATOLOGIST (CZE)
CESK DEMOGRAFIE 1985 27:18-21

KUCERA J
ACCUTANE - A NEW HUMAN TERATOGEN AS A CAUSE OF A NEW SYNDROME (CZE)
CESK PEDIATR 1985 40:358

KUCERA J
BIOLOGICAL STATUS OF THE OFFSPRING OF FEMALE HEALTH PERSONNEL (CZE)
CESK PEDIATR 1985 40:662-667

KUCERA J
ACCUTANE (ISOTRETINOIC ACID) - A NEW HUMAN TERATOGEN (CZE)
CESK GYNEKOL 1985 50:418-419

KUCERA J
CONGENITAL MALFORMATION SURVEILLANCE SYSTEMS (LETTER)
INT J EPIDEMIOL 1986 15:430

KUCERA J
EVALUATION OF DATA COLLECTED FOR THE MONITOR FOR CONGENITAL DEFECTS REGISTRY IN CZECHOSLOVAKIA 1983-1985 (CZE)
CESK PEDIATR 1987 42:111-115

KUCERA J
COMMENTS ON THE REGISTRY OF CONGENITAL DEFECTS IN CZECHOSLOVAKIA (CZE)
CESK PEDIATR 1987 42:498-499

KUCERA J
OFFSPRING OF WOMEN DELIVERING AFTER SUCCESSFUL TREATMENT OF THEIR PRIMARY STERILITY (CZE)
CESK PEDIATR 1988 43:212-215

KUCERA J
MYTHS AND TRUTH ABOUT INFANT MORTALITY IN THE CSR BETWEEN 1961 AND 1985 (CZE) IN: MORTALITY AND AGEING OF CZECHOSLOWAKIAN POPULATION KUCERA M (ED)
ACTA DEMOGRAPHICA 1988 1-205

KUCERA J
POPULATION TERATOLOGY (CZE)
PRAHA: AVICENUM 1989 1-238

KUCERA J
PREVENTION OF ABNORMAL OUTCOMES OF PREGNANCY USING NON-GENETICAL METHODS (CZE)
DEMOGRAFIE 1990 32:9-10

KUCERA J BENESOVA D
PORUCHY NITRODELOZNIHO VYVOJE CLOVEKA ZPUSOBENE POKUSEM O POTRAT
CESK PEDIATR 1962 17:483-9

KUCERA J DOLEZALOVA V
PRENATAL DEVELOPMENT OF MALFORMED FETUSES AT 28-42 WEEKS OF GESTATIONAL AGE (ANENCEPHALUS, HYDROCEPHALUS. DOWN'S SYNDROME, CLEFT LIP AND PALATE AND HYPOSPADIAS). I. WEIGHT GAINS.
BIOL NEONATE 1972 20:253-61

KUCERA J DOLEZALOVA V
PRENATAL DEVELOPMENT OF MALFORMED FETUSES AT 28-42 WEEKS OF GESTATIONAL AGE (ANENCEPHALUS, HYDROCEPHALUS, DOWN'S SYNDROME, CLEFT LIP AND PALATE, AND HYPOSPADIAS). II. LENGTH GAINS
BIOL NEONATE 1973 22:319-24

KUCERA J DUDORKINOVA D
SIGNS OF MULTIPLE SYNDROMES IN A SINGLE FETUS OF A DIABETIC MOTHER (CZE)
CESK PEDIATR 1983 38:21-4

KUCERA J HODR R
UVAHY NAD ETIOLOGII KAMPOMELICKEHO SYNDROMU
CESK PEDIATR 1974 29:156-9

KUCERA J HODR R VORISKOVA M STRAUSS J KOPECKY K
EPIDEMICS OF CONGENITAL HEART DEFECTS IN THE KLADNO DISTRICT IN 1972 (CZE)
CESK PEDIATR 1975 30:481-485

KUCERA J KUCERA J JR
MEDICAL AND POPULATION GENETICS PROBLEMS IN PRIMARY NON-TUBAL FEMALE STERILITY I PREGNANCY OUTCOME AFTER TREATMENT OF INFERTILITY WITH SPECIAL EMPHASIS ON THE QUALITY OF THE OFFSPRING (CZE)
CESK GYNECOL 1988 53:164-73

KUCERA J LENZ W
KAUDALE REGRESSION MIT OSOPHAGUSATRESIE UND NIERENAGENESIE - EIN SYNDROM?
Z KINDERHEILK 1967 98:326-9

KUCERA J LENZ W MAIER W
MISSBILDUNGEN DER BEINE UND DER KAUDALEN WIRBELSAULE BEI KINDERN DIABETISCHER MUTTER
DTSCH MED WSCHR 1965 90:901-5

KUCERA J PELESKOVA A
CETNOST A VYSKYT DOWNOVA SYNDROMU V CSR V LETECH 1961-66
CESK PEDIATR 1971 26:394-7

KUCERA J PELESKOVA A
INCIDENCE AND OCCURRENCE OF DOWN'S SYNDROME IN CSR IN THE YEARS 1961-1966 (CZE)
CESK PEDIATR 1971 26:397

KUCERA J PELESKOVA A
SECONDARY PREVENTION OF DOWN'S SYNDROME IN CZECHOSLOVAKIA 1975 (CZE)
CESK GYNECOL 1985 50:128-132

KUCERA J STRAUSS J KOPECKY K VORISKOV M HODRE R
HROMADNY VYSKYT VROZENYCH SRDEC NICH VAD U NOVOROZENCU NA KLADNE
CESK EPID MIKROBIOL IMUNOL 1976 25:1-9

KURPPA K HOLMBERG PC HERNBERG S RANTALA K RIALA R NURMINEN T
SCREENING FOR OCCUPATIONAL EXPOSURES AND CONGENITAL MALFORMATIONS
SCAND J WORK ENVIRON HEALTH 1983 9:89-93

KURPPA K HOLMBERG PC KUOSMA E SAXEN L
COFFEE CONSUMPTION DURING PREGNANCY (LETTER)
NEW ENG J MED 1982 306:1548-1549

KURPPA K HOLMBERG PC KUOSMA E SAXEN L
COFFEE CONSUMPTION DURING PREGNANCY AND SELECTED CONGENITAL MALFORMATIONS: A NATIONWIDE CASE-CONTROL STUDY
AM J PUBLIC HEALTH 1983 73:1397-1399

KURPPA K HOLMBERG PC RANTALA K NURMINEN T
BIRTH DEFECTS AND VIDEO DISPLAY TERMINALS (LETTER)
LANCET 1984 2:1339

KURPPA K HOLMBERG PC RANTALA K NURMINEN T SAXEN L
BIRTH DEFECTS AND EXPOSURE TO VIDEO DISPLAY TERMINALS DURING PREGNANCY A FINNISH CASE-REFERENT STUDY
SCAND J WORK ENVIRON HEALTH 1985 11:353-356

LA CAVA G GURRIERI F MASTROIACOVO P
LA SINDROME ORO-FACIO-DIGITALE TIPO II. DESCRIZIONE DI UN NUOVO CASO
PATHOLOGICA 1989 81:309-14

LAKOS P CZEIZEL E
A TERATOLOGICAL EVALUATION OF ANTICONVULSANT DRUGS
ACTA PAED ACAD SCI HUNG 1977 18:145

LAMMER EJ
ON THE PLAUSIBILITY OF RETINOIDS ADVERSELY INFLUENCING NEURAL CREST CELL ACTIVITY. IN: PROC GREENWOOD GENET CENTER SAUL RA (ED)
CLINTON SC: JACOBS PRESS 1985 29-32

LAMMER EJ CHEN DT HOAR RM AGNISH ND BENKE PJ BRAUN JT CURRY CJ FERNHOFF PM GRIX AW JR LOTT IT RICHARD JM
RETINOIC ACID EMBRYOPATHY
NEW ENG J MED 1985 313:837-841

LAMMER EJ CORDERO JF
TERATOGENICITY OF ANTICONVULSANT DRUGS (LETTER)
AM J MED GENET 1985 22:641-645

LAMMER EJ CORDERO JF
EXOGENOUS SEX HORMONE EXPOSURE AND THE RISK FOR MAJOR MALFORMATIONS
JAMA 1986 255:3128-3132

LAMMER EJ CORDERO JF KHOURY MJ
EXOGENOUS SEX HORMONE EXPOSURE AND THE RISK FOR VACTERL ASSOCIATION
TERATOLOGY 1986 34:165-9

LAMMER EJ EDMONDS LD
TRENDS IN PYLORIC STENOSIS INCIDENCE
J MED GENET 1987 24:482-7

LAMMER EJ SEVER LE OAKLEY GP JR
TERATOGEN UPDATE: VALPROIC ACID
TERATOLOGY 1987 35:465-73

LANCASTER PAL
HEALTH REGISTERS FOR CONGENITAL MALFORMATIONS AND IN VITRO FERTILIZATION
CLIN REPROD FERTIL 1986 4:27-37

LANCASTER PAL
CONGENITAL MALFORMATIONS AFTER IN VITRO FERTILISATION (LETTER)
LANCET 1987 2:1392-1393

LANCASTER PAL
TERATOGENICITY OF ISOTRETINOIN
LANCET 1988 2:1254-1255

LANCASTER PAL
BIRTH DEFECTS IN ABORIGINES
MED J AUST 1989 151:241-242

LANCASTER PAL ROGERS JG
ISOTRETINOIN USE IN PREGNANCY
MED J AUST 1988 146:654-655

LAYDE PM DOOLEY K ERICKSON JD
EDMONDS LD
AN EPIDEMIC OF VENTRICULAR SEPTAL
DEFECTS?(LETTER)
LANCET 1980 1:1297-8

LAYDE PM DOOLEY K ERICKSON JD
EDMONDS LD
IS THERE AN EPIDEMIC OF VENTRICULAR
SEPTAL DEFECTS IN THE USA?
LANCET 1980 1:407-408

LAYDE PM EDMONDS LD
EPIDEMIOLOGY OF BIRTH DEFECTS IN TWINS.
IN: PERSAUD TVN (ED) ADVANCES IN THE
STUDY OF BIRTH DEFECTS
ENGLAND: MTP PRESS 1982 197-203

LAYDE PM EDMONDS LD ERICKSON JD
MATERNAL FEVER AND NEURAL TUBE
DEFECTS
TERATOLOGY 1980 21:105-8

LAYDE PM ERICKSON JD FALEK A
MCCARTHY B
CONGENITAL MALFORMATIONS IN TWINS
AM J HUM GENET 1980 32:69-78

LAYDE PM GOLDBERG MF SAFRA MJ OAKLEY
GP JR
FAILED INTRAUTERINE DEVICE
CONTRACEPTION AND LIMB REDUCTION
DEFORMITIES: A CASE-CONTROL STUDY
FERT STERIL 1979 31:18-20

LENOIR G SIMON G BARBIER O MARTIN B
GOUJARD J
CYSTIC FIBROSIS IN FRANCE IN 1988 (FRE)
ANN PEDIATR (PARIS) 1988 35:623-5

LENZ W KUCERA J
L'ETIOLOGIE DE LA REGRESSION CAUDALE
(AGENESIE DU SACRUM)
MED HYG 1967 25:241-3

LIAN ZH ZACK MM ERICKSON JD
PATERNAL AGE AND THE OCCURRENCE OF
BIRTH DEFECTS
AM J HUM GENET 1986 39:648-60

LIE RT IRGENS LM SKJAERVEN R
SECULAR CHANGES IN PREVALENCE AT BIRTH
OF DOWN SYNDROME AMONG YOUNG
MOTHERS IN NORWAY, 1967-1986
EUR J EPIDEMIOL 1989 5:257

LINDBOHM ML HEMMINKI K KYYRONEN P
KILPIKARI I VAINIO H
SPONTANEOUS ABORTIONS AMONG RUBBER
WORKERS AND CONGENITAL MALFORMATIONS
IN THEIR OFFSPRING
SCAND J WORK ENVIRON HEALTH 1983 9:85-90

LINDBOHM ML TASKINEN H HEMMINKI K
REPRODUCTIVE HEALTH OF WORKING WOMEN:
SPONTANEOUS ABORTIONS AND CONGENITAL
MALFORMATIONS
PUBLIC HEALTH REV 1985 13:55-87

LINDHAM S
OMPHALOCELE AND GASTROSCHISIS IN
SWEDEN 1965 - 1976
ACTA PAEDIATR SCAND 1981 70:55-60

LISKER R MUTCHINICK O PEREZ BRICENO R
GOMEZ H NAVARRETE JI SALAZAR C
KOFMAN S SAAVEDRA D
DISTRIBUTION OF ABO BLOOD GROUPS AND
OTHER GENETIC MARKERS IN MOTHERS OF
INFANTS WITH CONGENITAL MALFORMATIONS
HUM HERED 1982 32:166-9

LISKER R MUTCHINICK O REYES ME SANTOS
MA FLORES T GARCIA RAMOS G
HERENCIA AUTOSOMICA RECESIVA EN UNA
FAMILIA MEXICANA CON DISTONIA DE
TORCION
REV INVEST CLIN 1984 36:265-8

LISKER R MUTCHINICK O SANTOS MA
RODARTE E LUFT M
TYPE A2 BRACHYDACTYLY IN A MEXICAN
FAMILY
ANN GENET 1983 26:177-9

LITTLE J NEVIN NC
CONGENITAL ANOMALIES IN TWINS IN
NORTHERN IRELAND I: ANOMALIES IN
GENERAL AND SPECIFIC ANOMALIES OTHER
THAN NEURAL TUBE DEFECTS AND OF THE
CARDIOVASCULAR SYSTEM 1974-79
ACTA GENET MED GEMEL (ROMA) 1989 38:1-16

LITTLE J NEVIN NC
CONGENITAL ANOMALIES IN TWINS IN
NORTHERN IRELAND II: NEURAL TUBE
DEFECTS 1974-79
ACTA GENET MED GEMEL (ROMA) 1989 38:17-25

LITTLE J NEVIN NC
CONGENITAL ANOMALIES IN TWINS IN
NORTHERN IRELAND III: ANOMALIES OF THE
CARDIOVASCULAR SYSTEM 1974-78
ACTA GENET MED GEMEL (ROMA) 1989 38:27-35

LITWIN A MERLOB P GRUNEBAUM M
COMPLETE ABSENCE OF EXTERNAL GENITALIA
IN LIMB-BODY WALL COMPLEX: TWO CASES
J MED GENET 1988 25:340-3

LYNBERG MC KHOURY MJ OAKLEY GP
THE CONTRIBUTION OF BIRTH DEFECTS TO
INFANT MORTALITY. UNITED STATES, 1986
MMWR 1989 38:633-5

MAC F KNUDSEN LB
CONGENITAL MALFORMATIONS AMONG NEWBORN CHILDREN BORN TO IMMIGRANTS IN DENMARK IN THE PERIOD 1983-87 (DAN)
UGESKR LAEGER 1989 151:1101-6

MACLER J STOLL C RENAUD R
ECHOGRAPHIC DETECTION OF FETAL MALFORMATIONS (EXPERIENCE OF AN AT-RISK PREGNANCY CENTER) (FRE)
J GENET HUM 1980 28:213-5

MAGNANI C CALZOLARI E COCCHI G RONCARATI E SALVIOLI GP VOLPATO S MORETTI M
GENITO-URINARY MALFORMATIONS IN A REGIONAL SURVEY IN EMILIA ROMAGNA
PEDIATR MED CHIR 1986 8:255-8

MAGNANI C COCCHI G MORINI MS RONCARATI E SCARPA P VIANI R
A FOLLOW-UP STUDY OF MALFORMED BABIES
EUR J EPIDEMIOL 1986 2:331

MAGNANI C COCCHI G RONCARATI E GARANI GP
THE VACTERL ASSOCIATION AND ITS NOSOLOGIC LIMITS (ITA)
PEDIATR MED CHIR 1982 4:505-8

MAGNUS P BERG K BJERKEDAL T
ASSOCIATION OF PARENTAL CONSANGUINITY WITH DECREASED BIRTH WEIGHT AND INCREASED RATE OF EARLY DEATH AND CONGENITAL MALFORMATIONS
CLINICAL GENETICS 1985 28:335-342

MAGNUS P BERG K BJERKEDAL T NANCE WE
THE HERITABILITY OF SMOKING IN PREGNANCY AND THE BIRTH WEIGHTS OF SMOKING-DISCORDANT TWINS
SCAND J SOC MED 1985 13:29-34

MAGNUS P BERG K BJERKEDAL T
ASSOCIATION OF PARENTAL CONSANGUINITY WITH DECREASED BIRTH WEIGHT AND INCREASED RATE OF EARLY DEATH AND CONGENITAL MALFORMATIONS
CLIN GENET 1985 28:335-342

MARTA V
FACIAL EFFECTS OF FETAL ALCOHOL EXPOSURE: ASSESSMENT BY PHOTOGRAPHS AND MORPOHOMETRIC ANALYSIS (LETTER)
AM J MED GENET 1987 28:1017-8

MARTIN L CHAVEZ GF ADAMS MJ MASON EE HANSON JW HADDOW JE CURRIER RW
GASTRIC BYPASS SURGERY AS A MATERNAL RISK FACTOR FOR NEURAL TUBE DEFECTS
LANCET 1988 I:640-1

MARTINEZ-FRIAS ML
BIRTH DEFECTS IN SPAIN: TEN YEARS OF EPIDEMIOLOGICAL SURVEILLANCE (SPA)
ESTUDIOS SANITARIOS MADRID: DIRRECCION GENERAL DE PLANIFICATION SANITARIA. MINISTERIO DE SANIDAD Y CONSUMO 1989

MARTINEZ-FRIAS ML
TERATOGENESIS: BIBLIOGRAPHICAL REVIEW AND SITUATION IN SPAIN (SPA)
MONOGRAFIAS TECNICAS NO 12 MADRID: DIRECCION GENERAL DE FARMACIA PRODUCTOS SANATARIOS 1989

MARTINEZ-FRIAS ML
PREVENTION OF BIRTH DEFECTS: EPIDEMIOLOGICAL RESEARCH PROGRAMME IN SPAIN (1976-1988) (SPA)
AN ESP PEDIATR 1989 31:97-99

MARTINEZ-FRIAS ML
ASSOCIATION OF HOLOPROSENCEPHALY AND DOWN SYNDROME (LETTER)
AM J MED GENET 1989 32:435

MARTINEZ-FRIAS ML FRIAS JL SALVADOR J
CLINICAL/EPIDEMIOLOGICAL ANALYSIS OF MALFORMATIONS
AM J MED GENET 1990 35:121-5

MARTINEZ-FRIAS ML HERRANZ I SALVADOR J PRIETO I RAMOS-ARROYO MA RODRIQUEZ-PINILLA E CORDERO JF
PREVALENCE OF DOMINANT MUTATIONS IN SPAIN: EFFECT OF CHANGES IN MATERNAL AGE DISTRIBUTION
AM J MED GENET 1988 31:845-52

MARTINEZ-FRIAS ML PARRALO JA SALVADOR J
SEX RATIOS IN NEURAL TUBE DEFECTS
LANCET 1986 2:871

MARTINEZ-FRIAS ML RAMOS-ARROYO MA SALVADOR J
THANATOPHORIC DYSPLASIA: AN AUTOSOMAL DOMINANT CONDITION?
AM J MED GENET 1988 31:815-20

MARTINEZ-FRIAS ML RODRIGUEZ-PINILLA E SALVADOR J
VALPROATE AND SPINA BIFIDA
LANCET 1989 1:611-2

MARTINEZ-FRIAS ML SALVADOR J
EPIDEMIOLOGY OF DOWN SYNDROME IN SPAIN I MATERNAL AGE APPLICABILITY OF THE RESULTS IN PRIMARY PREVENTION PROGRAMS (SPA)
REV SAN HIG PUB 1985 59:325-336

MARTINEZ-FRIAS ML SALVADOR J
MEGADOSE VITAMIN A AND TERATOGENICITY (LETTER)
LANCET 1988 1:236

MARTINEZ-FRIAS ML SALVADOR J
EPIDEMIOLOGICAL ASPECTS OF PRENATAL EXPOSURE TO HIGH DOSES OF VITAMIN A IN SPAIN
EUR J EPIDEMIOL 1990 6:118-23

MARTINEZ-FRIAS ML SALVADOR J PEQUE M ADAN A
ENVIRONMENTAL FACTORS AND BIRTH DEFECTS: EPIDEMIOLOGICAL ASPECTS (SPA)
REV ESP PEDIATR 1983 39:277-300

MARTINEZ-FRIAS ML SALVADOR J PRIETO L
SPANISH TOXIC OIL AND CONGENITAL MALFORMATIONS (LETTER)
LANCET 1982 2:1349

MARTINEZ-FRIAS ML SALVADOR J PRIETO L ZAPLANA J
INCIDENCE OF GASTROSCHISIS AND OMPHALOCELE IN SPAIN (SPA)
REV SAN HIG PUB 1982 56:107-118

MARTINEZ-FRIAS ML SALVADOR J PRIETO L ZAPLANA J
EPIDEMIOLOGICAL STUDY OF GASTROSCHISIS AND OMPHALOCELE IN SPAIN
TERATOLOGY 1984 29:377-82

MARTINEZ-FRIAS ML SALVADOR J TARAMONA A ALONSO MD PRIETO L
DESCRIPTIVE EPIDEMIOLOGIC STUDY OF CONGENITAL ANOMALIES OF THE CENTRAL NERVOUS SYSTEM IN SPAIN 1976-1982 (SPA)
AN ESP PEDIATR 1984 21 9:810-821

MARTINEZ-FRIAS ML RODRIGUEZ A SALGADO C MARCITLLACH ML CARA R SEARA ML GIL MT
THE STUDY OF BIRTH DEFECTS DURING THE FIRST THREE DAYS OF LIFE. EPIDEMIOLOGY AND PREVENTION (SPA)
PUBLICACIONES MINISTERIO SANIDAD Y SEGURIDAD SOCIAL, MADRID 1978

MARTINEZ-FRIAS ML SALVADOR J
MATERNAL AGE AND DOWN SYNDROME (MONGOLISM): SITUATION IN SPAIN QUANTIFICATION ON THE RISKS AND PREVENTION (SPA)
REV IBEROAMER FERT 1984 4:34-37

MARTINEZ-FRIAS ML SALVADOR J
MEDICAL AND SOCIAL RELEVANCE OF BIRTH DEFECTS (SPA). IN: CARRERA MACIA J ET AL. BARCELONA DIAGNOSTICO PRENATAL ED. SALVAT 1987 15-18

MARTINEZ-FRIAS ML SALVADOR J
ENCVIRONMENTAL FACTORS (SPA). IN: CARRERA MARCIA J ET AL.
BARCELONA DIAGNOSTICO PRENATAL ED. SALVAT 1987 71-80

MARTINEZ-FRIAS ML SALVADOR J ADAN A FRIAS JL
BIRTH DEFECTS FREQUENCY IN SPAIN: 1976-1983 (SPA)
AN ESP PEDIATR 1986 25:145-153

MASTROIACOVO P
DOWN'S SYNDROME IN ITALY: AN EPIDEMIOLOGICAL MULTICENTRE STUDY OF 21 MONTHS MATERIAL IN: TRISOMY 21 BRUGIO GR FRACCARD M TIEPOLO L WOLF U (EDS)
BERLIN: SPRINGER VERLAG, 1981 245-246

MASTROIACOVO P
THE ITALIAN BIRTH DEFECTS MONITORING SYSTEM: BASELINE RATES BASED ON 283,453 BIRTHS AND COMPARISON WITH OTHER REGISTRIES
PROG CLIN BIOL RES 1985 163B:17-21

MASTROIACOVO P
SURVEILLANCE OF CONGENITAL MALFORMATIONS (ITA)
PATHOLOGICA 1986 78:785-95

MASTROIACOVO P
DIFETTI CONGENITI DA AGENTI TERATOGENI (ITA)
PROSPETTIVE IN PEDIATRIA 1988 70:143-60

MASTROIACOVO P
EPIDEMIOLOGIA DELLA SINDROME DOWN IN ITALIA. IN: FERRI R SPAGNOLO A (EDS) LA SINDROME DOWN (ITA)
PENSIERO SCIENTIFICO, (ROMA) 1989 23-33

MASTROIACOVO P BERTOLLINI R CORCHIA C
SURVIVAL TRENDS IN DOWN SYNDROME
LANCET 1990 I:127B

MASTROIACOVO P BERTOLLINI R LICATA D
FETAL GROWTH IN THE OFFSPRING OF EPILEPTIC WOMEN: RESULTS OF AN ITALIAN MULTICENTRIC COHORT STUDY
ACTA NEUROL SCAND 1988 78:110-4

MASTROIACOVO P BERTOLLINI R MORANDINI S SEGNI G
MATERNAL EPILEPSY, VALPROATE EXPOSURE AND BIRTH DEFECTS (LETTER)
LANCET 1983 2:1499

MASTROIACOVO P BERTOLLINI R MUSACCHIO P
L'INDAGINE POLICENTRICA ITALIANA SULLE MALFORMAZIONI CONGENITE: UN PROGETTO COLLABORATIVO PILOTA FINALIZZATO ALLA SORVEGLIANZA DELLE MALFORMAZIONI CONGENITE (ITA)
PROSPETTIVE IN PEDIATRIA 1982 45:23-38

MASTROIACOVO P CALABRO A
AMNIOTIC-ADHESION MALFORMATIONS IN ITALY (LETTER)
LANCET 1980 2:801

MASTROIACOVO P CAMERA G
CONGENITAL DEFECTS CAUSED BY AMNIOTIC BANDS (ITA)
PATHOLOGICA 1984 76:719-721

MASTROIACOVO P DE ROSA G SATTA MA COLAVITA N PRIOLO F PASARGIKLIAN E
SYNDROME IDENTIFICATION CASE REPORT 90: MULTIPLE CRANIOFACIAL AND SKELETAL DEFECTS
J CLIN DYSMORPH 1983 1:13-5

MASTROIACOVO P PERSICHETTI B SPENNATI G
PERCHE' IL TASSO PIU' ELEVATO DI DIFETTI IN RIDUZIONE DEGLI ARTI E' REGISTRATO IN ABRUZZO?
OSS SANIT ABRUZZESE 1988 II/1:29

MASTROIACOVO P SPAGNOLO A MARNI E MEAZZA L BERTOLLINI R SEGNI G BORGNA-PIGNATTI C
BIRTH DEFECTS IN THE SEVESO AREA AFTER TCDD CONTAMINATION (PUBLISHED ERRATUM APPEARS IN JAMA 1988 AUG 12, 260:792)
JAMA 1988 259:1668-72

MATHERS CD FIELD B
SOME INTERNATIONAL TRENDS IN THE INCIDENCE OF NEURAL TUBE DEFECTS
COMMUN HEALTH STUD 1983 7:60-66

MAZZE RI KALLEN B
REPRODUCTIVE OUTCOME AFTER ANESTHESIA AND OPERATION DURING PREGNANCY: A REGISTRY STUDY OF 5405 CASES
AM J OBSTET GYNECOL 1989 161:1178-85

MEBERG A BROCH H WEFRING KW IRGENS LM
CEREBRAL PALSY IN VESTFOLD 1970-1984 (NOR)
TIDSSKR NOR LÆGEFOREN 1988 108:212-214

MEIRIK O KALLEN B GAUFFIN U ERICSON A
MAJOR MALFORMATIONS IN INFANTS BORN OF WOMEN WHO WORKED IN LABORATORIES WHILE PREGNANT (LETTER)
LANCET 1979 2:91

MENDEX JP ULLOA AGUIRRE A SANCHEZ J MUTCHINICK O PEREZ PALACIOS G
ENDOCRINE EVALUATION IN A PATIENT WITH MURCS ASSOCIATION AND OVARIAN AGENESIS
EUR J OBST GYNE REP 1986 22:161-9

MERLOB P AITKIN I
TIME TRENDS (1980-87) OF TEN SELECTED INFORMATIVE MORPHOGENETIC VARIANTS IN A NEWBORN POPULATION
CLIN GENET 1990 38:33-7

MERLOB P GRUNEBAUM M
SYNDACTYLY TYPE II OR SYNPOLYDACTYLY
J MED GENET 1986 23:237-41

MERLOB P GRUNEBAUM M REISNER SH
A NEWBORN INFANT WITH CRANIOFACIAL DYSMORPHISM AND POLYSYNDACTYLY (GREIG'S SYNDROME)
ACTA PAEDIATR SCAND 1981 70:275-7

MERLOB P GRUNEBAUM M REISNER SH
FAMILIAL OPPOSABLE TRIPHALANGEAL THUMB ASSOCIATED WITH DUPLICATION OF THE BIG TOE
J MED GENET 1985 22:78-80

MERLOB P LEVY Y SHUPER A
POSTAXIAL POLYDACTYLY ASSOCIATED WITH NEUROFIBROMATOSIS
CLINICAL GENETICS 1987 32:202-5

MERLOB P MOGILNER B MUHLBAUER B AITKIN I DULITZKY F
THE TIME TRENDS (1976-87) OF ANENCEPHALY AND SPINA BIFIDA IN 4 HOSPITALS AFFILIATED TO THE INTERNATIONAL CLEARINGHOUSE
ISR J MED SCI 1989 25:441-4

MERLOB P PAPIER CM KLINGBERG MA REISNER SH
INCIDENCE OF CONGENITAL MALFORMATIONS IN THE NEWBORN; PARTICULARLY MINOR ABNORMALITIES
PROG CLIN BIOL RES 1985 163C:51-5

MERLOB P SCHONFELD A GRUNEBAUM M MOR N REISNER SH
AUTOSOMAL DOMINANT CEREBRO-COSTO-MANDIBULAR SYNDROME: ULTRASONOGRAPHIC AND CLINICAL FINDINGS
AM J MED GENET 1987 26:195-202

MERLOB P SCHONFELD A OVADIA Y REISNER SH
REAL-TIME ECHO-DOPPLER DUPLEX SCANNER IN THE EVALUATION OF PATIENTS WITH POLAND SEQUENCE
EUR J OBST GYNE REP 1989 32:103-8

MERLOB P STEIER D REISNER SH
AUTOSOMAL DOMINANT ISOLATED (UNCOMPLICATED) MICROCEPHALY
J MED GENET 1988 25:750-3

MESZAROS M CZEIZEL A
POINT PREVALENCE AT BIRTH OF VENTRICULAR SEPTAL DEFECT IN HUNGARY
ACTA PAED ACAD SCI HUNG 1978 19:51-54

MESZAROS M NAGY A CZEIZEL A
INCIDENCE OF CONGENITAL HEART DISEASE IN HUNGARY
HUM HERED 1975 25:513-519

MESZAROS M NAGY A KRASZNAI G CZEIZEL A
BIRTH PREVALENCE OF CONGENITAL CARDIOVASCULAR MALFORMATIONS IN HUNGARY
ACTA PAED ACAD SCI HUNG 1980 21:221-5

METNEKI J CZEIZEL A
CONTRACEPTIVE PILLS AND TWINS
ACTA GENET MED GEMEL (ROMA) 1980 29:233-6

METNEKI J CZEIZEL A
GRISEOFULVIN TERATOLOGY (LETTER)
LANCET 1987 1:1042

METNEKI J CZEIZEL E
CONTRACEPTIVE PILLS AND TWIN PREGNANCIES (HUN)
ORV HETIL 1980 121:1125-1127

MIKKELSEN M
DOWN'S SYNDROME: CURRENT STAGE OF CYTOGENETIC EPIDEMIOLOGY
HUMAN GENETICS PART B: MEDICAL ASPECTS 1982 297-309

MIKKELSEN M
PARENTAL ORIGIN OF THE EXTRA CHROMOSOME IN DOWN'S SYNDROME
J MENT DEFIC RES 1982 26:143-151

MIKKELSEN M FISHER G HANSEN J PILGAARD B NIELSEN J
THE IMPACT OF LEGAL TERMINATION OF PREGNANCY AND OF PRENATAL DIAGNOSIS ON THE BIRTH PREVALENCE OF DOWN SYNDROME IN DENMARK
ANN HUM GENET 1983 47:123-131

MIKLOS M LASZLO B SCHMIDT K DETRE Z HERNADY T CZEIZEL A
A NEW VARIANT OF THE ACRORENAL SYNDROME ASSOCIATED WITH BILATERAL OLIGOMEGANEPHRONIC HYPOPLASIA
EUR J PEDIATR 1984 142:40-3

MILLER RW FLYNT JW JR
EPIDEMIOLOGICAL SURVEILLANCE IN: BRENT RL HARRIS MI (EDS) PREVENTION OF EMBRYONIC, FETAL AND PERINATAL DISEASE VOL 3
FOG INT SER PRE MED 1976 287-93

MIMOUNI F MERLOB P REISNER SH
OCCURRENCE OF SUPERNUMERARY NIPPLES IN NEWBORNS
AM J DIS CHILD 1983 137:952-3

MONTELEONE NETO R CASTILLA EE PAZ JE
HYPOSPADIAS: AN EPIDEMIOLOGICAL STUDY IN LATIN AMERICA
AM J MED GENET 1981 10:5-19

MORETTI M RONCARATI E COCCHI G MAGNANI C MASTELLA M ALTERTI R SCARPA P SALVIOLI GP VOLPATO S CAVAZZUTI GB
PROBLEMS OF DEVELOPMENT AND CARE OF CHILDREN BORN WITH SELECTED CONGENITAL MALFORMATIONS: DOWN'S SYNDROME CARDIOPATHY, CLEFT LIP AND PALATE, CLUBFOOT (ITA)
PEDIATR MED CHIR 1986 8:243-52

MORTENSEN ML SEVER LE OAKLEY GP JR
TERATOLOGY AND THE EPIDEMIOLOGY OF BIRTH DEFECTS IN: GABBE SG NIEBYL JR SIMPSON JL (EDS) OBSTETRICS: NORMAL AND PROBLEM PREGNANCIES
CHURCHILL LIVINGSTONE 1986 183-209

MULINARE J CORDERO JF ERICKSON JD BERRY RJ
PERICONCEPTIONAL USE OF MULTIVITAMINS AND THE OCCURRENCE OF NEURAL TUBE DEFECTS
JAMA 1988 260:3141-5

MULVIHILL JJ CZEIZEL A
PERSPECTIVES IN MUTATION EPIDEMIOLOGY 6. A 1983 VIEW OF SENTINEL PHENOTYPES
MUTAT RES 1983 123:345-61

MURPHY MF BOTTING BJ GEDELLA B
ANALYSIS OF PERINATAL AND INFANT MORTALITY ADJUSTED BY EXCLUSION OF DEATHS FROM CONGENITAL MALFORMATION
COMMUN MED 1987 9:129-40

MUTCHINICK O
MALFORMACIONES CONGENITAS EN EL LIBRO: GINECOLOGIA Y OBSTERICIA LEON J (ED)
BUENOS AIRES: EL ATENEO 1970

MUTCHINICK O
LIBRO SINDROMES DE ANOMALIAS CONGENITAS. LINEAMIENTOS DIAGNOSTICOS
MEXICO: SALUD PUBLICA MEX 1972

MUTCHINICK O
EPIDEMIOLOGIA DE LAS MALFORMACIONES CONGENITAS
TEMAS SELEC PED CLIN 1980 2:105-112

MUTCHINICK O
MALFORMACIONES CONGENITAS Y TERATOGENESIS EN: TRATADO DE MEDICINA INTERNA URIBE M (ED)
BUENOS AIRES: MEDICA PANAMERICANA 1988 2:C 298:2013-4

MUTCHINICK O LISKER R
ESTUDIOS SOBRE MUTAGENESIS AMBIENTAL. REGISTRO DE MALFORMACIONES CONGENITAS
GAC MED MEX 1980 115:117-180

MUTCHINICK O LISKER R
ENVIRONMENTAL MUTAGENESIS REGISTRATION OF CONGENITAL ABNORMALITIES (SPA)
GAC MED MEX 1980 116:177-180

MUTCHINICK O LISKER R BABINSKY V
REGISTRO Y VIGILANCIA EPIDEMIOLOGICA DE MALFORMACIONES CONGENITAS EXTERNAS 1 ASPECTOS METODOLOGICOS E INCIDENCIA
REV MED H GRAL 1982 45:287-93

MUTCHINICK O LISKER R BABINSKY V
PROGRAMA MEXICANO DE REGISTRO Y VIGILANCIA EPIDEMIOLOGICA DE MALFORMACIONES CONGENITAS EXTERNAS (RYVEMCE)
REV SALUD PUBL MEXICO 1988 30:88-100

MUTCHINICK O LISKER R BABINSKY V
WEIGHT LENGTH, HEAD CIRCUMFERENCE AND GESTATIONAL AGE IN NEWBORNS WITH DOWN SYNDROME
BRAIN DISFUNCTION 1989 2:189-95

MUTCHINICK O LISKER R BABINSKY V
SANTOS MA MEJIA F SAAVEDRA D
VILLANUEVA C
FETAL MORTALITY IN SIBSHIPS WITH ONE OR MORE AFFECTED MEMBERS WITH ORAL CLEFTS
AM J MED GENET 1985 20:317-23

MUTCHINICK O LISKER R RABINSKY V
THE MEXICAN PRORAM OF REGISTRATION AND EPIDEMIOLOGIC SURVEILLANCE OF EXTERNAL CONGENITAL MALFORMATIONS (SPA)
SALUD PUBLICA MEX 1988 30:88-100

MUTCHINICK O MATAYOSHI T
DOWN'S SYNDROME WITH XYY SEXUAL COMPLEMENT
REV INVEST CLIN 1979 4:377-9

MUTCHINICK O OROZCO E LISKER R
BABINSKY V Y NUNEZ C
FACTORES DE RIESGO ASOCIADOS A LOS DEFECTOS DE CIERRE DEL TUBO NEURAL: EXPOSICION DURANTE EL PRIMER TRIMESTRE DE LA GESTACION
GAC MED MEX 1990 126:227-33

NERI A OVADIA Y MERLOB P LIBAN E
ABRAMOVICI A
AMNIOTIC BAND SYNDROME
ISR J MED SCI 1982 18:505-7

NERI G MASTROIACOVO P (A CURA DI)
DIFETTI CONGENITI (ITA)
PROSPETTIVE IN PEDIATRIA 1988 70

NEVIN NC
RECURRENCE RISK OF NEURAL TUBE DEFECTS (LETTER)
LANCET 1980 1:1301-2

NEVIN NC
NEURAL TUBE DEFECTS (LETTER)
LANCET 1981 2:1290-1291

NEVIN NC
PREVENTION OF NEURAL TUBE DEFECTS IN AN AREA OF HIGH INCIDENCE DOBBING J (ED) PREVENTION OF SPINA BIFIDA AND OTHER NEURAL TUBE DEFECTS
LONDON: ACADEMIC PRESS, 1983 127-144

NEVIN NC
THE ROLE OF PERICONCEPTIONAL VITAMIN SUPPLEMENTATION IN THE PREVENTION OF NEURAL TUBE DEFECTS
PROG CLIN BIOL RES 1985 163B:389-96

NEVIN NC
PREVENTION AND AVOIDANCE OF CONGENITAL MALFORMATIONS
PHILOS TR R SOC LOND (BIOL) 1988 319:309-14

NEVIN NC JOHNSTON WP
A FAMILY STUDY OF SPINA BIFIDA AND ANENCEPHALUS IN BELFAST, NORTHERN IRELAND (1964-68)
J MED GENET 1980 17:203-11

NEVIN NC JOHNSTON WP
RISK OF RECURRENCE AFTER TWO CHILDREN WITH CENTRAL NERVOUS SYSTEM MALFORMATIONS IN AN AREA OF HIGH INCIDENCE
J MED GENET 1980 17:87-92

NEVIN NC JOHNSTON WP MERRETT JD
INFLUENCE OF SOCIAL CLASS ON THE RISK OF RECURRENCE OF ANENCEPHALUS AND SPINA BIFIDA
DEV MED CHILD NEUROL 1981 23:155-9

NEVIN NC MCDONALD JR WALBY AL
A COMPARISON OF NEURAL TUBE DEFECTS IDENTIFIED BY TWO INDEPENDENT ROUTINE RECORDING SYSTEMS FOR CONGENITAL MALFORMATIONS IN NORTHERN IRELAND
INT J EPIDEMIOL 1978 7:319-321

NEVIN NC SELLER MJ
PREVENTION OF NEURAL-TUBE-DEFECT RECURRENCES (LETTER)
LANCET 1990 335:178-9

NEVIN NC SELLER MJ SMITHELLS RW
PRODUCT LICENSE FOR PREGNATIVE FORTE F (LETTER)
LANCET 1987 2:516

NURMINEN M HOLMBERG PC
TEMPORAL CHARACTERISTICS RELATED TO LEAVE FROM WORK AND PREGNANCY AMONG MOTHERS WITH CONGENITALLY MALFORMED OFFSPRING
SCAND J SOC MED 1981 9:51-57

OAKLEY GP JR
BIRTH DEFECT SURVEILLANCE IN THE SEARCH FOR AND EVALUATION OF POSSIBLE HUMAN TERATOGENS. IN: BERGSMA D SCHIMKE RM (EDS) CYTOGENETICS, ENVIRONMENT AND MALFORMATION SYNDROMES. BIRTH DEFECTS
NEW YORK: ALAN R LISS INC 1976 1-6

OAKLEY GP JR
STRATEGIES IN EVALUATION OF UNCERTAIN CLAIMS OF ENVIRONMENTAL CAUSES OF BIRTH DEFECTS. IN: KELLY S HOOK EB JANERICH DT PORTER IH (EDS) BIRTH DEFECTS: RISKS AND CONSEQUENCES
NEW YORK: ACADEMIC PRESS INC 1976 185-91

OAKLEY GP JR
NATURAL SELECTION, SELECTION BIAS AND THE PREVALENCE OF DOWN'S SYNDROME
NEW ENG J MED 1978 299:1068-9

OAKLEY GP JR
BIRTH DEFECT SURVEILLANCE IN THE SEARCH FOR AND EVALUATION OF POSSIBLE HUMAN TERATOGENS
J ENV PATHOL TOXICOL 1978 2:211-216

OAKLEY GP JR
THREATENED ABORTION. HORMONE THERAPY AND MALFORMED EMBRYOS (LETTER)
TERATOLOGY 1979 20:481-2

OAKLEY GP JR
DRUG INFLUENCES ON MALFORMATIONS
CLIN PERINATOL 1979 6:403-14

OAKLEY GP JR
CAUSAL INFERENCE IN TERATOLOGY. IN: SCHWARZ RH YAFFE SJ (EDS) DRUG AND CHEMICAL RISKS TO THE FETUS AND NEWBORN
NEW YORK: ALAN R LISS INC 1980 33-9

OAKLEY GP JR
ANTENATAL DIAGNOSIS: POTENTIAL FOR MAJOR REDUCTION IN PEDIATRIC MORBIDITY
PEDIATRIC ANNALS 1981 10:61-6

OAKLEY GP JR
INCIDENCE AND EPIDEMIOLOGY OF BIRTH DEFECTS. IN: KABACK MM (ED) GENETIC ISSUES IN PEDIATRICS AND OBSTETRIC PRACTICE
CHICAGO: YEAR BOOK MEDICAL PUBLISHERS INC 1981 25-43

OAKLEY GP JR
SPERMICIDES AND BIRTH DEFECTS (EDITORIAL)
JAMA 1982 247:2405

OAKLEY GP JR
TERATOGENICITY OF PROGESTATIONAL AGENTS (LETTER)
TERATOLOGY 1984 29:131

OAKLEY GP JR
POPULATION AND CASE-CONTROL SURVEILLANCE IN THE SEARCH FOR ENVIRONMENTAL CAUSES OF BIRTH DEFECTS
PROG CLIN BIOL RES 1985 163B:27-32

OAKLEY GP JR
BIRTH DEFECTS EPIDEMIOLOGY AND SURVEILLANCE
PROG CLIN BIOL RES 1985 163B:71-90

OAKLEY GP JR
POPULATION AND CASE-CONTROL SURVEILLANCE IN THE SEARCH FOR ENVIRONMENTAL CAUSES OF BIRTH DEFECTS. IN: MAROIS M (ED) PREVENTION OF PHYSICAL AND MENTAL CONGENITAL DEFECTS PART B: EPIDEMIOLOGY
NEW YORK: ALAN R LISS INC 1985 27-32

OAKLEY GP JR
BIRTH DEFECTS EPIDEMIOLOGY AND SURVEILLANCE. IN: MAROIS M (ED) PREVENTION OF PHYSICAL AND MENTAL CONGENITAL DEFECTS PART A: THE SCOPE OF THE PROBLEM
NEW YORK: ALAN R LISS INC 1985 71-90

OAKLEY GP JR
FREQUENCY OF HUMAN CONGENITAL MALFORMATIONS
CLIN PERINATOL 1986 13:545-554

OAKLEY GP JR
EPIDEMIOLOGY OF DEVELOPMENTAL TOXICOLOGY
CONG ANOM 28 (SUPPL) 1988 81-8

OAKLEY GP JR ADAMS MJ JAMES LM
VITAMINS AND NEURAL TUBE DEFECTS (LETTER)
LANCET 1983 2:798-799

OAKLEY GP JR FLYNT JW JR FALEK A
HORMONAL PREGNANCY TESTS AND CONGENITAL MALFORMATIONS
LANCET 1973 2:256-257

OAKLEY GP JR FLYNT JW JR FALEK A
COMMUNITY SURVEILLANCE OF BIRTH DEFECTS IN: COHEN BH LILIENFELD AM HUANG PC (EDS) GENETIC ISSUES IN PUBLIC HEALTH AND MEDICINE
SPRINGFIELD: CHARLES C THOMAS 1978 235-48

OAKLEY GP JR GRANTLEY K CHEN ATL FERNHOFF PM GOLDBERG MF PRIEST JH TRUSLER S
A COMMUNITY APPROACH TO PRENATAL DIAGNOSIS IN: PORTER IH HOOK EB (EDS) SERVICE AND EDUCATION IN MEDICAL GENETICS
NEW YORK ACADEMIC PRESS INC 1979 163-82

OAKLEY GP JR JAMES LM EDMONDS LD
TEMPORAL TRENDS IN REPORTED MALFORMATION INCIDENCE FOR THE UNITED STATES - BIRTH DEFECTS MONITORING PROGRAM
CLIN PEDIATR (PHILA) 1984 23:246-247

OAKLEY GP JR STICKLE G HAY S
A COMMUNICATION FROM THE INTERNATIONAL CLEARINGHOUSE FOR BIRTH DEFECTS MONITORING SYSTEM
INT J EPIDEMIOL 1981 10:245-6

ORIOLI IM CASTILLA EE BARBOSA-NETO JG
THE BIRTH PREVALENCE RATES FOR THE SKELETAL DYSPLASIAS
J MED GENET 1986 23:328-332

ORIOLI IM CASTILLA EE CARVALHO WP
INBREEDING IN A SOUTH-AMERICAN NEWBORN SERIES
ACTA ANTHROPOGENET 1982 6:45-55

OSZTOVICS M KISS P
DOWN SYNDROME: CORRESPONDENCE OF CLINICAL DIAGNOSIS AND KARYOTYPE
ACTA PAED ACAD SCI HUNG 1982 23:261-282

OSZTOVICS M TOTH S WILHELM O
UNUSUAL CHROMOSOME ABERRATIONS IN 3 CHILDREN WITH DOWN SYNDROME
ACTA PAED ACAD SCI HUNG 1982 23:282-89

PAGANO M MASTROIACOVO P
LA PRESCRIZIONE DEI FARMACI IN GRAVIDANZA. GUIDA ALLA VALUTAZIONE DEL RISCHIO TERATOGENO (ITA)
MILANO: MACGRAW HILL 1988

PAPIER CM
PARENTAL OCCUPATION AND CONGENITAL MALFORMATIONS IN A SERIES OF 35,000 BIRTHS IN ISRAEL
PROG CLIN BIOL RES 1985 163B:291-294

PARKIN DM
THE EFFICIENCY OF NOTIFICATION OF CONGENITAL DISLOCATION OF THE HIP
PUBLIC HEALTH 1980 94:68-70

PATRIZI A COCCHI G NERI I MASINA M MORINI MS
A CASE OF HARLEQUIN FETUS (ITA)
G ITAL DERMATOL VENER 1988 123:47-50

PAZ JE CASTILLA EE MARTINEZ-FRIAS ML
HEREDABILIDAD DE LAS MALFORMACIONES DE MIEMBROS ENEL HOMBRE
MENDELIANA 1976 1:27-30

PAZ JE CASTILLA EE
FAMILIAL TOTAL ANOMALOUS PULMONARY VENOUS RETURN
J MED GENET 1971 8:312-314

PAZONYI I KUN A CZEIZEL A
CONGENITAL POSTURAL DEFORMITY ASSOCIATION
ACTA PAED ACAD SCI HUNG 1982 23:431-45

PICCHIO FM BACCARANI G PILU GL PEROLO A DALLACASA P COCCHI G ZANNINI L
PRENATAL DIAGNOSIS AND POSTNATAL FOLLOW-UP OF CONGENITAL HEART DISEASE. OUR EXPERIENCE WITH 57 CASES (ITA)
ACTA PAEDIATRICA LATINA 1989 42:144-48

PONS JC GOUJARD J DERBANNE C TOURNAIRE M
OUTCOME OF PREGNANCY IN PATIENTS EXPOSED IN UTERO TO DIETHYLSTILBESTROL. SURVEY BY THE NATIONAL COLLEGE OF FRENCH GYNECOLOGISTS AND OBSTETRICIANS (FRE)
J GYN OBST BIOL REPR 1988 17:307-16

RASMUSSEN S KHOURY MJ CORDERO JF
EPIDEMIOLOGY OF HOLOPROSENCEPHALY
PEDIATR RES 1990

RASMUSSEN SA MULINARE J KHOURY MJ MALONEY K
EVALUATION OF BIRTH DEFECT HISTORIES OBTAINED THROUGH MATERNAL INTERVIEWS
AM J HUM GENET 1990 46:478-85

REISNER SH SIVA Y NITZAN M MERLOB P
DETERMINATION OF ANTERIOR DISPLACEMENT OF THE ANUS IN NEWBORN INFANTS AND CHILDREN
PEDIATRICS 1984 73:216-7

RICHARDSON DE C Y MUTCHINICK O
CARACTERISTICAS CLINICAS Y GENETRICAS DE CIERTOS ENANISMOS DE MIEMBROS CORTOS EN EL RECIEN NACIDO
BOL MED HOSP INF MEX 1982 39:105-11

RINTALA A STEGARS T
INCREASING INCIDENCE OF CLEFTS IN FINLAND: RELIABILITY OF HOSPITAL RECORDS AND CENTRAL REGISTER OF CONGENITAL MALFORMATIONS
SCAND J PL REC SURG 1982 16:35-40

ROBERT E
VALPROIC ACID IN PREGNANCY - ASSOCIATION WITH SPINA BIFIDA: A PRELIMINARY REPORT
CLIN PEDIATR (PHILA) 1983 22:336

ROBERT E
SPINA BIFIDA APERTA-MYELOMENINGOCELE. ETIOLOGY AND GENETICS (FRE)
NEUROCHIRURGIE, 34 SUPPL 1988 1:16-28

ROBERT E
ISOTRETINOIN DOSE AND TERATOGENICITY (LETTER)
LANCET 1988 1:236

ROBERT E
VALPROIC ACID AS A HUMAN TERATOGEN
CONG ANOM 28 (SUPPL) 1988 28:71-80

ROBERT E
ANTIEPILEPTIC DRUGS AND CONGENITAL HEART DEFECTS
TERATOLOGY 1989 39:474

ROBERT E FRANCANNET C
COMMENTS ON TERATOGEN UPDATE ON LITHIUM
TERATOLOGY 1990 42:205

ROBERT E FRANCANNET C ROBERT JM
BIRTH DEFECTS AND DRUGS EXPERIENCE IN THE RHONE-ALPES-AUVERGNE REGION (FRE)
THERAPIE 1985 40:293-296

ROBERT E FRANCANNET C ROBERT JM
REGISTRIES OF MALFORMATIONS IN THE RHONE-ALPS/AUVERGNE REGION. VALUE AND LIMITS OF MONITORING TERATOGENESIS: 11 YEARS' EXPERIENCE (1976-86) (FRE)
J GYN OBST BIOL REPR 1988 17:601-7

ROBERT E GUIBAUD P
MATERNAL VALPROIC ACID AND CONGENITAL NEURAL TUBE DEFECTS (LETTER)
LANCET 1982 2:937

ROBERT E LARRIBE S COUDERT A
PEUT-ON ESPERER VOIR APPARAITRE UNE PREVENTION DU SPINA BIFIDA?
ANN KINESITH 1987 82:575-81

ROBERT E LOFKVIST E MAUGUIERE F
VALPROATE AND SPINA BIFIDA (LETTER)
LANCET 1984 2:1392

ROBERT E LOFKVIST E MAUGUIERE F ROBERT JM
EVALUATION OF DRUG THERAPY AND TERATOGENIC RISK IN A RHONE-ALPES DISTRICT POPULATION OF PREGNANT EPILEPTIC WOMEN
EUR NEUROL 1986 25:436-443

ROBERT E PRADAT E LAUMONT B
OVULATION INDUCTION AND NEURAL TUBE DEFECTS: A REGISTRY STUDY
REPR TOX 1991 5:83-84

ROBERT E ROBERT JM LAPRAS C
IS VALPROIC ACID TERATOGENIC? (FRE)
REV NEUROL (PARIS) 1983 139:445-7

ROBERT E ROCH-SUZUKI R BOGGIO D HAAG P
INCIDENCE OF MALFORMATIONS OF THE URINARY TRACT IN THE RHONE-ALPS AREA. A PROPOS 1,357 CASES OF AFFECTED INFANTS IDENTIFIED OVER A 7-YEAR PERIOD (1976-1982) (FRE)
J GENET HUM 1984 32:107-111

ROBERT E ROSA F
VALPROATE AND BIRTH DEFECTS (LETTER)
LANCET 1983 2:1142

ROBERT JM GUIBAUD P ROBERT E
A LOCAL OUTBREAK OF FEMORAL HYPOPLASIA OR APLASIA AND FEMORAL FIBULA-ULNAR-COMPLEX
J GENET HUM 1981 29:379-94

ROBERT JM ROBERT E FRANCANNET C
INTERNATIONAL CLEARINGHOUSE FOR BIRTH DEFECTS MONITORING SYSTEMS (ICBDMS) AN EXAMPLE OF EFFECTIVE INTERNATIONAL COOPERATION (FRE)
ARCH FR PEDIATR 1986 43:539-41

RODRIGUEZ-PINILLA E SALVADOR J GARCIA ALONSO F MARTINEZ-FRIAS ML
ANTICONVULSANTS AND BIRTH DEFECTS: STUDY ON A SPANISH POPULATION (1976-1983) (SPA)
FARMACOTERAPIA 1985 3:34-39

RODRIGUEZ-PINILLA E SALVADOR J ALONSO D MARTINEZ-FRIAS ML
RELATIONSHIP BETWEEN THE INTAKE OF BENZODIAZEPINES DURING PREGNANCY AND ORAL CLEFTS IN THE NEWBORN: A CASE CONTROL STUDY (SPA)
MED CLIN 1986 87:741-743

ROSENBERG L MITCHELL AA PARSELLS JL PASHAYAN H LOUIK C SHAPIRO S
LACK OF RELATION OF ORAL CLEFTS TO DIAZEPAM USE DURING PREGNANCY
N ENGL J MED 1983 309:1282-1285

ROTH M-P FEINGOLD J BAUMGARTEN A BIGEL P STOLL C
REEXAMINATION OF PATERNAL AGE EFFECT IN DOWN'S SYNDROME
HUM GENET 1983 63:149-152

ROTH MP DOTT B ALEMBIK Y STOLL C
CONGENITAL MALFORMATIONS IN A SERIES OF 66,068 CONSECUTIVE BIRTHS (FRE)
ARCH FR PEDIATR 1987 44:173-6

ROTH MP STOLL C TAILLEMITE JL GIRARD S BOUE A
PATERNAL AGE AND DOWN'S SYNDROME DIAGNOSED PRENATALLY: NO ASSOCIATION IN FRENCH DATA
PRENATAL DIAGNOSIS 1983 3:327-35

RUMEAU-ROUQUETTE C GOUJARD J ANCELIN C GRACCO DE LAY MO MAILLARD F
REGISTRES ET RECHERCHES IN: PREVENTION OF PHYSICAL AND MENTAL CONGENITAL DEFECTS PART B: EPIDEMIOLOGIE, EARLY DETECTION AND THERAPY AND ENVIRONMENTAL FACTORS MAROIS M (ED)
NEW YORK: ALAN R LISS INC 1985

RUMEAU-ROUQUETTE C GOUJARD J ANCELIN C GRACCO DE LAY MO MAILLARD F
REGISTERS AND RESEARCH (FRE)
PROG CLIN BIOL RES 1985 163B:23-6

RUTKAI K CZEIZEL A
OBSTETRIC FEATURES OF MOTHERS GIVING BIRTH TO INFANTS WITH POLYCYSTIC DISEASE OF THE KIDNEYS
ARCH GYNECOL 1982 231:235-40

SAFRA MJ OAKLEY GP ERICKSON JD
DESCRIPTIVE EPIDEMIOLOGY OF SMALL-BOWEL ATRESIA IN METROPOLITAN ATLANTA
TERATOLOGY 1976 14:143-149

SAFRA MJ OAKLEY GP JR
ASSOCIATION BETWEEN CLEFT LIP WITH OR WITHOUT CLEFT PALATE AND PRENATAL EXPOSURE TO DIAZEPAM
LANCET 1975 2:478-80

SAFRA MJ OAKLEY GP JR
VALIUM: AN ORAL CLEFT TERATOGEN?
CLEFT PALATE J 1976 13:198-200

SAFRA MJ OAKLEY GP JR
ASSOCIATION BETWEEN CLEFT LIP WITH OR WITHOUT CLEFT PALATE AND PRENATAL EXPOSURE TO DIAZEPAM
OB/GYN DIGEST 1976 7:56

SAINZ MP RODRIGUES PINILLA E MARTINEZ-FRIAS ML
HIGH-DOSE ESTTROGENS AND PROGESTAGENS (HORMONAL PREGNANCY TESTS): RISK OF DEVELOPMENT OF SPINA BIFIDA AND ANENCEPHALUS (SPA)
MED CLIN 1987 89:272-274

SALGADO LJ LOPEZ-CAMELO JS CASTILLA EE
EL BUSCA AND THE VALUE OF SIGNALS IN THE DIAGNOSIS OF DYSMORPHIC SYNDROMES: GOOD AND BAD HANDLES IN COMPUTER-ASSISTED DIFFERENTIAL DIAGNOSIS
J MED GENET 1990 27:446-450

SALVADOR J MARTINEZ FRIAS ML
MATERNAL AGE AND DOWN SYNDROME IN SPAIN (SPA)
REV ESP PEDIATR 1982 38:205-214

SALVADOR J MARTINEZ FRIAS ML RODRIQUEZ E
DRUG CONSUMPTION BY THE PREGNANT WOMEN IN SPAIN. ANALYSIS OF A SAMPLE DURING THE YEARS 1976-86 (SPA)
MONOGRAFIAS DE DIVULGACION NO 7 ED DIRECCION GENERAL DE FARMACIA Y PRODUCTOS 1989

SALVADOR J MARTINEZ-FRIAS ML
EPIDEMIOLOGICAL STUDY OF DOWN SYNDROME IN SPAIN (SPA)
ESTUDIOS SANATARIOS ED DIRECCION GENERAL DE PLANIFICATION SANITARIA, MADRID 1990

SALVADOR J MARTINEZ-FRIAS ML BORREGUERO M CEREIJO A ADAN A
EPIDEMIOLOGICAL DESCRIPTIVE STUDY ON BIRTH DEFECTS OF THE GENITOURINARY TRACT IN SPAIN (1976-1982) (SPA)
REV ESP PEDIATR 1985 41:53-62

SALVADOR J MARTINEZ-FRIAS ML
MECANISMS OF TERATOGENESIS (SPA). IN: CARRERA MACIA J ET AL.:
BARCELONA DIAGNOSTICO PRENATAL ED. SALVAT 1987 81-97

SALVAGGIO E MENONNA NM MASTROIACOVO P FUNDARO C AURITI C BIANCHI A D'ANDREA A SEGNI G
DESCRIPTIVE EPIDEMIOLOGY OF CONGENITAL MALFORMATIONS OF THE URINARY TRACT. AN ITALIAN MULTICENTER STUDY ON CONGENITAL MALFORMATIONS (ITA)
MINERVA PEDIATR 1986 38:739-49

SALVIOLI GP BOVICELLI L COCCHI G SANDRI F PILU G
PRENATAL DIAGNOSIS OF CONGENITAL MALFORMATIONS OF THE CENTRAL NERVOUS SYSTEM AND ITS IMPLICATIONS FOR CARE OF THE NEWBORN (FRE)
J GENET HUM 1986 24:348-53

SANDAHL B
SEASONAL INCIDENCE OF CLEFT LIPS AND CLEFT PALATES IN SWEDEN 1965-1974
SCAND J PL REC SURG 1977 11:39-43

SANDAHL B
SEASONAL INCIDENCE OF SOME CONGENITAL MALFORMATIONS IN THE CENTRAL NERVOUS SYSTEM IN SWEDEN 1965-1972
ACTA PAEDIATR SCAND 1977 66:65-72

SAVOLAINEN E SAKSELA E SAXEN L
TERATOGENIC HAZARDS OF ORAL CONTRACEPTIVES ANALYZED IN A NATIONAL MALFORMATION REGISTER
AM J OBSTET GYNECOL 1981 140:521-524

SAXEN I
CLEFT LIP AND PALATE IN FINLAND: PARENTAL HISTORIES, COURSE OF PREGNANCY AND SELECTED ENVIRONMENTAL FACTORS
INT J EPIDEMIOL 1974 3:263-270

SAXEN I
EPIDEMIOLOGY OF CLEFT LIP AND PALATE: AN ATTEMPT TO RULE OUT CHANCE CORRELATIONS
BR J PREV SOC MED 1975 29:103-110

SAXEN I
THE ASSOCIATION BETWEEN MATERNAL INFLUENZA, DRUG CONSUMPTION AND ORAL CLEFTS
ACTA ODONTOL SCAND 1975 33:259-267

SAXEN I
ASSOCIATIONS BETWEEN ORAL CLEFTS AND DRUGS TAKEN DURING PREGNANCY
INT J EPIDEMIOL 1975 4:37-44

SAXEN I LAHTI A
CLEFT LIP AND PALATE IN FINLAND: INCIDENCE SECULAR SEASONAL AND GEOGRAPHIC VARIATIONS
TERATOLOGY 1974 9:217-223

SAXEN I SAXEN L
ASSOCIATION BETWEEN MATERNAL INTAKE OF DIAZEPAM AND ORAL CLEFTS (LETTER)
LANCET 1975 2:498

SAXEN L
THE FINNISH REGISTER OF CONGENITAL MALFORMATIONS AND ITS APPLICATION TO EPIDEMIOLOGICAL STUDIES (FIN)
DUODECIM (HELSINKI) 1980 96:1390-1399

SAXEN L
THE FINNISH REGISTRY OF CONGENITAL MALFORMATIONS AND ITS APPLICATION IN EPIDEMIOLOGICAL STUDIES (FIN)
KATILOLEHTI 1981 86:53-60

SAXEN L HOLMBERG PC NURMINEN M KUOSMA E
SAUNA AND CONGENITAL DEFECTS
TERATOLOGY 1982 25:309-313

SAXEN L KARKINEN-JAASKELAINEN M SAXEN I
EPIDEMIOLOGIC METHODS IN TERATOLOGY (FIN)
DUODECIM (HELSINKI) 1974 90:1554-1564

SAXEN L KLEMETTI A
THE FINNISH REGISTER OF CONGENITAL MALFORMATIONS
ACTA UNIV CAROL (MED MONOGR , PRAHA) 1973 56:23-30

SAXEN L KLEMETTI A HARO AS
A MATCHED-PAIR REGISTER FOR STUDIES OF SELECTED CONGENITAL DEFECTS
AM J EPIDEMIOL 1974 100:297-306

SELEVAN SG HEMMINKI K LINDBOHM ML
LINKING DATA TO STUDY REPRODUCTIVE EFFECTS OF OCCUPATIONAL EXPOSURES
STATE ART REV OCCUP MED 1986 1:445-455

SELLER MJ
NEURAL TUBE DEFECTS AND SEX RATIOS (LETTER)
LANCET 1986 2:227

SELLER MJ NEVIN NC
PERICONCEPTIONAL VITAMIN SUPPLEMENTATION AND THE PREVENTION OF NEURAL TUBE DEFECTS IN SOUTH-EAST ENGLAND AND NORTHERN IRELAND
J MED GENET 1984 21:325-30

SEPE SJ OAKLEY GP MARKS JS MANLEY A
SCREENING FOR CYSTIC FIBROSIS (LETTER)
JAMA 1983 249:3175

SEVER LE
DEVELOPMENTAL TOXICITY RISK ASSESSMENT: TERATOLOGY AND HAZARD IDENTIFICATION
AM J EPIDEMIOL 1987 126:781-2

SEVER LE EDMONDS LD
RECENT ACTIVITIES IN BIRTH DEFECTS SURVEILLANCE
GREAT PLAINS GENETICS 1986 2:8 9

SEVER LE GILBERT ES HESSOL NA MCINTYRE JM
A CASE-CONTROL STUDY OF CONGENITAL MALFORMATIONS AND OCCUPATIONAL EXPOSURE TO LOW-LEVEL RADIATION
AM J EPIDEMIOL 1988 127:226-42

SEVER LE HESSOL NA GILBERT ES MCINTYRE JM
THE PREVALENCE AT BIRTH OF CONGENITAL MALFORMATIONS IN COMMUNITIES NEAR THE HANFORD SITE
AM J EPIDEMIOL 1988 127:243-54

SEVER LE STRASSBURG MA
EPIDEMIOLOGIC ASPECTS OF NEURAL TUBE DEFECTS IN THE UNITED STATES: CHANGING CONCEPTS AND THEIR IMPORTANCE FOR SCREENING AND PRENATAL DIAGNOSTIC PROGRAMS. IN: MIZEJEWSKI GJ PORTER IH (EDS) ALPHA-FETOPROTEIN AND CONGENITAL DISORDERS
NEW YORK: ACAD PRESS 1985 243-62

SHEPPARD S NEVIN NC SELLER MJ WILD J SMITHELLS RW READ AP HARRIS R FIELDING DW SCHORAH CJ
NEURAL TUBE DEFECT RECURRENCE AFTER 'PARTIAL' VITAMIN SUPPLEMENTATION
J MED GENET 1989 26:326-9

SHUPER A MERLOB P GRUNEBAUM M REISNER SH
THE INCIDENCE OF ISOLATED CRANIOSTENOSIS IN THE NEWBORN INFANT
AM J DIS CHILD 1985 139:85-86

SHUPER A MERLOB P WEITZ R VARSANO I
THE DIAGNOSIS OF DUBOWITZ SYNDROME IN THE NEONATAL PERIOD
EUR J PEDIATR 1986 145:151-2

SKJAERVEN R
DEPENDENCIES IN PERINATAL OUTCOME BETWEEN SUCCESSIVE SIBLINGS. INFLUENCE ON TRADITIONAL MEASURES IN PERINATAL EPIDEMIOLOGY ASSESSED ON THE BASIS OF BIRTHS IN NORWAY,1967-1984. THESIS
UNIVERSITY OF BERGEN 1989

SMITH ES DAFOE CS MILLER JR BANISTER P
AN EPIDEMIOLOGICAL STUDY OF CONGENITAL REDUCTION DEFORMITIES OF THE LIMBS
BR J PREV SOC MED 1977 31:39-41

SMITH ESO DAFOE C MILLER JR BANISTER P
POSSIBLE TERATOGENICITY OF TRICYCLIC ANTIDEPRESSANTS
LANCET 1972 1:838-839

SMITHELLS RW NEVIN NC SELLER MJ SHEPPARD S HARRIS R READ AP FIELDING DW WALKER S SCHORAH CJ WILD J
FURTHER EXPERIENCE OF VITAMIN SUPPLEMENTATION FOR PREVENTION OF NEURAL TUBE DEFECT RECURRENCES
LANCET 1983 1:1027-31

SMITHELLS RW SHEPPARD S SCHORAH CJ SELLER MJ NEVIN NC HARRIS R READ AP FIELDING DW
POSSIBLE PREVENTION OF NEURAL-TUBE DEFECTS BY PERICONCEPTIONAL VITAMIN SUPPLEMENTATION
LANCET 1980 1:339-40

SMITHELLS RW SHEPPARD S SCHORAH CJ SELLER MJ NEVIN NC HARRIS R READ AP FIELDING DW
APPARENT PREVENTION OF NEURAL TUBE DEFECTS BY PERICONCEPTIONAL VITAMIN SUPPLEMENTATION
ARCH DIS CHILD 1981 56:911-8

SMITHELLS RW SHEPPARD S SCHORAH CJ SELLER MJ NEVIN NC HARRIS R READ AP FIELDING DW WALKER S
VITAMIN SUPPLEMENTATION AND NEURAL TUBE DEFECTS (LETTER)
LANCET 1981 2:1425

SMITHELLS RW SHEPPARD S WILD J SCHORAH CJ FIELDING DW SELLER MJ NEVIN NC HARRIS R READ AP WALKER S
NEURAL-TUBE DEFECTS AND VITAMINS: THE NEED FOR A RANDOMIZED CLINICAL TRIAL (LETTER)
BR J OBSTET GYNAECOL 1985 92:185-8

SNIDER DE JR LAYDE PM JOHNSON MW LYLE MA
TREATMENT OF TUBERCULOSIS DURING PREGNANCY
AM REV RESPIR DIS 1980 122:65-79

SOKAL DC BYRD JR CHEN ATL GOLDBERG MF OAKLEY GP JR
PRENATAL CHROMOSOMAL DIAGNOSIS: RACIAL AND GEOGRAPHIC VARIATION FOR OLDER WOMEN IN GEORGIA
JAMA 1980 244:1355-7

SPIRA A GOUJARD J HENRION R LEMERLE J ROBEL P TCHOBROUTSKY C
ADMINISTRATING OF DIETHYLSTILBESTROL DURING PREGNANCY. A PUBLIC HEALTH PROBLEM (FRE)
REV EPIDEM SANTE PUBL 1983 31:249-72

STEPHENS TD SHEPARD TH
A REVIEW OF LIMB DEFECTS IN A LARGE FETUS COLLECTION
AM J HUM GENET 1983 35:508-519

STOCKBAUER JW HOFFMAN RE SCHRAM WF EDMONDS LE
REPRODUCTIVE OUTCOMES OF MOTHERS WITH POTENTIAL EXPOSURE TO 2 3 7 8-TETRACHLORODIBENZO-P-DIOXIN
AM J EPIDEMIOL 1988 128 2:410-19

STOLL C
THE NORTHEASTERN FRANCE BIRTH DEFECTS MONITORING SYSTEM
PROG CLIN BIOL RES 1985 163B:157-162

STOLL C ALEMBIK Y ROTH MP DOTT B DE GEETER B
RISK FACTORS IN CONGENITAL HEART DISEASE
EUR J EPIDEMIOL 1989 5:382-91

STOLL C CURIE P DOTT B FLOESSER J FLORI J GESCHICKT M MARZOLF G ROTH MP SUSSMANN M TREISSER A
CORRELATIONS BETWEEN PREGNANCY PATHOLOGY, STUDY OF THE PLACENTA, ANTENATAL ECHOGRAPHY AND EXAMINATION OF THE PRODUCT OF CONCEPTION IN A SERIES OF 175 CONGENITAL MALFORMATIONS (FRE)
J GENET HUM 1985 33:247-56

STOLL C DOTT B ROTH MP ALEMBIK Y
ETIOLOGIC AND EPIDEMIOLOGIC ASPECTS OF NEURAL TUBE DEFECTS
ARCH FR PEDIATR 1988 45:617-22

STOLL C DOTT B ROTH MP ALEMBIK Y
BIRTH PREVALENCE RATES OF SKELETAL DYSPLASIAS
CLIN GENET 1989 35:88-92

STOLL C ROTH M-P DOTT B BIGEL P
USEFULNESS OF A REGISTRY OF CONGENITAL MALFORMATIONS FOR GENETIC COUNSELING AND PRENATAL DIAGNOSIS
CLIN GENET 1986 29:204-210

STOLL C ROTH MP BIGEL P
A REEXAMINATION ON PARENTAL AGE EFFECT ON THE OCCURRENCE OF NEW MUTATIONS FOR ACHONDROPLASIA
PROG CLIN BIOL RES 1982 104:419-26

STOLL C ROTH MP DOTT B BIGEL P
DISCORDANCE FOR SKELETAL AND CARDIAC DEFECT IN MONOZYGOTIC TWINS
ACTA GENET MED GEMEL (ROMA) 1984 33:501-4

STRAUSS J KOPECKY K KUCERA J VORISKOVA M HODR L
MASS INCIDENCE OF CONGENITAL HEART DEFECTS IN NEONATES AT THE TOWN OF KLADNO IN 1972 (CZE)
CESK EPID MIKROBIOL IMUNOL 1976 25:1-9

SUREAU CI GERMAIN G FERRE F BREART G GOUJARD J UZAN M CEDARD L
THERAPEUTIC USE OF PROGESTERONE DURING THE LAST TWO TRIMESTERS OF PREGNANCY IN: PROGESTERONE AND PROGESTINS BARDIN CW MILGROM E MAUVAIS-JARVIS P
NEW YORK: RAVEN PRESS 1983 247-58

SWERDLOW AJ MELZER D
THE VALUE OF ENGLAND AND WALES CONGENITAL MALFORMATION NOTIFICATION SCHEME DATA FOR EPIDEMIOLOGY: MALE GENITAL TRACT MALFORMATIONS
J EPIDEMIOL COMMUNITY HEALTH 1988 42:8-13

SZENDREY T DANYI G CZEIZEL A
ETIOLOGICAL STUDY ON ISOLATED ESOPHAGEAL ATRESIA
HUM GENET 1985 70:51-58

TARAMONA A ZAPLANA J PEQUE M MARTINEZ FRIAS ML
INSTABILITY OF THE HIP GENETIC AND EPIDEMIOLOGICAL STUDY (SPA)
REV ESP PEDIATR 1982 5:327-336

THOMAS HF CZEIZEL A
SAFE AS 2 4 5-T? (LETTER)
NATURE 1982 295:276

THOMSON EJ CORDERO JF
THE NEW TERATOGENS: ACCUTANE AND OTHER VITAMIN-A ANALOGS
MATERNAL CHILD NURS J 1989 14:244-248

TOSOVSKY J KUCERA J
RELATIONSHIP BETWEEN FETAL WEIGHT IN CERTAIN CONGENITAL ANOMALIES FROM THE 28TH TO 42ND WEEK OF GESTATION
FOLIA MORPHOL (PRAHA) 1978 26:343-350

TREISSER A DREYFUS M OLIVIER D RENAUD R STOLL C PHILLIPPE E
EARLY BIOPSY OF CHORIONIC VILLI. PERSONAL EXPERIENCE AND REVIEW OF THE LITERATURE (FRE)
REV FR GYNECOL OBSTET 1985 80:397-412

TUSNADY G CZEIZEL A TELEGDI L
ML-FITTING OF MULTIFACTORIAL THRESHOLD MODELS
PERIOD MATHEMAT HUNG 1981 12:205-16

URIOSTE M PINEL I GOMAR JL MARTINEZ-FRIAS ML
DIPLOID/TETRAPLOID MOSAICISM IN A STILLBORN INFANT WITH PRUNE BELLY ANOMALY
ANN GENET 1990 33:49-51

URIOSTE M VALCARCEL E GOMEZ MA PINEL I GARCIA DE LEON R DIAZ DE BUSTAMANTE A TEBAR R MARTINEZ-FRIAS ML
HOLOPROSENCEPHALY AND TRISOMY 21 IN A CHILD BORN TO A NONDIABETIC MOTHER
AM J MED GENET 1988 30:925-8

VITEZ A KORANYI G GONCZY E RUDAS T CZEIZEL A
A SEMIQUANTITATIVE SCORE SYSTEM FOR EPIDEMIOLOGIC STUDIES OF FETAL ALCOHOL SYNDROME
AM J EPIDEMIOL 1983 119:3

VITEZ M KORANYI G GONCZY E RUDAS T CZEIZEL A
ORIGINAL CONTRIBUTIONS. A SEMIQUANTITATIVE SCORE SYSTEM FOR EPIDEMIOLOGICASTUDIES OF FETAL ALCOHOL SYNDROME
AMER J EPID 1984 119:301-8

VOLLSET SE
OVULATION INDUCTION AND NEURAL TUBE DEFECTS (LETTER)
LANCET 1990 335:178

WAN CHONGHUA
THE SINGLE SAMPLE SCHEME AND ITS APPLICATION IN BIRTH DEFECTS MONITORING (CHI)
CHINESE J HEALTH STATISTICS 1990 7:19-21

WEATHERALL JAC
REPORTS ON CONGENITAL ABNORMALITIES (LETTER)
LANCET 1968 2:1040

WEATHERALL JAC
THE DETECTION OF INCIDENCE OF CONGENITAL MALFORMATIONS IN THE COMMUNITY
PROC R SOC MED 1970 63:1251-1252

WEATHERALL JAC
EPIDEMIOLOGICAL REGISTERS - THE WAY AHEAD HEALTH AND SAFETY AT WORK: THE UNBORN CHILD: EFFECTS ON OFFSPRING OF PARENTAL OCCUPATIONAL EXPOSURE
LONDON: SOC OCCUP MED 1980 23-27

WEATHERALL JAC GREENBERG G
MATERNAL DRUG USAGE AND CONGENITAL MALFOMATIONS. A CASE CONTROL STUDY CONTRIBUTIONS TO EPIDEMIOLOGY AND BIOSTATISTICS VOL 1 EPIDEMIOLOGIC METHODS FOR THE DETECTION OF TERATOGENS
BASEL:KARGER, 1979 71-77

WEATHERALL JAC HASKEY JC
SURVEILLANCE OF MALFORMATIONS
BR MED BULL 1976 32:39-44

WILD J READ AP SHEPPARD S SELLER MJ SMITHELLS RW NEVIN NC SCHORAH CJ FIELDING DW WALKER S HARRIS R
RECURRENT NEURAL TUBE DEFECTS RISK FACTORS AND VITAMINS
ARCH DIS CHILD 1986 61:440-4

WINDHAM GC BJERKEDAL T
MALFORMATION FREQUENCIES IN SIBS OF ATRESIA CASES (LETTER)
LANCET 1982 2:816-817

WINDHAM GC BJERKEDAL T
SECULAR TRENDS OF NEURAL TUBE DEFECTS BY DEMOGRAPHIC SUBGROUPS IN NORWAY 1967-81
NIPH ANN 1982 5:57-67

WINDHAM GC BJERKEDAL T
MALFORMATIONS IN TWINS AND THEIR SIBLINGS NORWAY 1967-79
ACTA GENET MED GEMEL (ROMA) 1984 33:87-95

WINDHAM GC BJERKEDAL T SEVER LE
THE ASSOCIATION OF TWINNING AND NEURAL TUBE DEFECTS: STUDIES IN LOS ANGELES CALIFORNIA AND NORWAY
ACTA GENET MED GEMEL (ROMA) 1982 31:165-172

WINDHAM GC EDMONDS LD
CURRENT TRENDS IN THE INCIDENCE OF NEURAL TUBE DEFECTS
PEDIATRICS 1982 70:333-7

WOLFE MS CORDERO JF
SAFETY OF CHLOROQUINE IN CHEMOSUPPRESSION OF MALARIA DURING PREGNANCY
BR MED J 1985 290:1466-1467

XIAO KZ
A PEDIGREE OF SYNDACTYLY AND TRIPHALANGEAL THUMB IN THREE CONSECUTIVE GENERATIONS (CHI)
NAT MED J CHINA 1981 61:758-61

XIAO KZ
A SURVEY OF BIRTH DEFECTS AMONG 11,230 CHILDREN IN CHENGDU AREA (CHI)
NAT MED J CHINA 1984 64:236

XIAO KZ
THE CORRELATION BETWEEN THE POSITION OF AXIAL TRIRADIUS AND AGE (CHI)
NAT MED J CHINA 1984 64:450

XIAO KZ
A MONITORING FOR BIRTH DEFECTS IN 100 HOSPITALS IN SICHUAN PROVINCE (A PRELIMINARY REPORT)(CHI)
HEREDITY DIS 1985 2:5

XIAO KZ
CLINIC PERINATOLOGY (CHAPTER: BIRTH DEFECTS)(CHI)
SICHUAN PUBL HOUSE TEC 1986

XIAO KZ
THREE YEAR MONITORING FOR SOME RISKY BIRTH DEFECTS IN SICHUAN PROVINCE (CHI)
HEREDITY DIS 1988 5:65

XIAO KZ
CURRENT STATUS OF BIRTH DEFECTS MONITORING IN CHINA AND ABROAD (CHI)
J PRAC OBSTET GYNECOL 1989 5:1-3

XIAO KZ
RAISE THE EFFICIENCY OF SURVEILLANCE AND RESEARCH OF BIRTH DEFECTS IN CHINA TO A NEW LEVEL (CHI)
NAT MED J CHINA 1989 69:183-4

XIAO KZ
EPIDEMIOLOGY OF NEURAL TUBE DEFECTS IN CHINA (CHI)
NAT MED J CHINA 1989 69:189-91

XIAO KZ
EPIDEMIOLOGY OF CLEFT LIP AND CLEFT PALATE IN 18 REGIONS OF SICHUAN PROVINCE (CHI)
W CHINA J STOMATOL 1989 7:240

XIAO KZ
ATLAS OF BIRTH DEFECTS IN CHINA (CHI)
CHENGDU MAP PUBLISHING HOUSE 1990

XIAO KZ
SEASONAL INCIDENCE OF NTDS IN SICHUAN CHINA (CHI)
CHINESE J HEALTH STATISTICS 1990 7:1-4

XIAO KZ LANG ZC CHENG JH ET AL
MONITORING FOR BIRTH DEFECTS IN 100 HOSPITALS OF SICHUAN PROVINCE (A PRELIMINARY REPORT) (CHI)
HERED DIS 1985 2:5-8

XIAO KZ TIAN ZJ ZHAN SQ ET AL
NEONATAL DEFECTS IN 18,158 PARTURITIONS IN THE CHENGDU AREA (CHI)
NAT MED J CHINA 1985 65:104-106

YIANG SQ XIAO KZ
THE CUMULATIVE SUM (CUSUM) TECHNIQUE FOR BIRTH DEFECTS MONITORING (CHI)
CHINESE J HEALTH STATISTICS 1989 6:1